SpringerWienNewYork

Acta Neurochirurgica
Supplements

Editor: H.-J. Steiger

Cerebral Hemorrhage

Edited by
L.-F. Zhou, G. Xi, X.-C. Chen, R. F. Keep,
F.-P. Huang, Y. Hua, Y.-C. Lu, K. M. Muraszko

Acta Neurochirurgica
Supplement 105

SpringerWienNewYork

Liang-Fu Zhou
Xian-Cheng Chen
Feng-Ping Huang
Department of Neurosurgery, School of Medicine, Huashan Hospital, Fudan University, Shanghai, China

Guohua Xi
Richard F. Keep
Ya Hua
Karin Muraszko
Department of Neurosurgery, University of Michigan, Ann Arbor, MI, USA

Yi-Cheng Lu
Department of Neurosurgery, Shanghai Changzheng Hospital, Shanghai, China

© 2008 Springer-Verlag/Wien
Printed in Austria
Springer-Verlag Wien New York is a part of Springer Science + Business Media
springer.at

Typesetting: Thomson Press, Chennai, India
Printing and Binding: Druckerei Theiss GmbH, St. Stefan, Austria, www.theiss.at

Printed on acid-free and chlorine-free bleached paper
SPIN: 11976097

Library of Congress Control Number: 2008938112

With 73 Figures (thereof 3 coloured)

ISSN 0065-1419
ISBN 978-3-211-09468-6 SpringerWienNewYork

Acta Neurochir Suppl (2008) 105: V
© Springer-Verlag 2008
Printed in Austria

Preface

These are the proceedings of the 2nd International Symposium on Cerebral Hemorrhage, which was held on November 10–11th, 2007 in Shanghai, China. This symposium followed the successful first symposium held in Ann Arbor, Michigan, USA, in 2005. The aim of the conference was to bring together experts on cerebral hemorrhage from throughout the world to present and discuss data on this understudied form of stroke. The conference covered both clinical and basic science studies on cerebral hemorrhage and particularly intracerebral hemorrhage. Papers from the conference in these proceedings cover the full gamut, from molecular biology to clinical trials and epidemiology. They show that our knowledge of cerebral hemorrhage has greatly expanded in recent years and there is hope that this will be translated into new therapies for the clinic.

The symposium in Shanghai was a joint collaboration between Fudan University and the University of Michigan. It was to have been co-chaired by Professors Liang-Fu Zhou and Julian T. Hoff. Unfortunately, Professor Hoff died prior to the meeting and his presence was sorely missed by all. This volume includes a paper on Professor Hoff and his contributions to the field of cerebral hemorrhage research by Dr. Karin Muraszko, who succeeded Dr. Hoff as Chair of Neurosurgery at the University of Michigan.

With the success of the 1st and 2nd symposia, there was a unanimous desire for these meetings to continue. The 3rd International Symposium on Cerebral Hemorrhage will be held in Palm Springs, USA, under the direction of Professors John Zhang and Austin Colohan of Loma Linda University. Symposium attendees look forward to a successful meeting in that city in November 2009. Plans are also underway to host a 4th meeting in Newcastle, England, in 2011.

The editors wish to thank Ms. Holly Wagner and the staff of Springer-Verlag for the commitment and editorial skills necessary to prepare these proceedings.

Liang-Fu Zhou, Guohua Xi,
Xian-Cheng Chen, Richard F. Keep,
Feng-Ping Huang, Ya Hua, Yi-Cheng Lu,
Karin M. Muraszko

Acta Neurochir Suppl (2008) 105: VI
© Springer-Verlag 2008
Printed in Austria

Acknowledgments

The Editors would like to express their sincere thanks to those who made the 2nd International Symposium on Cerebral Hemorrhage possible. Thanks are due especially to the International Advisory Board and the Local Asian Organizing Committee.

International Advisory Board

Jaroslaw Aronowski
Daniel F. Hanley, Jr.
Julian T. Hoff
Richard F. Keep
Toshihiko Kuroiwa
Eng H. Lo
Neil A. Martin
Stephan A. Mayer
A. David Mendelow
Lewis B. Morgenstern
Seigo Nagao
Frank R. Sharp
Akira Tamura
Stella E. Tsirka
Kenneth R. Wagner
Guohua Xi
John H. Zhang

Local Asian Organizing Committee

Xian-Cheng Chen
Yong Gu Chung
Zhen Hong
Feng-Ping Huang
Ru-Xun Huang
Cengiz Kuday
Liang-Shong Lee
Yi-Cheng Lu
Zhuan-Zhen Lv
Ying Mao
Wai S. Poon
Jian-Kang Shen
Yong-Kwang Tu
Wen-Zhi Wang
Tao Xu
Qi-Wu Xu
Su-Ming Zhang
Xiang Zhang
Ji-Zong Zhao
Ding-Biao Zhou
Fan-Min Zhou
Liangfu Zhou (Chair)
Jian-Hong Zhu

Contents

Experimental intracerebral hemorrhage – other mechanisms

Experimental intracerebral hemorrhage – model development and characterization

Human intracerebral hemorrhage

Experimental intracranial hemorrhage (non-intracerebral hemorrhage)

Human intracranial hemorrhage (non-intracerebral hemorrhage)

Listed in Current Contents

Acta Neurochir Suppl (2008) 105: XI–XII
© Springer-Verlag 2008
Printed in Austria

Julian Theodore (Buz) Hoff 1936–2007

K. Muraszko

Department of Neurosurgery, University of Michigan Health System, MI, USA

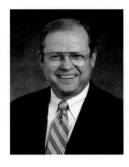

On April 16, 2007 the world of neurosurgery lost one of its great leaders, Julian T. (Buz) Hoff. He passed away after a 7-month battle with acute leukemia and died peacefully at home with the comfort of his loving family. Although his life seemed to be cut short, it was a life well-lived and he will be missed.

Dr. Hoff was a graduate of Caldwell High School in Caldwell, Idaho. He received his A.B. degree from Stanford University and he attended Cornell Medical College, graduating in 1962. He completed his neurosurgical training at New York Hospital in 1970 and went on to the University of California at San Francisco where he quickly rose to the rank of professor. Dr. Hoff left San Francisco in 1981 to assume the position as head of the neurosurgery section here at the University of Michigan. He was appointed Richard C. Schneider Professor in 1992 and the section became the Department of Neurosurgery in 2001. Dr. Hoff served as the first chairman of the Department of Neurosurgery at the University of Michigan Health System from 2001 until 2005.

Buz had a distinguished career in neurosurgery, having served on the editorial boards of the major neurosurgical journals and as co-chair of the Editorial Board for the Journal of Neurosurgery from 1997 to 1999. He maintained continuous NIH funding from 1972 until the present day. His most recent R01 focused on mechanisms of brain edema after intracerebral hemorrhage. He received the prestigious Jacob Javitz Award for Neuroscience Research twice, and was a member of the Institute of Medicine National Academy of Sciences since 1999. He received the Cushing Medal from the American Association of Neurological Surgeons, the Grass Prize from the Society of Neurological Surgeons, and was the honored guest of the Congress of Neurological Surgeons. He received the Distinguished Alumni Award from Caldwell High School in Caldwell, Idaho. He also received the Distinguished Service Award from the Society of Neurological Surgeons. He was the author of numerous papers, book chapters, plus the editor of several books.

Buz's research career was a distinguished one. His first publication was on cerebral hemangioblastomas in a patient with Von Hippel–Lindau disease. As he progressed through his residency he continued to publish. In his early career he became very interested in cerebral edema, and specifically, intracerebral hemorrhage. In the 1970s he published a series of papers looking at the effects of alpha-adrenergic blockade on cerebral circulation as well as the effect of hypoxia on the Cushing reflex in intracranial pressure. He looked at various mechanisms to abate injury secondary to cerebral edema. His research interests focused on intracranial pressure and the effects of hematoma, both intraparenchymal as well as subdural, in patients with head injury. As a result of his outstanding research, he was awarded the Grass Award by the Society of Neurological Surgeons in 2002. The selection committee particularly commented on his sustained interest in cerebral edema and the important contributions he and his laboratory made to our understanding of cerebral edema under a variety of circumstances.

Correspondence: Karin Muraszko, M.D., Department of Neurosurgery, University of Michigan Health System, 1500 E. Medical Center Drive, Room 3552 Taubman Center, Ann Arbor, MI 48109-5338, USA.
e-mail: karinm@umich.edu

Buz's contributions within the laboratory were also notable for his significant ability to mentor young faculty as well as residents in the pursuit of academic careers. At present, there are 5 chairs of neurosurgical departments who trained under Buz and who received mentoring and tutelage from him with respect to their academic careers. He sponsored numerous residents in the laboratory and consistently provided protected time for laboratory work during residency training. Numerous residents went on to win awards by the Congress of Neurological Surgeons as well as the American Association of Neurological Surgeons. Many also received funding from the Neurosurgery Research and Education Foundation (NREF).

Buz served in executive positions in every major neurosurgical society including the American Academy of Neurological Surgeons, as president of the American Association of Neurological Surgeons, and as vice-president of the Congress of Neurological Surgeons. He was a member of the Residency Review Committee for neurosurgery from 1987 to 1993 and continued to serve on the appeals panel for neurosurgery. Within the University of Michigan he served on a variety of committees. Whenever a complex job needed to be done, Buz was always selected to perform that job, and he did so with wisdom and an affable personality.

An Eagle Scout in his early life, Dr. Hoff was particularly beloved for his strong leadership abilities that were displayed in a collegial and kind fashion. In choosing residents, he often indicated that he employed the lessons learned in his early life with the Boy Scouts. A strong advocate of resident education, he sought to create a collegial environment in which even the most complex political and scientific issues could be discussed in a manner of warmth and openness.

Dr. Hoff was particularly pleased that in 2006, the Department of Neurosurgery completed an endowed chair honoring him. Dr. Karin Muraszko serves as the first Julian T. Hoff Professor of Neurosurgery and Chair of the Department of Neurosurgery. The Department has also established a Resident Education and Research Fund in Dr. Hoff's name to continue his outstanding legacy of leadership in academic neurosurgery and his longstanding support of residency education. A Hoff Lectureship has now been established in the Department of Neurosurgery and is associated with a Hoff Alumni Day. Dr. John McGillicuddy will give the first Hoff Lectureship this summer.

Dr. Hoff is survived by his wife of 45 years, Diane (Shanks) Hoff, and by 3 children, Paul Hoff, MD (Donna Hoff, MD), Allison Hoff, MA, and Julia Haughey, MSW (Michael Haughey). He leaves 5 grandchildren, Lauren Hoff, Kiersten Hoff, Kathryn Haughey, Kelly Haughey, and Charles Haughey.

A memorial service at the First Presbyterian Church in Ann Arbor, Michigan on May 19, 2007 celebrated Dr. Hoff's outstanding life. It was a time in which friends from around the world gathered in memory of a truly outstanding leader and great friend to neurosurgery. All who have had the privilege of knowing Dr. Hoff will remember him for his wonderful smile, his bright eyes, and his unfailingly pleasant personality. Behind all this was a blazing intellect that has left behind a legacy of outstanding scholarship, strong national leadership, and a personal ethical and moral compass to which we all aspire. Dr. Hoff's legacy goes beyond a summary of his many accomplishments and is reflected by a generation of scientists, residents, colleagues, patients, and friends who felt honored and privileged to know him, and who lead lives that will forever be influenced by his presence.

Acta Neurochir Suppl (2008) 105: XIII
© Springer-Verlag 2008
Printed in Austria

Hoff Fellowships

To honor the memory of Dr. Julian T. Hoff and his contributions to the field of intracerebral hemorrhage research, a number of fellowships were established to allow young scientists and clinicians to attend and present at the 2nd International Symposium on Cerebral Hemorrhage in Shanghai. The awardees are to be applauded for their research. They were as follows:

Xuhui Bao, Department of Neurosurgery, Fudan University, China

Tim Lekic, Department of Physiology, Loma Linda University, USA

Timothy Morgan, Department of Neurology, Johns Hopkins University, USA

Molly E. Ogle, Department of Pathology, Laboratory Medicine, Medical University of South Carolina, USA

Qing Xie, Department of Neurosurgery, Fudan University, China

Feng Zhou, Department of Neurosurgery, 2nd Affiliated Hospital, Zhejiang University, China

Experimental intracerebral hemorrhage – iron, hemoglobin and free radicals

Acta Neurochir Suppl (2008) 105: 3–6
© Springer-Verlag 2008
Printed in Austria

Deferoxamine therapy for intracerebral hemorrhage

Y. Hua, R. F. Keep, J. T. Hoff, G. Xi

Department of Neurosurgery, University of Michigan Medical School, Ann Arbor, MI, USA

Summary

Intracerebral hemorrhage (ICH) is a subtype of stroke with very high mortality. Experiments have indicated that clot lysis and iron play an important role in ICH-induced brain injury. Iron overload occurs in the brain after ICH in rats. Intracerebral infusion of iron causes brain edema and neuronal death.

Deferoxamine, an iron chelator, is an FDA-approved drug for the treatment of acute iron intoxication and chronic iron overload due to transfusion-dependent anemia. Deferoxamine can rapidly penetrate the blood–brain barrier and accumulate in the brain tissue in significant concentration after systemic administration. We have demonstrated that deferoxamine reduces ICH-induced brain edema, neuronal death, brain atrophy, and neurological deficits. Iron chelation with deferoxamine could be a new therapy for ICH.

Keywords: Brain edema; cerebral hemorrhage; deferoxamine; iron; neuronal death.

Introduction

Spontaneous intracerebral hemorrhage (ICH) is a common and often fatal stroke subtype. If the patient survives the ictus, the resulting hematoma within brain parenchyma triggers a series of events leading to secondary insults and severe neurological deficits [23, 39]. Although the hematoma in humans gradually resolves, the neurological deficits in ICH patients are usually permanent and disabling.

Iron plays an important role in brain injury after ICH [31]. Our recent studies suggest that iron overload occurs in the brain following ICH, which results in brain damage [18, 35]. In particular, we have found that an iron chelator, deferoxamine, can reduce ICH-induced

Correspondence: Guohua Xi, MD, Department of Neurosurgery, University of Michigan Medical School, 109 Zina Pitcher Place, R5018 Biomedical Science Research Building, Ann Arbor, MI 48109-2200, USA. e-mail: guohuaxi@umich.edu

brain edema, neuronal death and neurological deficits in rats [5, 7, 18, 19].

Erythrocyte lysis and brain edema

Brain edema around the hematoma is commonly observed during the acute and subacute stages following ICH, contributing to poor outcomes [25, 41]. Although the mechanisms of edema formation following ICH are not fully resolved, several mechanisms are responsible for edema development. These include hydrostatic pressure during hematoma formation and clot retraction, coagulation cascade activation and thrombin production, hemoglobin and iron toxicity, complement activation, mass effect, secondary perihematomal ischemia, reperfusion brain injury, and blood–brain barrier (BBB) disruption [6, 13, 15, 16, 30, 36–38]. Various animal models of ICH have allowed detailed study of these mechanisms and their roles in the pathophysiological events that occur in brain tissue after ICH.

Edema around a hematoma reaches its peak several days after the ictus [3, 17, 29]. In rats, the edema peak occurs on the third or the fourth day after experimental ICH [36, 40]. In contrast, thrombin-induced brain edema peaks within 48 h [36]. This difference in time course led us to examine whether there might be a third phase (after 3 days) of injury involving red blood cell (RBC) lysis and hemoglobin-induced neuronal toxicity. Infusion of packed erythrocytes caused edema after about 3 days, suggesting that RBCs are associated with delayed edema formation [36]. A clinical study of edema and ICH indicated that delayed brain edema is related to significant midline shift after ICH in humans [41]. This delayed brain edema formation (in the second or third weeks after onset in human) is probably due to RBC lysis and hemoglobin degradation products.

Hemoglobin, hemoglobin degradation products, and brain injury

Hemoglobin causes brain damage through its degradation products [39]. Heme from hemoglobin is degraded by heme oxygenase in the brain into iron, carbon monoxide, and biliverdin. Biliverdin is then converted to bilirubin by biliverdin reductase [12]. Our previous studies demonstrated that an intracerebral infusion of hemoglobin and its degradation products, hemin, iron, and bilirubin, cause the formation of brain edema within 24 h. Hemoglobin itself induces heme oxygenase-1 (HO-1) upregulation in the brain and heme oxygenase inhibition by tin-protoporphyrin (SnPP) reduces hemoglobin-induced brain edema. In addition, an intraperitoneal injection of a large dose of deferoxamine (an iron chelator) attenuates brain edema induced by hemoglobin. These results indicate that hemoglobin causes brain injury by itself and through its degradation products, particularly iron [9].

Iron toxicity and neuronal death

Iron is essential for normal brain function, but iron overload may have devastating effects [1]. Iron overload contributes to many kinds of brain injury including hemorrhagic and ischemic stroke [8]. Clot lysis and iron release from heme occurs within the first week after ICH in animal studies, and this appears to contribute to acute brain edema formation [36]. However, brain atrophy occurs several weeks later, suggesting that iron exposure causes cell damage that results in delayed cell death. For example, iron may cause sufficient damage that the cell cannot repair itself. If such death occurs in cells that are storing iron released from the hematoma, the new iron release may affect nearby cells leading to amplification of the lesion. Alternately, the iron stored in cells after resolution of the clot may be naturally released for clearance across the BBB or through cerebrospinal fluid, but with potential for causing further tissue damage.

After erythrocyte lysis, iron concentrations in the brain can reach very high levels. Our recent data showed a 3-fold increase in brain non-heme iron content after ICH in rats, and it remains high for at least 28 days [35]. Intracerebral infusion of iron causes brain edema and an iron chelator reduces hematoma-and hemoglobin-induced edema, suggesting that iron plays an important role in edema formation after ICH [9, 18].

Iron-induced brain damage may result from oxidative stress. Cortical iron injections cause focal epileptiform paroxysmal discharges [4, 33]. Iron and lipid peroxidation also have an important role in hemoglobin-induced brain injury. For example, a subpial injection of $FeCl_2$ induces brain edema and lipid peroxidation in the brain [34]. Iron can also stimulate the formation of free radicals leading to neuronal damage. It is known that ferrous (Fe^{2+}) and ferric (Fe^{3+}) iron react with lipid hydroperoxides to produce free radicals [27]. Antioxidants block neuronal toxicity induced by hemoglobin and iron [24, 32].

Iron transport and storage proteins in the brain

A number of proteins, including transferrin (Tf), transferrin receptor (TfR), and ferritin are involved in maintaining brain iron homeostasis. We found that brain Tf, TfR, and ferritin levels are increased after ICH [35]. Tf, an 80-kDa protein, is a major iron distributor in the brain. Cellular uptake of Tf-bound iron is achieved by binding to the TfR. In normal brain, TfR is expressed at very high levels at the BBB, where it is involved in iron uptake into brain. However, a recent report indicates that there is rapid efflux of Tf from brain to blood across the BBB [42], suggesting that Tf could contribute to iron clearance when there is brain iron overload. TfR is normally only expressed on brain parenchymal cells at low levels but it can be increased under pathophysiological conditions. The brain can produce ferritin, the iron storage protein. Ferritin has 2 subunits, heavy-ferritin (21 kDa) and light-ferritin (19 kDa) [2]. Ferritin is found mainly in glial cells but not neurons.

Deferoxamine therapy

Deferoxamine, an iron chelator, is a Food and Drug Administration (FDA)-approved drug for the treatment of acute iron intoxication and of chronic iron overload due to transfusion-dependent anemias. Its molecular weight is 657. Deferoxamine can rapidly penetrate the BBB and accumulate in brain tissue in significant concentration after systemic administration [11, 20]. The terminal half-life of deferoxamine after intravenous infusion is 3.05 h [21]. Deferoxamine chelates iron by forming a stable complex that prevents the iron from entering into further chemical reactions. It readily chelates iron from ferritin and hemosiderin but not readily from transferrin. *In vivo*, deferoxamine can reduce hematoma- and hemoglobin-induced brain edema [9, 18]. Our recent studies show that deferoxamine reduces ICH-induced neuronal death, brain atrophy, and neurological deficits [5, 7, 28].

Deferoxamine binds ferric iron and prevents the formation of hydroxyl radical via the Fenton/Haber-Weiss reaction. Deferoxamine reduces hemoglobin-induced brain Na^+/K^+ ATPase inhibition and neuronal toxicity [24, 26]. Favorable effects of iron chelator therapy have been reported in various cerebral ischemia models [10, 14].

Although deferoxamine is an iron chelator, it can have other effects. Thus, it can act as a direct free radical scavenger [10, 14] and it can induce ischemic tolerance in the brain [22]. The latter has been demonstrated *in vivo* and *in vitro*, and it may be related to a deferoxamine induction of hypoxia-inducible transcription factor-1 binding to DNA [22].

Deferoxamine, however, may cause hypersensitivity reactions, systemic allergic reactions, cardiovascular, hematologic, and neurological adverse reactions. Serious adverse reactions include significant hypotension and marked body weight loss. In addition, deferoxamine may cause cytotoxicity because deferoxamine inhibits DNA synthesis *in vitro*.

Remarks

At present, there is no effective treatment that attenuates brain edema and improves long-term outcome in ICH. Our previous studies have shown that iron plays an important role in edema formation, neuronal death, brain atrophy, and behavioral deficits. Iron chelation with deferoxamine could be a new therapy for ICH. Such a therapy would be of great benefit, not only to the patients, but also to their caregivers and to society in general by reducing the cost of care for hemorrhagic stroke patients.

Deferoxamine has just entered Phase I clinical trial in humans.

Acknowledgment

This study was supported by grants NS-017760, NS-39866, NS-047245, and NS-052510 from the National Institutes of Health (NIH) and Grant-in-Aid 075571Z from American Heart Association (AHA). The content is solely the responsibility of the authors and does not necessarily represent the official views of the NIH or AHA.

References

1. Chiueh CC (2001) Iron overload, oxidative stress, and axonal dystrophy in brain disorders. Pediatr Neurol 25: 138–147
2. Connor JR, Menzies SL, Burdo JR, Boyer PJ (2001) Iron and iron management proteins in neurobiology. Pediatr Neurol 25: 118–129
3. Enzmann DR, Britt RH, Lyons BE, Buxton JL, Wilson DA (1981) Natural history of experimental intracerebral hemorrhage: sonography, computed tomography and neuropathology. Am J Neuroradiol 2: 517–526
4. Hammond EJ, Ramsay RE, Villarreal HJ, Wilder BJ (1980) Effects of intracortical injection of blood and blood components on the electrocorticogram. Epilepsia 21: 3–14
5. He Y, Wan S, Hua Y, Keep RF, Xi G (2008) Autophagy after experimental intracerebral hemorrhage. J Cereb Blood Flow Metab 28: 897–905
6. Hua Y, Xi G, Keep RF, Hoff JT (2000) Complement activation in the brain after experimental intracerebral hemorrhage. J Neurosurg 92: 1016–1022
7. Hua Y, Nakamura T, Keep RF, Wu J, Schallert T, Hoff JT, Xi G (2006) Long-term effects of experimental intracerebral hemorrhage: the role of iron. J Neurosurg 104: 305–312
8. Hua Y, Keep RF, Hoff JT, Xi G (2007) Brain injury after intracerebral hemorrhage: the role of thrombin and iron. Stroke 38(2 Suppl): 759–762
9. Huang FP, Xi G, Keep RF, Hua Y, Nemoianu A, Hoff JT (2002) Brain edema after experimental intracerebral hemorrhage: role of hemoglobin degradation products. J Neurosurg 96: 287–293
10. Hurn PD, Koehler RC, Blizzard KK, Traystman RJ (1995) Deferoxamine reduces early metabolic failure associated with severe cerebral ischemic acidosis in dogs. Stroke 26: 688–695
11. Keberle H (1964) The biochemistry of desferrioxamine and its relation to iron metabolism. Ann NY Acad Sci 119: 758–768
12. Kutty RK, Maines MD (1981) Purification and characterization of biliverdin reductase from rat liver. J Biol Chem 256: 3956–3962
13. Lee KR, Betz AL, Kim S, Keep RF, Hoff JT (1996) The role of the coagulation cascade in brain edema formation after intracerebral hemorrhage. Acta Neurochir (Wien) 138: 396–401
14. Liachenko S, Tang P, Xu Y (2003) Deferoxamine improves early postresuscitation reperfusion after prolonged cardiac arrest in rats. J Cereb Blood Flow Metab 23: 574–581
15. Mayer SA, Lignelli A, Fink ME, Kessler DB, Thomas CE, Swarup R, Van Heertum RL (1998) Perilesional blood flow and edema formation in acute intracerebral hemorrhage: a SPECT study. Stroke 29: 1791–1798
16. Mendelow AD (1993) Mechanisms of ischemic brain damage with intracerebral hemorrhage. Stroke 24(12 Suppl): I115–I119
17. Mun-Bryce S, Kroh FO, White J, Rosenberg GA (1993) Brain lactate and pH dissociation in edema: 1H- and 31P-NMR in collagenase-induced hemorrhage in rats. Am J Physiol 265: R697–R702
18. Nakamura T, Keep RF, Hua Y, Schallert T, Hoff JT, Xi G (2004) Deferoxamine-induced attenuation of brain edema and neurological deficits in a rat model of intracerebral hemorrhage. J Neurosurg 100: 672–678
19. Nakamura T, Keep RF, Hua Y, Hoff JT, Xi G (2005) Oxidative DNA injury after experimental intracerebral hemorrhage. Brain Res 1039: 30–36
20. Palmer C, Roberts RL, Bero C (1994) Deferoxamine posttreatment reduces ischemic brain injury in neonatal rats. Stroke 25: 1039–1045
21. Porter JB (2001) Deferoxamine pharmacokinetics. Semin Hematol 38(1 Suppl 1): 63–68
22. Prass K, Ruscher K, Karsch M, Isaev N, Megow D, Priller J, Scharff A, Dirnagl U, Meisel A (2002) Desferrioxamine induces delayed

tolerance against cerebral ischemia in vivo and in vitro. J Cereb Blood Flow Metab 22: 520–525

23. Qureshi AI, Tuhrim S, Broderick JP, Batjer HH, Hondo H, Hanley DF (2001) Spontaneous intracerebral hemorrhage. N Engl J Med 344: 1450–1460

24. Regan RF, Panter SS (1993) Neurotoxicity of hemoglobin in cortical cell culture. Neurosci Lett 153: 219–222

25. Ropper AH, King RB (1984) Intracranial pressure monitoring in comatose patients with cerebral hemorrhage. Arch Neurol 41: 725–728

26. Sadrzadeh SM, Anderson DK, Panter SS, Hallaway PE, Eaton JW (1987) Hemoglobin potentiates central nervous system damage. J Clin Invest 79: 662–664

27. Siesjö BK, Agardh CD, Bengtsson F (1989) Free radicals and brain damage. Cerebrovasc Brain Metab Rev 1: 165–211

28. Song S, Hua Y, Keep RF, Hoff JT, Xi G (2007) A new hippocampal model for examining intracerebral hemorrhage-related neuronal death: effects of deferoxamine on hemoglobin-induced neuronal death. Stroke 38: 2861–2863

29. Tomita H, Ito U, Ohno K, Hirakawa K (1994) Chronological changes in brain edema induced by experimental intracerebral hematoma in cats. Acta Neurochir Suppl (Wien) 60: 558–560

30. Wagner KR, Xi G, Hua Y, Kleinholz M, de Courten-Myers GM, Myers RE, Broderick JP, Brott TG (1996) Lobar intracerebral hemorrhage model in pigs: rapid edema development in perihematomal white matter. Stroke 27: 490–497

31. Wagner KR, Sharp FR, Ardizzone TD, Lu A, Clark JF (2003) Heme and iron metabolism: Role in cerebral hemorrhage. J Cereb Blood Flow Metab 23: 629–652

32. Wang X, Mori T, Sumii T, Lo EH (2002) Hemoglobin-induced cytotoxicity in rat cerebral cortical neurons: caspase activation and oxidative stress. Stroke 33: 1882–1888

33. Willmore LJ, Sypert GW, Munson JV, Hurd RW (1978) Chronic focal epileptiform discharges induced by injection of iron into rat and cat cortex. Science 200: 1501–1503

34. Willmore LJ, Rubin JJ (1982) Formation of malonaldehyde and focal brain edema induced by subpial injection of $FeCl_2$ into rat isocortex. Brain Res 246: 113–119

35. Wu J, Hua Y, Keep RF, Nakamura T, Hoff JT, Xi G (2003) Iron and iron-handling proteins in the brain after intracerebral hemorrhage. Stroke 34: 2964–2969

36. Xi G, Keep RF, Hoff JT (1998) Erythrocytes and delayed brain edema formation following intracerebral hemorrhage in rats. J Neurosurg 89: 991–996

37. Xi G, Wagner KR, Keep RF, Hua Y, de Courten-Myers GM, Broderick JP, Brott TG, Hoff JT (1998) The role of blood clot formation on early edema development following experimental intracerebral hemorrhage. Stroke 29: 2580–2586

38. Xi G, Hua Y, Keep RF, Younger JG, Hoff JT (2001) Systemic complement depletion diminishes perihematomal brain edema in rats. Stroke 32: 162–167

39. Xi G, Keep RF, Hoff JT (2006) Mechanisms of brain injury after intracerebral haemorrhage. Lancet Neurol 5: 53–63

40. Yang GY, Betz AL, Chenevert TL, Brunberg JA, Hoff JT (1994) Experimental intracerebral hemorrhage: relationship between brain edema, blood flow, and blood–brain barrier permeability in rats. J Neurosurg 81: 93–102

41. Zazulia AR, Diringer MN, Derdeyn CP, Powers WJ (1999) Progression of mass effect after intracerebral hemorrhage. Stroke 30: 1167–1173

42. Zhang Y, Pardridge WM (2001) Rapid transferrin efflux from brain to blood across the blood–brain barrier. J Neurochem 76: 1597–1600

Acta Neurochir Suppl (2008) 105: 7–12
© Springer-Verlag 2008
Printed in Austria

Bilirubin oxidation products, oxidative stress, and intracerebral hemorrhage

J. F. Clark[1], M. Loftspring[1], W. L. Wurster[1], S. Beiler[2], C. Beiler[2], K. R. Wagner[1,2], G. J. Pyne-Geithman[1]

[1] Department of Neurology, University of Cincinnati, and the Medical Research Service, Cincinnati, OH, USA
[2] Department of Veterans Affairs Medical Center, Cincinnati, OH, USA

Summary

Hematoma and perihematomal regions after intracerebral hemorrhage (ICH) are biochemically active environments known to undergo potent oxidizing reactions. We report facile production of bilirubin oxidation products (BOXes) *via* hemoglobin/Fenton reaction under conditions approximating putative *in vivo* conditions seen following ICH.

Using a mixture of human hemoglobin, physiological buffers, unconjugated solubilized bilirubin, and molecular oxygen and/or hydrogen peroxide, we generated BOXes, confirmed by spectral signature consistent with known BOXes mixtures produced by independent chemical synthesis, as well as HPLC-MS of BOX A and BOX B. Kinetics are straightforward and uncomplicated, having initial rates around 0.002 μM bilirubin per μM hemoglobin per second under normal experimental conditions. In hematomas from porcine ICH model, we observed significant production of BOXes, malondialdehyde, and superoxide dismutase, indicating a potent oxidizing environment. BOX concentrations increased from 0.084 ± 0.01 in fresh blood to 22.24 ± 4.28 in hematoma at 72 h, and were 11.22 ± 1.90 in adjacent white matter (nmol/g). Similar chemical and analytical results are seen in ICH *in vivo*, indicating the hematoma is undergoing similar potent oxidations.

This is the first report of BOXes production using a well-defined biological reaction and *in vivo* model of same. Following ICH, amounts of unconjugated bilirubin in hematoma can be substantial, as can levels of iron and hemoglobin. Oxidation of unconjugated bilirubin to yield bioactive molecules, such as BOXes, is an important discovery, expanding the role of bilirubin in pathological processes seen after ICH.

Keywords: Bilirubin oxidation products; edema; reactive oxygen species; pathology; stroke.

Introduction

Radical processes are well-known in biochemistry and are proposed to occur in living organisms, creating many known disease states. Oxidation of common metabolic products by oxygen, hydrogen peroxide, free iron, and other simple compounds have been widely studied and reported [16, 21–23]. The nature of these oxidation products is not well understood, even though they may have significant physiological impact and lead to subsequent tissue damage. There is growing interest in the oxidations that occur in intracerebral hematoma after intracerebral hemorrhage (ICH), because there appears to be a compromised region around the hematoma that is refractory to current therapies or even hematoma evacuation [6, 9, 20, 22, 26].

We previously reported that bilirubin is oxidized in a hemorrhagic medium and *in vivo* [4, 8, 12, 17]. Bilirubin oxidation products (BOXes), 1-(1,5-dihydropyrrole-2-ylidene) acetamide and related compounds, are small vasoactive molecules with demonstrated clinical importance [17]. They are found in the cerebrospinal fluid of patients who have had hemorrhagic strokes such as subarachnoid and intracerebral hemorrhage. These compounds exhibit biological activity *in vivo* and *in vitro* and have been postulated to be a major contributor to cerebral vasospasm, a pathological constriction of arteries. BOXes have been synthesized *in vitro* by the oxidation of unconjugated bilirubin at room temperature with a large excess of hydrogen peroxide. The conversion of bilirubin to BOXes is associated with a biochemical state that may cause or contribute to pathological sequelae after ICH. In this report, we outline the conversion of unconjugated (free) bilirubin and other relevant compounds to compounds well-known to have physiological and pathological effects. This was achieved using an *in vitro* system for modeling chemical oxidations, and *in vivo* using a porcine ICH model. Our results suggest that potent oxidations occur in the hematoma, and that the oxidized products penetrate into the perihematomal region with possible detrimental effects.

Correspondence: Joseph F. Clark, Ph.D., Department of Neurology, University of Cincinnati, Cincinnati, OH 45267-0536, USA. e-mail: Joseph.clark@uc.edu

Experimental methods

Reagents and chemicals

All reagents were American Chemical Society grade or better. Chemicals and biomaterials were purchased from Sigma-Aldrich Co. (St. Louis, MO) unless otherwise stated. BOXes were prepared as previously described [4, 8, 12]. Gasses used were technical grade or better. Optical spectra were obtained on a micro-Quant microwell plate reader using ultraviolet transparent 96-well plates. All optical densities (OD) are reported as uncorrected for plate. Aliquots of the reaction mixture were taken directly and read for OD within a short period of time from sampling and analyzed for kinetics data. Reaction mixture consisted of 100 μM solubilized bilirubin, 1 g sodium carbonate, 200 mL deionized water, 1 mg human hemoglobin, μM oxygen, and/or 100 μL of 30% hydrogen peroxide. Figure 1 is a schematic of how the in vitro system was designed. Figures 2A and B show data collected using this reaction system.

Pig surgery and tissue sampling

Animal procedures were approved by the Institutional Animal Care and Use Committee at the University of Cincinnati. Methods to induce ICH have been previously described [18–20]. Briefly, 3 mL of autologous blood was infused into frontal hemispheric white matter of pentobarbital-anesthetized pigs. Brains were frozen *in situ* with liquid nitrogen at various time points up to 72 h. Approximately 20 mg of perihematomal, edematous white matter was sampled and homogenized in 200 μL of homogenization buffer, as previously described [11].

Bilirubin determination

Total bilirubin was assayed using a method based on those developed by Michaelsson *et al.* [14] and adapted for use in a microtiter plate, as previously described [17]. Briefly, bilirubin in the sample is first treated with a caffeine solution to release all bilirubin moieties, followed by a diazo reagent to yield a colored product. This is then alkalized until the color is in a range that is not overlapping the absorption range of hemoglobin, and the absorption is recorded at 600 nm. Sample absorbance is compared to a concomitantly run standard curve constructed from commercially available bilirubin standard solutions (Wako Chemicals USA, Inc., Richmond, VA) to determine total bilirubin concentrations.

BOXes determination

BOXes were quantified by spectroscopic analysis at 320 nm, as previously described [17]. Chemically prepared BOXes were used to construct a standard curve. Samples were subjected to a chloroform extraction and evaporation, and re-suspended in 0.9% saline for analysis.

Hemoglobin determination

The sample was exposed to Drabkin's reagent ($NaHCO_3$:$K_3Fe(CN)_6$: KCN, 100:20:5) in order to convert all hemoglobin moieties into cyanomethemoglobin [5]. A surfactant (Brij-35) was added to prevent protein- or lipid-induced turbidity. Concentration of cyanomethemoglobin is determined by comparison to a standard curve constructed with commercially available lyophilized hemoglobin (Sigma-Aldrich), treated with Drabkin's reagent, and the absorbance read at 540 nm.

Malondialdehyde (MDA) determination

MDA was assessed using a commercially available assay kit from Calbiochem (San Diego, CA). Briefly, MDA reacts with N-methyl-2-phenylindole in acetonitrile and ferric ions to form a colored molecule that has maximum absorbance at 568 nm [5].

Superoxide dismutase (SOD) assay

SOD activity was measured using a commercially available kit (Fluka, St. Louis, MO) according to the manufacturer's instructions. Upon reac-

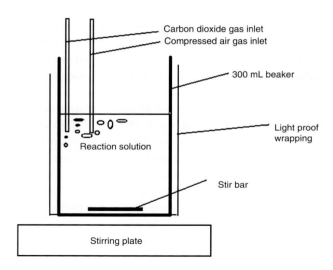

Fig. 1. Simple oxidization reaction vessel showing *in vitro* system for modeling the oxidizing environment in porcine hematoma

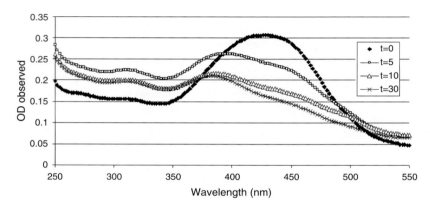

Fig. 2A. A solution of 1 g sodium carbonate, 105 μM solubilized bilirubin, saturating levels of carbon dioxide gas and compressed air, 1 mg human hemoglobin, and 42 mM hydrogen peroxide were allowed to react with constant stirring in an open system. Aliquots of reaction were taken at 0 min (*square*), 5 min (*triangle*), 10 min (*X*), and 30 min (*diamond*). Optical density was followed in the visible region. The pH of this reaction is 6.8

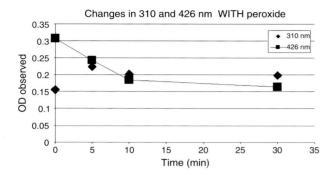

Fig. 2B. The apparent kinetics of bilirubin degradation and BOX production using visible spectroscopy and extinction coefficients for bilirubin and BOXes. The rise in BOXes is apparent within 10 min and plateaus at about 10 min, reaching a steady state. Bilirubin falls at 426 nm, mirroring the production of BOXes

tion with superoxide, Donjino's tetrazolium salt, WST-1, produces a water soluble formazan dye with an absorbance of 450 nm [27, 28]. Samples were treated with Donjino's and xanthine oxidase to produce superoxide. The percent inhibition of formazan formation by SOD was measured.

Total protein determination

Total protein was determined using the BCA protein assay (Pierce Biotechnology, Rockford, IL). Side chains of several amino acids reduce cupric copper to the cuprous oxidation state, and this change is measured at 562 nm. The total protein concentration is interpolated from a standard curve using bovine serum albumin as the standard.

Statistics

Statistical differences were determined using ANOVA or Student t-test where indicated. A p-value of ≤ 0.05 was considered statistically significant.

Results

Figures 2A and B indicate the facile conversion of bilirubin (loss of OD at 425 nm) and conversion to BOXes (OD at 310 nm). This conversion is rapid and takes only 5 min at room temperature under the experimental conditions described (Fig. 2B). This indicates that the small molecules of BOXes have extreme membrane permeability and high biological activity, and appear to be formed in the model system under pseudo-physiological conditions. Both peroxide and hemoglobin are necessary for the reaction to occur. Carbon monoxide significantly inhibits the reaction; thus, the reaction involves the heme moiety in the hemoglobin (Fig. 3). These observations are indicative of a free radical reaction. Also, deferoxamine has little effect on the reaction, indicating that free iron is not involved in, or essential for, the reaction. Thus, this *in vitro* reaction produces significant amounts of BOXes in about 10 min. Figure 3 shows that there are both activators and inhibitors of this simple reaction.

Table 1 summarizes the production of BOXes as well as related metabolites produced in and around the hematoma after ICH. Of note is that concentrations of BOXes reach substantial levels in hematoma and perihematomal white matter on the ipsilateral side. Bilirubin levels are increased in the hematoma as well as perihematomal region and have not reached a plateau at 72 h. Production of MDA appears to plateau at 24 h and is present in both ipsilateral and contralateral brain. SOD activity was consistently highest in the hematoma brain and was relatively constant following hemorrhage. The

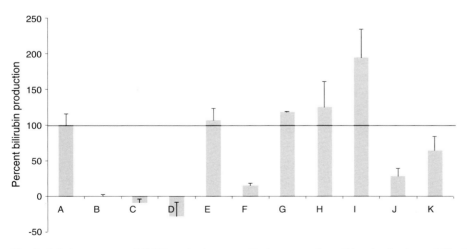

Fig. 3. Relative amounts of BOX production normalized to control condition A. A = hemoglobin (0.64 μM), bilirubin (105 μM), peroxide (383 mM); B = incubation A without hemoglobin; C = incubation without hemoglobin and peroxide; D = incubation A without peroxide; E = incubation A with added deferoxamine (65 mM); F = incubation A with carbon monoxide; G = incubation A with benzoic acid (1.2 mM); H = incubation A with added potassium cyanide (6.5 mM); I = incubation A with added arachidonic acid (4.3 mM); J = incubation A with added oxalic acid (550 mM); K = incubation A with added thiourea (110 mM). Error bars are standard deviation. $N = 3$ or more for all conditions. Reactions were performed in phosphate-buffered saline at pH 7.5

Table 1. *Metabolites present post ICH*

	Malondialdehyde (mM/mg protein)	Superoxide dismutase (% activity/mg/mL protein)	Bilirubin (mg/dL)	Bilirubin oxidation products (nmol/g)
Fresh blood	0.37 ± 0.06		4.18 ± 0.08	0.084 ± 0.01
Sham ipsilateral	0.51 ± 0.041	0.16 ± 0.010		
Sham contralateral	0.54 ± 0.021	0.17 ± 0.011		
1 h hematoma	0.088 ± 0.034	0.029 ± 0.0021		
1 h contralateral	1.15 ± 0.45	0.19 ± 0.041		
1 h ipsilateral	0.86 ± 0.030	0.16 ± 0.040		
8–12 h hematoma	0.56 ± 0.038		13.6 ± 0.98	3.44 ± 0.37
24 h hematoma	0.082 ± 0.036	0.039 ± 0.011	20.31 ± 3.32	
24 h contralateral	0.99 ± 0.33	0.174 ± 0.017	0.71	0.78
24 h ipsilateral	0.47 ± 0.14	0.181 ± 0.012	10.35	3.10
48 h hematoma	0.11 ± 0.097	0.034 ± 0.011		11.22 ± 1.90
48 h ipsilateral	0.39 ± 0.20	0.18 ± 0.025		
48 h contralateral	0.96 ± 0.23	0.16 ± 0.030		
72 h hematoma	0.098 ± 0.011	0.027 ± 0.002	40.72 ± 3.03	22.24 ± 4.28
72 h ipsilateral	0.63 ± 0.07	0.25 ± 0.060		
72 h contralateral	0.88 ± 0.16	0.17 ± 0.002		

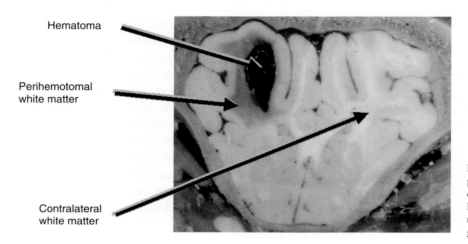

Hematoma

Perihemotomal white matter

Contralateral white matter

Fig. 4. Representative cross-section of porcine brain 16 h after ICH. Breakdown of blood–brain barrier is indicated by Evans blue perfusion. Arrows indicate relative areas of sampling for use in generating data presented in Table 1

relative location for obtaining samples presented in Table 1 can be seen in Fig. 4, where we show a representative section of pig brain demonstrating the hematoma, perihematomal region, and contralateral white matter. The edema present in the porcine brain after ICH is visible at 1 h and appears to peak at 48 h (Fig. 5).

Discussion

ICH is a devastating event, with high mortality from the initial hemorrhage. and a tragically high death and disability rate for patients who survive the initial ictus. Complications after ICH include, but are not limited to, increased intracranial pressure, breakdown of blood–brain barrier, clot mass effect, hydrocephalus, necrosis, atrophy, activation of complement, spreading depression, ischemia, and death [2, 7, 9, 10, 15, 24, 25].

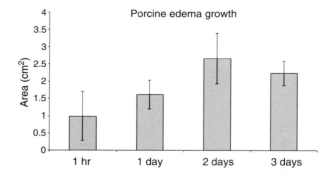

Fig. 5. Edema in the pig brain after ICH is evident in 8 h after hemorrhage and appears to peak at 2 days

Less than 30% of patients who survive an ICH return to normal, and many of the survivors require dependent care [1]. Thus, ICH and complications after ICH are a substantial health burden to the nation and to the families of survivors. Better understanding of the mechanisms associated with the complications will be important in treating these patients and providing hope for improved outcomes.

Our findings include: 1) the chemical environment found after ICH produces a potent oxidizing environment; 2) oxidations in the hematoma produce a cocktail of dangerous metabolites; and 3) these metabolites are quickly found in the perihematomal white matter. Taken together, these data suggest that the chemical environment of the hematoma is a substantial cause of the pathological sequelae seen after ICH, and that damage from the hematoma manifests rapidly after ICH. These 3 major findings and how they contribute to the body of evidence concerning the toxic environment produced by the hematoma are discussed below.

The chemical environment produces BOXes and toxic metabolites

In solution, we found that bilirubin is quickly oxidized in minutes, using several single electron reactions. We were able to confirm significant production of BOXes in the presence of the Fenton reaction as well as a carbon dioxide/carbonate 1-electron donor system (Fig. 3). Importantly, but not surprisingly, we found that there was an apparent pH optimum for this reaction of 6.8. This is a pH that is quite plausible after ICH. Reactive oxygen species can also produce an oxidizing environment to produce BOXes and other metabolites. We found that BOXes are produced with a similar time course when hydrogen peroxide is added to the system as compared to a 1-electron donor system. These data suggest that reactive oxygen species, single electron oxidations, and some radical reactions will produce BOXes. Should BOXes and other toxic metabolites be oxidized in this way, we believe that this oxidizing environment may cause or contribute to the pathological sequelae seen after ICH by allowing these compounds to leech into the perihematomal region and have their toxic effects.

Oxidations in the hematoma produce a cocktail of dangerous metabolites

The potent oxidizing environment seen in the hematoma after ICH can produce substantial concentrations of BOXes and other oxidized metabolites relatively quickly after ICH. These concentrations are in the range that has been reported previously [12, 13, 17], and are associated with toxicity responses *in vitro* [13]. We also found that substantial amounts of MDA, SOD,

and BOXes are produced in the hematoma at 1 h after ICH. These molecules are associated with oxidative damage and are considered to be indicators of hemorrhagic complications. Some of these are also directly biologically active [3].

Metabolites are found in the perihematomal white matter soon after ictus

If one believes that there are toxic compounds produced in the hematoma and that these toxic compounds cause or contribute to the pathological sequelae seen after ICH, it is necessary to assume that these compounds are diffusing out of the hematoma into the surrounding parenchyma. Therefore, we closely examined the concentration of metabolites and compounds in the perihematomal white matter. Ipsilateral brain consistently had elevated levels of BOXes, MDA, and SOD in our studies, with variations in the time course of these metabolites. It is unclear from our data whether the edema and breakdown of the blood–brain barrier is caused by the diffusion of these compounds out of the hematoma, or if these compounds are contributing to this breakdown. There does, nonetheless, seem to be a positive correlation of oxidative damage, oxidative stress, and BOXes with some of the pathological sequelae seen after ICH.

We also believe it is significant that substantial changes in histopathology as well as chemistry can occur within minutes and are manifested within hours. This might be highly relevant when designing strategies to treat these patients. Our data suggests that damage to the perihematomal white matter is occurring in as little as an hour after ICH, and that simple evacuation strategies might be less than successful if they do not address the harmful metabolites that have already diffused from the hematoma.

Conclusions

In this study, we found that a potent oxidizing environment exists in the hematoma after ICH, and that oxidative stress produces a cadre of compounds, some of which are known to be toxic and biologically active. These compounds diffuse into perihematomal white matter and may cause or contribute to the pathological sequelae seen after ICH. The time course for these chemical changes is also quite rapid (many seen in less than 24 h), suggesting that ultra-early intervention may be needed to prevent damage caused by the hematoma after ICH.

Acknowledgment

This work was supported by grants NS050569, NS042308, NS049428 and NS30652 from the National Institutes of Health. ML is supported by the Physician Scientist Training Program PSTP.

References

1. Butcher K, Laidlaw J (2003) Current intracerebral haemorrhage management. J Clin Neurosci 10: 158–167
2. Chen M, Regan RF (2007) Time course of increased heme oxygenase activity and expression after experimental intracerebral hemorrhage: correlation with oxidative injury. J Neurochem 103: 2015–2021
3. Cheng J, Ou JS, Singh H, Falck JR, Narsimhaswamy D, Pritchard KA Jr, Schwartzman ML (2008) 20-hydroxyeicosatetraenoic acid causes endothelial dysfunction via eNOS uncoupling. Am J Physiol Heart Circ Physiol 294: H1018–H1026
4. Clark JF, Loftspring M, Wurster WL, Pyne-Geithman GJ (2008) Chemical and biochemical oxidations in spinal fluid after subarachnoid hemorrhage. Front Biosci 13: 1806–1812
5. Esterbauer H, Cheeseman KH (1990) Determination of aldehydic lipid peroxidation products: malonaldehyde and 4-hydroxynonenal. Methods Enzymol 186: 407–421
6. Fayad PB, Awad IA (1998) Surgery for intracerebral hemorrhage. Neurology 51: S69–S73
7. Karwacki Z, Kowiański P, Witkowska M, Karwacka M, Dziewiatkowski J, Moryś J (2006) The pathophysiology of intracerebral haemorrhage. Folia Morphol (Warsz) 65: 295–300
8. Kranc KR, Pyne GJ, Tao L, Claridge TD, Harris DA, Cadoux-Hudson TA, Turnbull JJ, Schofield CJ, Clark JF (2000) Oxidative degradation of bilirubin produces vasoactive compounds. Eur J Biochem 267: 7094–7101
9. Lapchak PA, Araujo DM (2007) Advances in hemorrhagic stroke therapy: conventional and novel approaches. Expert Opin Emerg Drugs 12: 389–406
10. Lodhia KR, Shakui P, Keep RF (2006) Hydrocephalus in a rat model of intraventricular hemorrhage. Acta Neurochir Suppl 96: 207–211
11. Loftspring MC, Beiler S, Beiler C, Wagner KR (2006) Plasma proteins in edematous white matter after intracerebral hemorrhage confound immunoblots: an ELISA to quantify contamination. J Neurotrauma 23: 1904–1911
12. Loftspring MC, Wurster WL, Pyne-Geithman GJ, Clark JF (2007) An in vitro model of aneurysmal subarachnoid hemorrhage: oxidation of unconjugated bilirubin by cytochrome oxidase. J Neurochem 102: 1990–1995
13. Lyons MA, Shukla R, Zhang K, Pyne GJ, Singh M, Biehle SJ, Clark JF (2004) Increase of metabolic activity and disruption of normal contractile protein distribution by bilirubin oxidation products in vascular smooth-muscle cells. J Neurosurg 100: 505–511
14. Michaelsson M, Nosslin B, Sjolin S (1965) Plasma bilirubin determination in the newborn infant. A methodological study with especial reference to the influence of hemolysis. Pediatrics 35: p925–p931
15. Mun-Bryce S, Wilkerson AC, Papuashvili N, Okada YC (2001) Recurring episodes of spreading depression are spontaneously elicited by an intracerebral hemorrhage in the swine. Brain Res 888: 248–255
16. Nakamura T, Keep RF, Hua Y, Nagao S, Hoff JT, Xi G (2006) Iron-induced oxidative brain injury after experimental intracerebral hemorrhage. Acta Neurochir Suppl 96: 194–198
17. Pyne-Geithman GJ, Morgan CJ, Wagner K, Dulaney EM, Carrozzella J, Kanter DS, Zuccarello M, Clark JF (2005) Bilirubin production and oxidation in CSF of patients with cerebral vasospasm after subarachnoid hemorrhage. J Cereb Blood Flow Metab 25: 1070–1077
18. Wagner KR, Xi G, Hua Y, Kleinholz M, de Courten-Myers GM, Myers RE, Broderick JP, Brott TG (1996) Lobar intracerebral hemorrhage model in pigs: rapid edema development in perihematomal white matter. Stroke 27: 490–497
19. Wagner KR, Xi G, Hua Y, Kleinholz M, de Courten-Myers GM, Myers RE (1998) Early metabolic alterations in edematous perihematomal brain regions following experimental intracerebral hemorrhage. J Neurosurg 88: 1058–1065
20. Wagner KR, Xi G, Hua Y, Zuccarello M, de Courten-Myers GM, Broderick JP, Brott TG (1999) Ultra-early clot aspiration after lysis with tissue plasminogen activator in a porcine model of intracerebral hemorrhage: edema reduction and blood–brain barrier protection. J Neurosurg 90: 491–498
21. Wagner KR, Packard BA, Hall CL, Smulian AG, Linke MJ, De Courten-Myers GM, Packard LM, Hall NC (2002) Protein oxidation and heme oxygenase-1 induction in porcine white matter following intracerebral infusions of whole blood or plasma. Dev Neurosci 24: 154–160
22. Wagner KR, Sharp FR, Ardizzone TD, Lu A, Clark JF (2003) Heme and iron metabolism: role in cerebral hemorrhage. J Cereb Blood Flow Metab 23: 629–652
23. Wang J, Doré S (2007) Heme oxygenase-1 exacerbates early brain injury after intracerebral haemorrhage. Brain 130: 1643–1652
24. Xi G, Wagner KR, Keep RF, Hua Y, de Courten-Myers GM, Broderick JP, Brott TG, Hoff JT (1998) Role of blood clot formation on early edema development after experimental intracerebral hemorrhage. Stroke 29: 2580–2586
25. Yang S, Nakamura T, Hua Y, Keep RF, Younger JG, He Y, Hoff JT, Xi G (2006) The role of complement C3 in intracerebral hemorrhage-induced brain injury. J Cereb Blood Flow Metab 26: 1490–1495
26. Zuccarello M, Andaluz N, Wagner KR (2002) Minimally invasive therapy for intracerebral hematomas. Neurosurg Clin N Am 13: 349–354
27. Zhou JY, Prognon P (2006) Raw material enzymatic activity determination: A specific case for validation and comparison of analytical methods – the example of superoxide dismutase (SOD). J Pharm Biomed Anal 40: 1143–1148
28. Peskin AV, Winterbourn CC (2000) A microtiter plate assay for superoxide dismutase using a water-soluble tetrazolium salt (WST-1). Clin Chim Acta 293: 157–166

Acta Neurochir Suppl (2008) 105: 13–18
© Springer-Verlag 2008
Printed in Austria

Deferoxamine reduces brain swelling in a rat model of hippocampal intracerebral hemorrhage

S. Song[1,2], **Y. Hua**[1], **R. F. Keep**[1], **Y. He**[1], **J. Wang**[2], **J. Wu**[1,2], **G. Xi**[1]

[1] Department of Neurosurgery, University of Michigan Medical School, Ann Arbor, MI, USA
[2] The Second Affiliated Hospital, Zhejiang University Medical School, China

Summary

In this study, we examine the effects of deferoxamine on hemoglobin-induced brain swelling in a newly developed hippocampal model of intracerebral hemorrhage (ICH). There were 2 parts to the experiments in this study. In the first part, male Sprague-Dawley rats received a 10-μL infusion of either packed red blood cells (RBC), lysed RBC, hemoglobin, ferrous iron, or saline, into the hippocampus. In the second part, rats received a 10-μL infusion of hemoglobin and then were treated with either deferoxamine (100 mg/kg, intraperitoneally, given immediately after hemoglobin injection, then every 12 h for 24 h) or vehicle. Rats were then killed to obtain hippocampus size and DNA damage measurements. We found that lysed RBC induced marked brain swelling in the hippocampus. Compared to saline, hemoglobin or iron injection caused swelling. Systemic use of deferoxamine reduced hemoglobin-induced brain swelling (6.14 ± 0.45 vs. $7.11 \pm 0.58 \, \text{mm}^2$ in the vehicle group, $p < 0.05$). In addition, deferoxamine reduced hemoglobin-induced DNA damage. These results indicate that iron has a key role in hemoglobin-induced brain swelling. Deferoxamine may be a useful treatment for ICH patients.

Keywords: Brain edema; cerebral hemorrhage; deferoxamine; hemoglobin; iron.

Introduction

Intracerebral hemorrhage (ICH) is a subtype of stroke with a high rate of mortality [10, 20]. To understand the underlying mechanisms of ICH-induced brain injury and to evaluate therapeutic interventions, a number of animal models of ICH in different species, including mouse, rat, dog, and pig, have been developed [1, 14, 19, 23, 25, 29, 33, 37, 38]. A reproducible ICH model in the rat, involving infusion of autologous whole blood, has been used extensively to study mechanisms of brain injury, especially brain edema and blood–brain barrier disruption

[36]. Recently, delayed brain atrophy has been found in a rat model of ICH [3, 8], but ICH-induced neuronal death seems diffuse and it has been difficult to quantify. It is very important to develop an ICH model for quantification of neuronal loss. For this purpose, we developed a hippocampal ICH model in rats [24].

Both *in vivo* and *in vitro* experiments have demonstrated that hemoglobin and its degradation products, especially iron, contribute to brain injury after ICH [27, 36]. *In vivo* studies have demonstrated the role of red blood lysis, hemoglobin release, and iron toxicity in perihematomal edema formation [13, 33]. Recent studies have also shown iron overload occurs in the brain after ICH and contributes to ICH-induced DNA damage and brain atrophy [8, 15, 31, 32].

Deferoxamine, an iron chelator, can reduce cerebrospinal fluid (CSF) free iron levels following ICH [28]. Our previous studies have shown that ICH-induced brain edema, oxidative DNA damage, brain atrophy, and neurological deficits are less in deferoxamine-treated group compared with those in vehicle-treated group [8, 13]. Deferoxamine also can reduce hemoglobin-induced brain edema *in vivo* [9] and neuronal death *in vitro* [21, 22].

In the present study, the effects of systemic use of deferoxamine on hemoglobin-induced brain swelling were investigated in the newly developed hippocampal ICH model.

Materials and methods

Animal preparation and intracerebral infusion

The University of Michigan Committee on the Use and Care of Animals approved the protocols for these animal studies. Adult male Sprague-Dawley rats ($n = 78$; 275–350 g; Charles River Laboratories, Portage,

---

Correspondence: Guohua Xi, MD, Department of Neurosurgery, University of Michigan Medical School, R5018 Biomedical Science Research Building, 109 Zina Pitcher Place, Ann Arbor, MI 48109-2200, USA. e-mail: guohuaxi@umich.edu

MI) were used for the experiments. Aseptic precautions were utilized in all surgical procedures. Animals were anesthetized with pentobarbital (45 mg/kg, intraperitoneally (i.p.); Abbott Laboratories, North Chicago, IL). The right femoral artery was catheterized for blood pressure monitoring and blood sampling. Blood was obtained from the catheter for analysis of blood gases, blood pH, hematocrit, and glucose concentration. The animal was placed in a stereotactic frame (Model 5000, Kopf Instrument, Tujunga, CA), a cranial burr-hole (1 mm) was drilled into the skull at the injection site, and a 26-gauge needle was inserted stereotaxically into the right hippocampus (coordinates: 3.8 mm posterior, 3.2 mm ventral and 3.5 mm lateral to the bregma). Saline, hemoglobin, $FeCl_2$, packed red blood cells (RBC), and lysed RBC were infused at a rate of 1 μL per minute into the right hippocampus using a micro-infusion pump (World Precision Instruments Inc., Sarasota, FL). The needle remained in place for 2 min after completion of injection and was then removed. The skin incision was closed with sutures. Throughout the surgery, the core body temperature was maintained at 37.5 °C using a rectal probe feedback-controlled heating pad.

Experiment groups

There were 2 parts to this study. In the first part, rats ($n = 6$, each group) received an intrahippocampal 10-μL injection of either saline, bovine hemoglobin, $FeCl_2$, packed RBC, or lysed RBC, and were killed at 24 h. Brains were used for histology and DNA damage measurement. Packed RBCs (hematocrit = $87 \pm 1\%$) were obtained by centrifuging unclotted blood. Packed RBCs were frozen in liquid nitrogen for 5 min followed by thawing at 37 °C to obtain lysed RBCs. In the second part, rats ($n = 6$ each group) received an intracerebral 10-μL infusion of bovine hemoglobin (150 mg/mL) and were treated with either deferoxamine (100 mg/kg in 1 mL saline, i.p., given immediately after hemoglobin injection, then every 12 h) or the same amount of vehicle. Rats were killed 24 h later, and the brains were used for histology and DNA damage measurement.

Histological studies

Histological studies were performed as previously described [7]. Briefly, rats were anesthetized with pentobarbital (60 mg/kg, i.p.) followed by intracardiac perfusion with 4% paraformaldehyde in 0.1 M, pH 7.4 phosphate-buffered saline (PBS). Brains were removed quickly and further

fixed with the same fixation solution at 4 °C overnight. Post-fixed brains were dehydrated with 30% sucrose for 3–4 days at 4 °C. The brains were embedded in O.C.T. compound (Sakura Finetek USA Inc., Torrance, CA) and underwent coronal serial sectioning (18 μm thick) in the area covering dorsal hippocampus (−3.0 to −4.5 mm from bregma) on a cryostat. The sections were dehydrated with ethanol at graded concentrations of 50–100% (v/v), and hematoxylin and eosin (H & E) was used for staining.

The brain sections from 1 mm posterior to the blood injection site were scanned and the hippocampus was outlined on a computer by a blinded observer. The hippocampal areas were measured using the NIH Image software (Image Version 1.63, National Institutes of Health).

Terminal deoxynucleotidyl transferase-mediated dUTP nick end-labeling (TUNEL)

The TUNEL technique was performed. Brain slides were obtained for the histological studies at 1, 3, and 7 days after the infusion of saline, hemoglobin, and iron. The brain sections from 1 mm anterior to the blood injection site were used for TUNEL staining. The ApopTag Peroxidase Kit (Intergen Co., Purchase, NY) was used in this study. First, 3% hydrogen peroxide in 0.1 M PBS was applied to the specimens for 5 min to quench endogenous peroxidases. After washing with PBS and equilibrating with the solution supplied, the specimens were incubated with TdT enzyme at 37 °C for 1 h. The reaction was stopped by washing with buffer for 10 min. Anti-digoxigenin peroxidase conjugate was then applied to the slide for 30 min at room temperature. We used 3,3' diaminobenzidine (DAB) to visualize. Omission of the terminal deoxynucleotidyl transferase was used as the negative control [31]. TUNEL-positive cells in the hippocampus were counted.

Statistical analysis

All data in this study are presented as mean $\pm$ SD. Data were analyzed by ANOVA test or Student *t*-test. A level of $p < 0.05$ was considered statistically significant.

Results

Physiological parameters were recorded immediately before intrahippocampal injections. The mean arterial

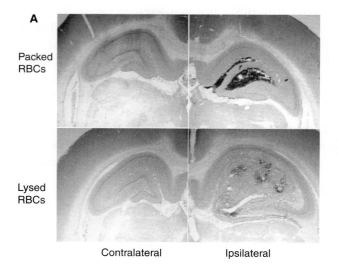
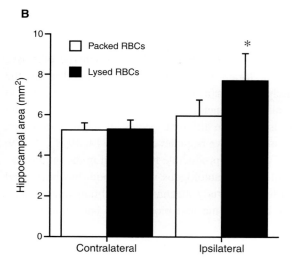

Fig. 1. Contralateral and ipsilateral hippocampal size 24 h after intracerebral 10-μL injection of either packed RBC or lysed RBC into the right hippocampus. Values are mean $\pm$ SD, $n = 6$, *$p < 0.05$ vs. packed RBC group

blood pressure (MABP), blood pH, blood gases, hematocrit, and blood glucose were controlled within normal ranges (MABP, 80–120 mmHg; pO_2, 80–120 mmHg; pCO_2, 35–45 mmHg; hematocrit, 38–42%; blood glucose, 80–120 mg/dL).

Hippocampal swelling

Lysed RBC rather than packed RBC caused marked hippocampal swelling (Fig. 1). To investigate the effects of hemoglobin and iron on brain swelling in the hippocampus, rats received an intrahippocampal injection of either hemoglobin or $FeCl_2$. Control rats had an injection of saline. Brains were perfused 24 h after infusion and H&E staining was used to measure hippocampal sizes. We found that hippocampal infusion of hemoglobin caused swelling in the ipsilateral hippocampus compared with that in the control group (6.83 ± 0.53 vs. 5.38 ± 0.34 mm^2, $p < 0.01$; Fig. 2). $FeCl_2$ injection mimicked hemoglobin's effect and caused significant

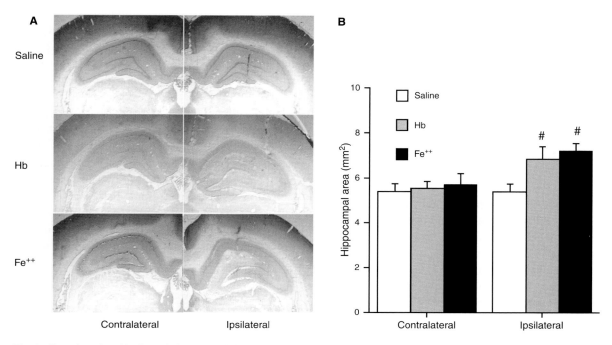

Fig. 2. Contralateral and ipsilateral hippocampal size 24 h after 10-μL intracerebral injection of either saline, hemoglobin (Hb), or ferrous iron (Fe^{++}) into right hippocampus. Values are mean $\pm$ SD, $n = 6$, $^{\#}p < 0.01$ vs. saline group

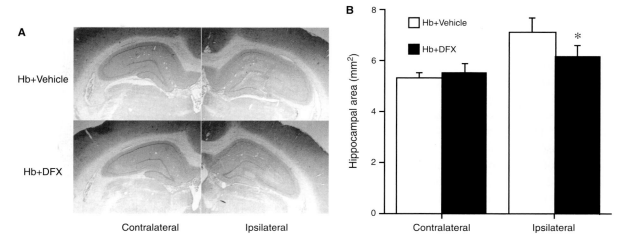

Fig. 3. Contralateral and ipsilateral hippocampal size 24 h after 10-μL intracerebral injection of hemoglobin with or without deferoxamine treatment. Values are mean $\pm$ SD, $n = 6$, $^{*}p < 0.05$ vs. Hb + Vehicle group

swelling in the hippocampus ($7.19 \pm 0.36\,mm^2$, Fig. 2), and desferrioxamine (DFX) reduced hippocampal swelling induced by hemoglobin (6.14 ± 0.45 vs. $7.10 \pm 0.58\,mm^2$ in the vehicle-treated group, $p < 0.05$; Fig. 3).

Double-strand DNA damage

To detect double-strand DNA damage, TUNEL staining was performed at 24 h after an intrahippocampal injection of hemoglobin, FeCl$_2$, and saline. TUNEL-positive cells were found in the ipsilateral hippocampus 1 day after injections of hemoglobin (171 ± 111 cells/slice) or FeCl$_2$ (173 ± 54 cells/slice), but not saline.

To examine the effects of DFX on hemoglobin-induced DNA damage, DFX was given immediately after hemoglobin injection. DFX reduced TUNEL-positive cells in the ipsilateral hippocampus (43 ± 19 vs. 247 ± 116 cells/slice in the vehicle-treated group; $p < 0.05$).

Discussion

Our previous study demonstrated lysed RBCs but not packed RBCs result in marked brain edema at 24 h in a caudate ICH model [33]. This study demonstrates that intrahippocampal infusion of lysed RBCs results in brain swelling by 24 h. This swelling appears to be hemoglobin mediated, since hemoglobin infusion also can cause brain swelling in the hippocampus.

Brain swelling in the hippocampus was also found after iron injection. As the iron chelator, DFX, reduces brain swelling induced by hemoglobin, iron appears to be an important factor in hemoglobin-induced injury. Cellular edema may contribute to brain swelling, but the main form of edema formation after ICH is vasogenic brain edema [35]. Studies have shown that hemoglobin can cause death of endothelial cells [16] and a significant disruption of the blood–brain barrier [34]. Whether or not DFX can reduce blood–brain barrier disruption should be investigated further.

Hemoglobin is a major component of a hematoma and is neurotoxic. Hemoglobin and its degradation products all can cause brain damage [27, 36]. An intracerebral infusion of hemoglobin degradation products, hemin, iron, and bilirubin, cause brain edema formation within 24 h, and heme oxygenase (HO) inhibition reduces hemoglobin-induced brain edema [9]. In a porcine ICH model, perihematomal edema is reduced by tin-mesoporphyrin, a HO inhibitor [26]. In addition, tin-mesoporphyrin reduces neuronal loss in a rabbit

ICH model [11]. Our recent data show that another HO inhibitor, zinc protoporphyrin, can also reduce ICH-induced brain injury [4]. However, hemoglobin itself rather than its breakdown products may activate lipid peroxidation and cause brain injury [6]. Hemoglobin-induced toxicity in neuronal cell cultures is blocked by the 21-aminosteroid U74500A, and the antioxidant Trolox [21].

An intrahippocampal injection of hemoglobin or iron results in significant DNA damage. DNA damage has a key role in hemoglobin- and iron-induced neuronal death in the hippocampus. Both endonuclease-mediated DNA fragmentation and oxidative injury can cause DNA damage [5]. Several pieces of evidence suggest that oxidative stress may play a key role in DNA damage following ICH. First, 2 oxidative DNA injury markers, 8-hydroxyl-2′-deoxyguanosine (8-OHdG) and apurinic/apyrimidinic (AP) sites, are markedly increased in the perihematomal zone [15]. Second, DFX reduces brain 8-OHdG levels and ameliorates a decrease in AP endonuclease/redox effector factor-1, a DNA repair enzyme, after ICH [13]. Third, hemoglobin activates caspases in neurons, but caspase inhibition does not reduce hemoglobin neurotoxicity [30]. Fourth, antioxidants reduce hemoglobin-induced neuronal death and caspase-3 activation in primary neuronal cultures [30].

In the present study, we detected double-strand breaks by TUNEL staining. Abundant TUNEL-positive cells were found 1 day after hemoglobin or iron injection. Iron-induced DNA damage may result from oxidative stress. It is known that reactive oxygen species can attack DNA directly, forming oxidative base damage and strand breaks [12]. DNA damage by reactive oxygen species can be greatly amplified in the presence of free iron [2].

Another important finding of this study was that systemic use of DFX reduces DNA damage induced by hemoglobin. DFX is an iron chelator that can pass the blood–brain barrier rapidly after systemic administration [17]. Deferoxamine chelates iron from ferritin and hemosiderin by forming a stable complex that prevents the iron from entering into further chemical reactions. Our previous studies have demonstrated that DFX given systemically reduces brain edema formation, neurological deficits, and brain atrophy following ICH [8, 13]. Here, we confirmed that DFX can attenuate brain edema and brain atrophy in a new model of ICH. Although DFX can protect brain through non-iron-chelation mechanisms [18], we believe DFX-related neuronal protection is due to its effect on iron chelation, since DFX reduces free iron levels in the CSF and brain ferritin immunoreactivity after ICH [8, 28].

In conclusion, iron has a key role in hemoglobin-induced tissue swelling and cell death. Systemic deferoxamine blocked these effects of hemoglobin, suggesting that it may be a useful treatment for ICH patients.

Acknowledgments

This study was supported by grants NS-017760, NS-039866, NS-047245 and NS-052510 from the National Institutes of Health (NIH), and 0755717Z and 0840016N from American Heart Association (AHA). The content is solely the responsibility of the authors and does not necessarily represent the official views of the NIH or AHA.

References

1. Andaluz N, Zuccarello M, Wagner KR (2002) Experimental animal models of intracerebral hemorrhage. Neurosurg Clin N Am 13: 385–393
2. Aruoma OI, Halliwell B, Dizdaroglu M (1989) Iron ion-dependent modification of bases in DNA by the superoxide radical-generating system hypoxanthine/xanthine oxidase. J Biol Chem 264: 13024–13028
3. Felberg RA, Grotta JC, Shirzadi AL, Strong R, Narayana P, Hill-Felberg SJ, Aronowski J (2002) Cell death in experimental intracerebral hemorrhage: the "black hole" model of hemorrhagic damage. Ann Neurol 51: 517–524
4. Gong Y, Tian H, Xi G, Keep RF, Hoff JT, Hua Y (2006) Systemic zinc protoporphyrin administration reduces intracerebral hemorrhage-induced brain injury. Acta Neurochir Suppl 96: 232–236
5. Graham SH, Chen J (2001) Programmed cell death in cerebral ischemia. J Cereb Blood Flow Metab 21: 99–109
6. Gutteridge JM (1987) The antioxidant activity of haptoglobin towards haemoglobin-stimulated lipid peroxidation. Biochim Biophys Acta 917: 219–223
7. Hua Y, Schallert T, Keep RF, Wu J, Hoff JT, Xi G (2002) Behavioral tests after intracerebral hemorrhage in the rat. Stroke 33: 2478–2484
8. Hua Y, Nakamura T, Keep RF, Wu J, Schallert T, Hoff JT, Xi G (2006) Long-term effects of experimental intracerebral hemorrhage: the role of iron. J Neurosurg 104: 305–312
9. Huang FP, Xi G, Keep RF, Hua Y, Nemoianu A, Hoff JT (2002) Brain edema after experimental intracerebral hemorrhage: role of hemoglobin degradation products. J Neurosurg 96: 287–293
10. Kase CS, Caplan LR (1994) Intracerebral hemorrhage. Butterworth-Heinemann, Boston
11. Koeppen AH, Dickson AC, Smith J (2004) Heme oxygenase in experimental intracerebral hemorrhage: the benefit of tin-mesoporphyrin. J Neuropathol Exp Neurol 63: 587–597
12. Nagayama T, Lan J, Henshall DC, Chen D, O'Horo C, Simon RP, Chen J (2000) Induction of oxidative DNA damage in the peri-infarct region after permanent focal cerebral ischemia. J Neurochem 75: 1716–1728
13. Nakamura T, Keep RF, Hua Y, Schallert T, Hoff JT, Xi G (2004) Deferoxamine-induced attenuation of brain edema and neurological deficits in a rat model of intracerebral hemorrhage. J Neurosurg 100: 672–678
14. Nakamura T, Xi G, Hua Y, Schallert T, Hoff JT, Keep RF (2004) Intracerebral hemorrhage in mice: model characterization and application for genetically modified mice. J Cereb Blood Flow Metab 24: 487–494
15. Nakamura T, Keep RF, Hua Y, Hoff JT, Xi G (2005) Oxidative DNA injury after experimental intracerebral hemorrhage. Brain Res 1039: 30–36
16. Ogihara K, Zubkov AY, Bernanke DH, Lewis AI, Parent AD, Zhang JH (1999) Oxyhemoglobin-induced apoptosis in cultured endothelial cells. J Neurosurg 91: 459–465
17. Palmer C, Roberts RL, Bero C (1994) Deferoxamine posttreatment reduces ischemic brain injury in neonatal rats. Stroke 25: 1039–1045
18. Prass K, Ruscher K, Karsch M, Isaev N, Megow D, Priller J, Scharff A, Dirnagl U, Meisel A (2002) Desferrioxamine induces delayed tolerance against cerebral ischemia in vivo and in vitro. J Cereb Blood Flow Metab 22: 520–525
19. Qureshi AI, Wilson DA, Hanley DF, Traystman RJ (1999) No evidence for an ischemic penumbra in massive experimental intracerebral hemorrhage. Neurology 52: 266–272
20. Qureshi AI, Tuhrim S, Broderick JP, Batjer HH, Hondo H, Hanley DF (2001) Spontaneous intracerebral hemorrhage. N Engl J Med 344: 1450–1460
21. Regan RF, Panter SS (1993) Neurotoxicity of hemoglobin in cortical cell culture. Neurosci Lett 153: 219–222
22. Regan RF, Rogers B (2003) Delayed treatment of hemoglobin neurotoxicity. J Neurotrauma 20: 111–120
23. Rosenberg GA, Mun-Bryce S, Wesley M, Kornfeld M (1990) Collagenase-induced intracerebral hemorrhage in rats. Stroke 21: 801–807
24. Song S, Hua Y, Keep RF, Hoff JT, Xi G (2007) A new hippocampal model for examining intracerebral hemorrhage-related neuronal death: effects of deferoxamine on hemoglobin-induced neuronal death. Stroke 38: 2861–2863
25. Wagner KR, Xi G, Hua Y, Kleinholz M, de Courten-Myers GM, Myers RE, Broderick JP, Brott TG (1996) Lobar intracerebral hemorrhage model in pigs: rapid edema development in perihematomal white matter. Stroke 27: 490–497
26. Wagner KR, Hua Y, de Courten-Myers GM, Broderick JP, Nishimura RN, Lu SY, Dwyer BE (2000) Tin-mesoporphyrin, a potent heme oxygenase inhibitor, for treatment of intracerebral hemorrhage: in vivo and in vitro studies. Cell Mol Biol (Noisy-le-grand) 46: 597–608
27. Wagner KR, Sharp FR, Ardizzone TD, Lu A, Clark JF (2003) Heme and iron metabolism: role in cerebral hemorrhage. J Cereb Blood Flow Metab 23: 629–652
28. Wan S, Hua Y, Keep RF, Hoff JT, Xi G (2006) Deferoxamine reduces CSF free iron levels following intracerebral hemorrhage. Acta Neurochir Suppl 96: 199–202
29. Wang J, Tsirka SE (2005) Neuroprotection by inhibition of matrix metalloproteinases in a mouse model of intracerebral haemorrhage. Brain 128: 1622–1633
30. Wang X, Mori T, Sumii T, Lo EH (2002) Hemoglobin-induced cytotoxicity in rat cerebral cortical neurons: caspase activation and oxidative stress. Stroke 33: 1882–1888
31. Wu J, Hua Y, Keep RF, Schallert T, Hoff JT, Xi G (2002) Oxidative brain injury from extravasated erythrocytes after intracerebral hemorrhage. Brain Res 953: 45–52
32. Wu J, Hua Y, Keep RF, Nakamura T, Hoff JT, Xi G (2003) Iron and iron-handling proteins in the brain after intracerebral hemorrhage. Stroke 34: 2964–2969
33. Xi G, Keep RF, Hoff JT (1998) Erythrocytes and delayed brain edema formation following intracerebral hemorrhage in rats. J Neurosurg 89: 991–996

34. Xi G, Hua Y, Bhasin RR, Ennis SR, Keep RF, Hoff JT (2001) Mechanisms of edema formation after intracerebral hemorrhage: effects of extravasated red blood cells on blood flow and blood–brain barrier integrity. Stroke 32: 2932–2938

35. Xi G, Keep RF, Hoff JT (2002) Pathophysiology of brain edema formation. Neurosurg Clin N Am 13: 371–383

36. Xi G, Keep RF, Hoff JT (2006) Mechanisms of brain injury after intracerebral haemorrhage. Lancet Neurol 5: 53–63

37. Xue M, Del Bigio MR (2000) Intracortical hemorrhage injury in rats: relationship between blood fractions and brain cell death. Stroke 31: 1721–1727

38. Zhao X, Zhang Y, Strong R, Grotta JC, Aronowski J (2006) 15d-Prostaglandin J2 activates peroxisome proliferator-activated receptor-gamma, promotes expression of catalase, and reduces inflammation, behavioral dysfunction, and neuronal loss after intracerebral hemorrhage in rats. J Cereb Blood Flow Metab 26: 811–820

Acta Neurochir Suppl (2008) 105: 19–21
© Springer-Verlag 2008
Printed in Austria

The antioxidant effects of melatonin after intracerebral hemorrhage in rats

H. Rojas[1], **T. Lekic**[1], **W. Chen**[1], **V. Jadhav**[1], **E. Titova**[1], **R. D. Martin**[1], **J. Tang**[1], **J. Zhang**[1,2,3]

[1] Department of Physiology and Pharmacology, Loma Linda University, Loma Linda, CA, USA
[2] Department of Neurosurgery, Loma Linda University, Loma Linda, CA, USA
[3] Department of Anesthesiology, Loma Linda University, Loma Linda, CA, USA

Summary

Free radical mechanisms are involved in secondary brain injury after intracerebral hemorrhage (ICH). Since melatonin is a potent free radical scavenger and indirect antioxidant, the objective of this study was to evaluate whether melatonin administration would attenuate oxidative stress, brain edema, and neurological deficits in a rat model of ICH. Animals were assigned into groups consisting of sham (needle trauma), vehicle, and melatonin (15 or 150 mg/kg). All injections occurred through the intraperitoneal route, at either 15 min or 3 h after collagenase ICH induction. Then, lipid peroxidation, neurological scoring (18-point system), and brain water content were evaluated at 24 h post-ICH. Results demonstrated dramatically increased lipid peroxidation after collagenase-induced ICH; however, melatonin treatment effectively attenuated this lipid peroxidation. Nonetheless, neurological scoring and brain water content in the right basal ganglia was without significant difference between any treatment regimens (15 or 150 mg/kg of melatonin) or time points of drug administration (15 min or 3 h post-ICH). Therefore, melatonin reduced oxidative stress but did not change extent of brain edema or neurologic deficits.

Keywords: Melatonin; intracerebral hemorrhage; rats; collagenase.

Introduction

Intracerebral hemorrhage (ICH) is a devastating event that accounts for approximately 5 to 15% of all strokes [2, 13]. It is more than twice as common as subarachnoid hemorrhage and much more likely to result in major disability or death than subarachnoid hemorrhage or ischemic stroke [1]. Spontaneous ICH predominantly occurs in ganglionic areas of the brain (putamen, caudate, and thalamus) followed by lobar, and then cerebellar or pontine areas [2]. Treatment of ICH is primarily supportive, without conclusive evidence indicating an effective strategy for treatment [6, 13]. Therefore,

animal models have been important for investigating and understanding the pathophysiology of ICH and potentially preventing the event or improving outcome after the event, with treatment strategies aimed at the important factors that contribute to severe brain damage in this condition. We used the collagenase-induced ICH rat model originally described by Rosenberg *et al.* [15].

Free radical-related mechanisms have been linked to secondary brain injury after ICH [16]. A number of free radical scavengers and antioxidants have been shown to attenuate neurological deficits in the rat ICH model [10]. Melatonin (N-acetyl-5-methoxytryptamine) is a potent free radical scavenger and an indirect antioxidant that has shown neuroprotective effects in both *in vitro* and *in vivo* ischemic-hypoxia models [3, 4, 12, 14]. However, nothing to date has been published on the possible neuroprotective effect of melatonin in the rat ICH model. Our study examined whether melatonin reduces oxidative stress and consequently reduces brain edema and neurological deficits after collagenase-induced ICH in rats.

Materials and methods

All the procedures used in our studies were in compliance with the *Guide for the Care and Use of Laboratory Animals* and approved by the Animal Care and Use Committee at Loma Linda University. Aseptic technique was used for all surgeries, and rats were allowed free access to food and water. Male Sprague-Dawley rats (290–395 g; Harlan, Indianapolis, IN, USA) were used for this study. Rats were anaesthetized with isoflurane and placed prone in a stereotaxic frame (Kopf Instruments, Tujunga, CA, USA). Then, using a collagenase injection ICH model similar to that described previously in rats [15], we used the following stereotactic coordinates to localize the right basal ganglia: 0.2 mm anterior, 5.6 mm ventral, and 2.9 mm lateral to the bregma. A posterior cranial burr hole (1 mm) was drilled over the right cerebral hemisphere, into which a 27-gauge needle was inserted at a rate of 1 mm/min. A microinfusion pump (Harvard Apparatus, Holliston,

---

Correspondence: John H. Zhang, MD, PhD, Department of Physiology and Pharmacology, Loma Linda University School of Medicine, Loma Linda, CA 92354, USA. e-mail: Johnzhang3910@yahoo.com

MA, USA) infused the bacterial collagenase (VII-S; Sigma-Aldrich, St Louis, MO, USA) (0.2 U in 1 μL saline) through a Hamilton syringe at a rate of 0.2 μL/min. The needle remained in place for an additional 10 min after injection to prevent "back-leakage." To maintain a core temperature within $37.0 \pm 0.5 \,°C$, an electronic thermostat-controlled warming blanket was used throughout the operation. After needle removal, the burr hole was sealed with bone wax, the incision sutured closed, and the animals were allowed to recover. Sham surgeries consisted of needle insertion alone. Animals were euthanized 24 h after surgery, when brain water content (BWC), neurological deficits, and lipid peroxidation were examined.

Experimental groups

All drug administration was done by intraperitoneal injection, and consisted of vehicle (10% ethanol in 0.9% normal saline), or low-dose (15 mg/kg) or high-dose (150 mg/kg) melatonin. For neurological and BWC testing, drug administration occurred at either 15 min (low-dose) or 3 h (low- and high-dose) post-ICH, and rats were subdivided randomly into 5 groups: (a) sham, (b) untreated-ICH, (c) vehicle-ICH, (d) low-dose melatonin-ICH, and (e) high-dose melatonin-ICH. For lipid peroxidation measurements (malondialdehyde assay [MDA]), all drug administration occurred at 3 h post-ICH induction, and rats were subdivided into 3 groups: (a) sham, (b) vehicle-ICH, and (c) low-dose melatonin-ICH (15 mg/kg). All parameters (lipid peroxidation, BWC, and neurologic function) were assessed 24 h after ICH induction.

Brain water content

Brain edema was measured by methods described previously [16]. Briefly, under deep anesthesia, rats were decapitated and brains were removed immediately, and then divided into 5 parts: ipsilateral and contralateral basal ganglia, ipsilateral and contralateral cortex, and cerebellum. These tissue samples were weighed on an electronic analytical balance (model AE 100; Mettler-Toledo Inc., Columbus, OH, USA) to the nearest 0.01 mg to obtain the wet weight (WW), and then the tissue was dried at $100 \,°C$ for 24 h to determine the dry weight (DW). Finally, percent of BWC was calculated as $(WW - DW)/WW \times 100$.

Neurological function

Neurological testing was performed at 24 h after ICH. The scoring system consisted of 6 tests with possible scores of 0–3 for each test (0 = worst; 3 = best). The minimum neurological score was 0 and the maximum was 18; greater detail has been described elsewhere [5]. Rats were evaluated using 6 individual tests: (a) spontaneous activity, (b) symmetry of movement, (c) forepaw outstretching, (d) climbing, (e) body proprioception, and (f) response to vibrissae touch. The score given to each rat at completion of the evaluation was the summation of all 6 individual test scores. The examiner had no specific knowledge as to the extent of neurological injury, procedure, or treatment of each rat.

Lipid peroxidation

The animals were anesthetized and brain samples were collected at 24 h after ICH. The level of lipid peroxidation products (MDA) in the right cerebral cortex was measured using an LPO-586 kit (OxisResearch, Portland, OR, USA) as previously described [8]. Brain tissue was homogenized in 20 mmol/L phosphate buffer (pH 7.4) with 0.5 M butylated hydroxytoluene in acetonitrile. These homogenates were then centrifuged at $20,800 \, g$ for 10 min at $4\,°C$ and the supernatants collected. The protein concentration was measured using a DC protein assay (Bio-Rad Laboratories, Hercules, CA, USA) and these samples were reacted with a chromogenic reagent at $45\,°C$ for 60 min. After incubation, the samples were centrifuged at $20,800 \, g$ for 10 min at $4\,°C$ and supernatants

were measured at 586 nm. The level of MDA was calculated as picomoles per milligram of protein according to the derived standard curve.

Statistical analysis

All data are presented as $\pm$ standard error. BWC, behavioral tests, and lipid peroxidation assay were analyzed using analysis of variance (ANOVA). The *t*-test or Mann–Whitney rank sum tests were used when appropriate. Statistical significance was considered as $p < 0.05$.

Results

Lipid peroxidation (MDA) was significantly lower in the sham group ($n = 4$; 6.6 ± 0.5) compared to ICH with vehicle ($n = 4$; 21.8 ± 1.4) and ICH with 15 mg/kg melatonin treatment (i.p. 15 min after ICH; $n = 4$; 17.4 ± 1.1). Furthermore, melatonin treatment led to significantly lower lipid peroxidation compared to treatment with vehicle alone ($p < 0.05$). BWC in the right (ipsilateral) basal ganglia of the sham group ($n = 4$; $77.7 \pm 0.4\%$) was significantly lower than all ICH groups ($p < 0.05$). Intraperitoneal injection (15 min post-ICH induction) of vehicle ($n = 4$; 82.4 ± 0.9) or 15 mg/kg melatonin ($n = 4$; 81.2 ± 0.8) resulted in no differences ($p > 0.05$) in brain edema formation, as compared to untreated ICH rats ($n = 4$; 82.6 ± 0.7). Similarly, at 3 h post-ICH induction, the intraperitoneal injection of vehicle ($n = 4$; 82.8 ± 0.6) and 15 mg/kg melatonin ($n = 4$; 81.8 ± 0.7) did not result in any significant amelioration of BWC ($p > 0.05$). Furthermore, an increased melatonin dose to 150 mg/kg at 3 h post-ICH ($n = 4$; 81.9 ± 0.4), did not lead to an improvement either. The neurological score of the sham group ($n = 4$; 17.5 ± 0.5) was significantly higher than all ICH groups ($p < 0.05$). Intraperitoneal injection (15 min post-ICH induction) of vehicle ($n = 4$; $11.5.0 \pm 1.0$) or 15 mg/kg melatonin (9.3 ± 0.5) resulted in no differences ($p > 0.05$) in ICH-induced neurological deficits, as compared to the untreated rats ($n = 4$; 11.8 ± 1.5). Similarly, at 3 h post-ICH induction, the intraperitoneal injection of vehicle ($n = 4$; 11.5 ± 1.7) and 15 mg/kg melatonin ($n = 4$; 9.8 ± 1.0), did not result in any significant amelioration of the neurological score ($p > 0.05$). Additionally, an increased melatonin dose to 150 mg/kg at 3 h post-ICH ($n = 4$; 11.8 ± 0.8), did not lead to an improvement either.

Conclusion

Lipid peroxidation was reduced by 15 mg/kg of melatonin 3 h after ICH induction. These results support the previously described antioxidant effects of melatonin in multiple rat cerebral injury and *in vitro* neuronal studies

[3, 4, 12, 14]. Although others reported improvements in neurological function after treatment with an ICH free radical trapping agent [10], we did not. This could be partially explained by differences in the drug delivery system; specifically, their use of a continuous, subcutaneous mini-pump, as compared to our intraperitoneal method. Furthermore, the known reduction in infarct volume, as previously shown in a model of middle cerebral artery occlusion [12], did not translate into a reduction of brain edema in our collagenase ICH model. Likely, the antioxidant effects of melatonin were either functionally insignificant, or this effect was attenuated by other mechanisms of collagenase-induced brain injury, such as: rebleeding from massive blood brain barrier rupture [7], other inflammatory mediators such as cytokines [11], or from direct toxicity of red blood cell degradation lysates (hemoglobin, iron, bilirubin, carbon monoxide, and hemin) [9]. Further studies should evaluate these mechanisms in order to clarify the role of melatonin in the progression of molecular outcomes after ICH.

Acknowledgements

Funding provided by National Institutes of Health to Jiping Tang (Grant NS52492) and John Zhang (Grant NS53407).

References

1. Broderick JP, Brott T, Tomsick T, Miller R, Huster G (1993) Intracerebral hemorrhage more than twice as common as subarachnoid hemorrhage. J Neurosurg 78: 188–191
2. Caplan LR (1994) General symptoms and signs. In: Kase CS, Caplan LR (eds) Intracerebral hemorrhage. Butterworth-Heinemann, Boston
3. Cazevieille C, Safa R, Osborne NN (1997) Melatonin protects primary cultures of rat cortical neurones from NMDA excitotoxicity and hypoxia/reoxygenation. Brain Res 768: 120–124
4. Cho S, Joh TH, Baik HH, Dibinis C, Volpe BT (1997) Melatonin administration protects CA1 hippocampal neurons after transient forebrain ischemia in rats. Brain Res 755: 335–338
5. Garcia JH, Wagner S, Liu KF, Hu XJ (1995) Neurological deficit and extent of neuronal necrosis attributable to middle cerebral artery occlusion in rats. Statistical validation. Stroke 26: 627–635
6. Juvela S, Heiskanen O, Poranen A, Valtonen S, Kuurne T, Kaste M, Troupp H (1989) The treatment of spontaneous intracerebral hemorrhage. A prospective randomized trial of surgical and conservative treatment. J Neurosurg 70: 755–758
7. Kitaoka T, Hua Y, Xi G, Hoff JT, Keep RF (2002) Delayed argatroban treatment reduces edema in a rat model of intracerebral hemorrhage. Stroke 33: 3012–3018
8. Kusaka I, Kusaka G, Zhou C, Ishikawa M, Nanda A, Granger DN, Zhang JH, Tang J (2004) Role of AT1 receptors and NAD(P)H oxidase in diabetes-aggravated ischemic brain injury. Am J Physiol Heart Circ Physiol 286: H2442–H2451
9. Masuda T, Hida H, Kanda Y, Aihara N, Ohta K, Yamada K, Nishino H (2007) Oral administration of metal chelator ameliorates motor dysfunction after a small hemorrhage near the internal capsule in rat. J Neurosci Res 85: 213–222
10. Peeling J, Del Bigio MR, Corbett D, Green AR, Jackson DM (2001) Efficacy of disodium 4-[(tert-butylimino)methyl]benzene-1,3-disulfonate N-oxide (NXY-059), a free radical trapping agent, in a rat model of hemorrhagic stroke. Neuropharmacology 40: 433–439
11. Peeling J, Yan HJ, Corbett D, Xue M, Del Bigio MR (2001) Effect of FK-506 on inflammation and behavioral outcome following intracerebral hemorrhage in rat. Exp Neurol 167: 341–347
12. Pei Z, Pang SF, Cheung RT (2003) Administration of melatonin after onset of ischemia reduces the volume of cerebral infarction in a rat middle cerebral artery occlusion stroke model. Stroke 34: 770–775
13. Qureshi AI, Tuhrim S, Broderick JP, Batjer HH, Hondo H, Hanley DF (2001) Spontaneous intracerebral hemorrhage. N Engl J Med 344: 1450–1460
14. Reiter RJ (1998) Oxidative damage in the central nervous system: protection by melatonin. Prog Neurobiol 56: 359–384
15. Rosenberg GA, Mun-Bryce S, Wesley M, Kornfeld M (1990) Collagenase-induced intracerebral hemorrhage in rats. Stroke 21: 801–807
16. Tang J, Liu J, Zhou C, Ostanin D, Grisham MB, Neil Granger D, Zhang JH (2005) Role of NADPH oxidase in the brain injury of intracerebral hemorrhage. J Neurochem 94: 1342–1350

Acta Neurochir Suppl (2008) 105: 23–27

Poly(ADP-ribose) polymerase activation and brain edema formation by hemoglobin after intracerebral hemorrhage in rats

X. Bao, G. Wu, S. Hu, F. Huang

Department of Neurosurgery, Huashan Hospital, Fudan University, Shanghai, China

Summary

Brain edema induced by intracerebral hemorrhage (ICH) is a serious problem in the treatment of ICH. However, the mechanisms of brain edema formation following ICH are not well-understood. We have found that hemoglobin plays an important role in edema development after ICH. In this study, we sought to explore the mechanism of brain edema formation caused by hemoglobin.

Hemoglobin was infused into the right basal ganglia of male Sprague-Dawley rats. The animals were killed 24 h later to detect brain water and ion content. Meanwhile, Western blot analysis and immunohistochemical studies were applied for Poly(ADP-ribose) polymerase (PARP) measurement. The effect of the iron chelator, deferoxamine, on PARP activation was also examined. We found that intracerebral infusion of hemoglobin caused an increase in brain water content at 24 h. At the same time, PARP was activated after hemoglobin infusion. Deferoxamine (500 mg/kg, i.p.) reduced hemoglobin-induced brain edema and activation of PARP.

These results demonstrate that hemoglobin can cause brain edema and activate PARP in rat brain.

Keywords: Poly(ADP-ribose) polymerase; hemoglobin; intracerebral hemorrhage; brain edema.

Introduction

Intracerebral hemorrhage (ICH) is a subtype of stroke with high morbidity and mortality. As perihematomal brain edema develops immediately after ICH and peaks several days later, many patients with ICH deteriorate progressively [3, 19]. However, the mechanisms of brain edema formation following ICH are not well understood. Previous studies have found that hemoglobin and its breakdown products play an important role in edema development after ICH [3, 8].

Iron, a hemoglobin degradation product, is associated with free radical formation in the brain after ICH. Several previous studies have indicated that iron accumulation and oxidative stress in brain contribute to secondary brain damage after ICH. The overwhelming production of free radicals, which include reactive oxygen species (ROS) and reactive nitrogen species (RNS), results in tissue damage, lipid peroxidation of cell membranes, protein oxidation, and changes in DNA (strand breaks and base modifications). Deferoxamine, an iron chelator, can reduce brain edema after ICH [8].

Poly(ADP-ribose) polymerase (PARP), also known as poly(ADP-ribose) synthetase and poly(ADP-ribose) transferase, is an abundant nuclear enzyme present in eukaryotes, which functions as a DNA nick-sensor enzyme. Upon binding to DNA breaks, activated PARP cleaves NAD^+ into nicotinamide and ADP-ribose and polymerizes the latter onto nuclear acceptor proteins including histones, transcription factors, and PARP itself. Poly (ADP-ribosylation) contributes to DNA repair and to maintenance of genomic stability. On the other hand, oxidative stress-induced over-activation of PARP consumes NAD^+ and consequently ATP, culminating in cell dysfunction or necrosis. This cellular suicide mechanism has been implicated in the pathomechanism of stroke, myocardial ischemia, diabetes, diabetes-associated cardiovascular dysfunction, shock, traumatic central nervous system injury, arthritis, colitis, allergic encephalomyelitis, and various other forms of inflammation [14].

In this study we examined changes in PARP and brain edema induced by hemoglobin through immunohistochemical studies and Western blot analysis. The

Correspondence: Fengping Huang, M.D., Ph.D., #12 Wulumuqi Zhong Road, Shanghai 200040, China. e-mail: fphuang@hsh.stn.sh.cn effect of deferoxamine on PARP activation was also examined.

Materials and methods

Animal preparation and intracerebral infusion

A total of 56 males Sprague-Dawley rats (Shanghai Experimental Animal Center, China) weighing 300–420 g were used in this study. The animals were anesthetized with 40 mg/kg pentobarbital administered intraperitoneally. The right femoral artery was catheterized for continuous blood pressure monitoring and blood sampling. Blood was obtained from the catheter for analysis of pH, PaO_2, $PaCO_2$, hematocrit, and blood glucose. Core temperature was maintained at $37\,°C \pm 0.5\,°C$. The rats were positioned in a stereotactic head frame (David Kopf Instruments, Tujunga, CA), and a 1-mm burr hole was made on the right coronal suture 4 mm lateral to the bregma. A variety of solutions (30 μL) were infused with a microinfusion pump into the right caudate nucleus through a 26-gauge needle (coordinates: 0.2 mm anterior, 5.5 mm ventral, and 4 mm lateral to the bregma) at a rate of 2 μL/min. The needle was removed 10 min after infusion and the skin closed with sutures.

Experimental groups

There were 5 parts to this study.

Part I. Ten rats were randomly divided into 2 groups (5 rats per group). Rats received 30-μL intracerebral infusion of either saline or bovine hemoglobin (300 mg/mL in saline). The animals were anesthetized again and decapitated 24 h after infusion. Brain water and ion contents were measured.

Part II. Six groups of 3 rats each received 30-μL bovine hemoglobin (300 mg/ml in saline) infusion. The rats were killed 1, 6, 12, 24, 48, and 72 h later for Western blot analysis.

Part III. Two groups of 6 rats each received a 30-μL infusion of either saline or bovine hemoglobin (300 mg/mL in saline). The rats were killed 24 h later for Western blot analysis (3 rats per group) or immunohisto-chemical studies (3 rats per group).

Part IV. Two groups of 5 rats each were studied in this part. All rats received a 30-μL infusion of bovine hemoglobin (300 mg/mL in normal saline), followed immediately by intraperitoneal infusion of 1 mL saline or 500 mg/kg deferoxamine (dissolved in 1 mL saline). The animals were decapitated 24 h later to determine brain water and ion content.

Part V. Two groups of 3 rats each were examined in this part. All rats received a 30-μL infusion of bovine hemoglobin (300 mg/mL in saline), followed immediately by intraperitoneal injection of 1 mL saline or 500 mg/kg deferoxamine (dissolved in 1 mL saline). The rats were killed 24 h later for Western blot analysis.

Measurement of brain water and ion content

Animals were re-anesthetized 24 h later with 60 mg/kg pentobarbital administered intraperitoneally and killed by decapitation. Brains were removed and a 3-mm thick coronal brain slice was cut with a blade approximately 4 mm from the frontal pole. The brain slice was separated into ipsilateral and contralateral cortex, and ipsilateral and contralateral basal ganglia. The cerebellum served as a control specimen. Brain samples were immediately weighed on an electronic analytical balance for wet weight (WW), and were dried at 95 °C for 24 h to obtain the dry weight (DW). Water content was determined as (WW − DW)/WW. The dehydrated samples were then digested in 1 mL of 1 M

nitric acid for more than 7 days and the sodium content of this solution was measured with an automatic flame photometer. Ion content was expressed in milliequivalents per kilogram of dehydrated brain tissue (mEq/kg DW).

Western blot analysis

Animals were re-anesthetized and underwent transcardiac perfusion with normal saline. Brain tissues were sampled as described above. The rats were decapitated and a coronal brain slice was cut as described above. Ipsilateral brain tissues were immersed in 1 mL of 0.05 mol/L Tris/HCl (pH 7.4; 0.01% PMSF) and homogenized in ice. The samples then were centrifuged at $1000 \times g$ for 20 min 2 h later at 4 °C. Ipsilateral brain tissue protein (25 μg) was run on 7.5% polyacrylamide gels with a 5% stacking gel after boiling for 5 min at 100 °C. The protein was transferred to pure nitrocellulose membrane, and membranes were probed with a 1:500 dilution of the primary antibody (rabbit anti-PARP antibody, Trevigen Inc., Gaithersburg, MD) overnight at room temperature, and then incubated for 1 h in a 1:1000 dilution of the second antibody (peroxidase-conjugated goat anti-rabbit immunoglobulin-G). Finally, protein bands were then visualized by incubating membranes with ECL Plus detecting reagents (Amersham Biosciences, Piscataway, NJ). Grey values of 89 kDa PARP protein bands were analyzed to represent the activity of PARP.

Immunohistochemical studies

The rats were re-anesthetized with 60 mg/kg pentobarbital administered intraperitoneally and perfused with 4% paraformaldehyde in 0.1 M phosphate-buffered saline (pH 7.4). Brains were removed and kept in 4% paraformaldehyde for 6 h, then immersed in 25% sucrose for 3 to 4 days at 4 °C. Brains were embedded in optimal cutting temperature compound and 10-μm thick sections were made with a cryostat. The sections were incubated according to the avidin-biotin complex method [18]. The primary antibody was mouse anti-PAR IgG (1:300 dilution; Trevigen Inc.). Normal mouse immunoglobulin-G was used as negative control.

Statistical analysis

All data in this study are presented as mean ± SD. Data from different animal groups were analyzed using analysis of variance with a Student *t*-test. Differences were considered significant at probability values less than 0.05.

Results

Brain water content was increased in the ipsilateral basal ganglia 24 h after intracerebral infusion of hemoglobin ($82.2 \pm 1.3\%$ vs. $77.9 \pm 0.2\%$ in saline control; $p < 0.01$; Fig. 1A). Edema formation after hemoglobin infusion was associated with an accumulation of sodium ion (Fig. 1B).

Deferoxamine treatment reduced hemoglobin-induced brain edema in ipsilateral basal ganglia ($80.5 \pm 1\%$ vs. $82.4 \pm 1.1\%$; $p < 0.01$) and in the cortex ($80 \pm 0.2\%$ vs. $82.3 \pm 1.3\%$ in control) (Fig. 1C).

After an infusion of hemoglobin, 89-kDa cleaved PARP was detected in ipsilateral basal ganglia at 1, 6, 12, 24, 48, and 72 h. Compared with saline control group, 89-kDa PARP contents in ipsilateral brain tissue

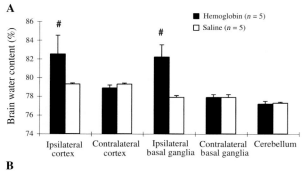

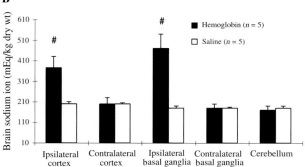

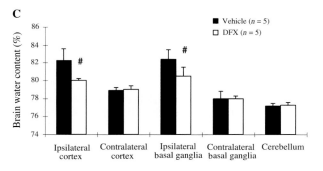

Fig. 1. (A) Brain water and (B) sodium ion content 24 h after 30-μL infusion of hemoglobin. (C) Brain water content in rats 24 h after 30-μL infusion of hemoglobin, immediately followed by intraperitoneal injections of either 1 mL saline (*control*) or 500 mg/kg deferoxamine (in 1 mL normal saline). Values are expressed as mean ± SD; # $p < 0.01$

were significantly increased 24 h after hemoglobin injection (ratio of [PARP/β-actin]: 1.594 ± 0.663 vs. 0.305 ± 0.017, $p < 0.05$, Fig. 2A). Deferoxamine blocked hemoglo-

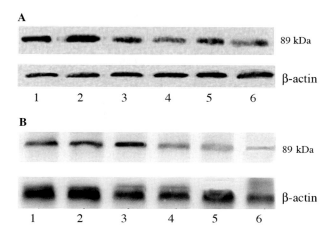

Fig. 2. (A) Western blots of 89 kDa cleaved PARP levels 24 h after either intracerebral infusion of hemoglobin (*1–3*) or saline control (*4–6*). (B) Western blots of 89 kDa PARP levels 24 h after intracerebral infusion of hemoglobin followed immediately by intraperitoneal injections of either 1 mL saline (control, *1–3*) or 500 mg/kg deferoxamine (in 1 mL normal saline, *4–6*)

bin-induced PARP activation (ratio of [PARP/β-actin]: 0.482 ± 0.193 vs. 1.214 ± 0.146; $p < 0.05$; Fig. 2B).

Immunohistochemical studies detected numerous PAR-positive cells in ipsilateral hemisphere 24 h after hemoglobin infusion. A few PAR-positive cells were found in the ipsilateral hemisphere after saline injection (Fig. 3).

Discussion

In this study, we confirmed that an intracerebral infusion of hemoglobin induced PARP activation in the brain along with the formation of brain edema within 24 h. We demonstrated that an intraperitoneal injection of a large dose (500 mg/kg) of deferoxamine not only attenuated brain edema induced by hemoglobin but also downregulated PARP activation in the brain.

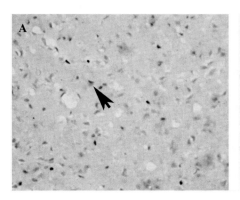

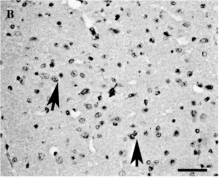

Fig. 3. Photomicrographs of rat brain sections showing PAR immunoactivity in ipsilateral basal ganglia after (A) saline infusion and (B) hemoglobin infusion. Examples of PAR-positive cells are indicated by *arrows*. Scale bar = 40 μm

Studies have shown that hemoglobin had deleterious effects on the brain. For example, an intracortical hemoglobin injection in rats produced chronic focal spike activity and gliosis [12]. Furthermore, hemoglobin itself could also inhibit Na^+/K^+ adenosine triphosphate activity [13], activate lipid peroxidation [1], exacerbate excitotoxic injury in cortical cells [11], and induce depolarization in hippocampal CA1 neurons [21]. Koenig and Meyerhoff [5] found that hemoglobin at a concentration of 25 nM induced the death of 50% of forebrain neurons in culture within 8 h, and 72% within 24 h. Another previous study in humans indicated that delayed brain edema after ICH was associated with a significant midline shift [22], and it was later determined that this delayed edema was probably due to erythrocyte lysis and hemoglobin-induced brain damage [3].

Deferoxamine reduced hemoglobin-induced brain edema, indicating that iron has a role in brain edema formation induced by hemoglobin. Free-iron levels within the cerebrospinal fluid increase after ICH in rats and the excess iron was not cleared for at least 28 days [16]. Rat studies have shown up to a 3-fold increase in brain non-heme iron [2, 17] with a concurrent increase in ferritin [2, 6, 15]. Iron toxicity is largely based on Fenton chemistry, where iron reacts with reactive oxygen intermediates, including hydrogen peroxide (H_2O_2) and the superoxide anion (O_2^-) – both byproducts of aerobic metabolism – to produce highly reactive free radical species such as the hydroxyl radical (OH).

The overwhelming production of free radicals, as well as lipid peroxidation induced by hemoglobin itself and its breakdown product, iron, which includes ROS and RNS, results in tissue damage, lipid peroxidation of cell membranes, and protein oxidation. Excessive generation of peroxynitrite and other free radicals can also cause massive DNA damage, resulting in PARP over-activation. Over-activated PARP transforms NAD^+ into long polymers of poly(ADP-ribose) leading to depletion of NAD^+ and subsequent drastic decrease in cellular ATP pool. This energy depletion can cause serious brain injury [4]. Narasimhan *et al.* [9] found scavenging of superoxide radicals by SOD1 inhibited the formation of peroxynitrite and the activation of PARP. In our study, we found deferoxamine downregulates the expression of PARP in rat brain after hemoglobin injection.

Activation of PARP causes endothelial dysfunction and cell death via a variety of pathways [10]. A recent study demonstrated that permeability of the blood–brain barrier increased after ischemia-reperfusion and PJ34, a PARP inhibitor, reduces blood–brain barrier disruption and attenuates brain edema after global cerebral ischemia [7]. On the other hand, necrosis or apoptosis of neurons and astrocytes by NAD^+ depletion and energy failure could be mediated by PARP activation [20].

Conclusion

In summary, our results showed that hemoglobin, through one of its degradation products, iron, causes brain edema and PARP activation.

Acknowledgments

This study was supported by a grant from National Natural Science Foundation, China (No.30571905).

References

1. Gutteridge JM (1987) The antioxidant activity of haptoglobin towards haemoglobin-stimulated lipid peroxidation. Biochim Biophys Acta 917: 219–223
2. Hua Y, Nakamura T, Keep RF, Wu J, Schallert T, Hoff JT, Xi G (2006) Long-term effects of experimental intracerebral hemorrhage: the role of iron. J Neurosurg 104: 305–312
3. Huang FP, Xi G, Keep RF, Hua Y, Nemoianu A, Hoff JT (2002) Brain edema after experimental intracerebral hemorrhage: role of hemoglobin degradation products. J Neurosurg 96: 287–293
4. Kaundal RK, Shah KK, Sharma SS (2006) Neuroprotective effects of NU1025, a PARP inhibitor in cerebral ischemia are mediated through reduction in NAD depletion and DNA fragmentation. Life Sci 79: 2293–2302
5. Koenig ML, Meyerhoff JL (1997) Neurotoxicity resulting from prolonged exosure [sic] to hemoglobin. Abstr Soc Neurosci 23: 1935
6. Koeppen AH (1995) The history of iron in the brain. J Neurol Sci 134(Suppl): 1–9
7. Lenzsér G, Kis B, Snipes JA, Gáspár T, Sándor P, Komjáti K, Szabó C, Busija DW (2007) Contribution of poly(ADP-ribose) polymerase to postischemic blood–brain barrier damage in rats. J Cereb Blood Flow Metab 27:1318–1326
8. Nakamura T, Keep RF, Hua Y, Schallert T, Hoff JT, Xi G (2004) Deferoxamine-induced attenuation of brain edema and neurological deficits in a rat model of intracerebral hemorrhage. J Neurosurg 100: 672–678
9. Narasimhan P, Fujimura M, Noshita N, Chan PH (2003) Role of superoxide in poly(ADP-ribose) polymerase upregulation after transient cerebral ischemia. Brain Res Mol Brain Res 113: 28–36
10. Pacher P, Szabó C (2005) Role of poly(ADP-ribose) polymerase-1 activation in the pathogenesis of diabetic complications: endothelial dysfunction, as a common underlying theme. Antioxid Redox Signal 7: 1568–1580
11. Regan RF, Panter SS (1996) Hemoglobin potentiates excitotoxic injury in cortical cell culture. J Neurotrauma 13: 223–231
12. Rosen AD, Frumin NV (1979) Focal epileptogenesis after intracortical hemoglobin injection. Exp Neurol 66: 277–284

13. Sadrzadeh SM, Anderson DK, Panter SS, Hallaway PE, Eaton JW (1987) Hemoglobin potentiates central nervous system damage. J Clin Invest 79: 662–664

14. Virág L, Szabó C (2002) The therapeutic potential of poly(ADP-ribose) polymerase inhibitors. Pharmacol Rev 54: 375–429

15. Wagner KR, Sharp FR, Ardizzone TD, Lu A, Clark JF (2003) Heme and iron metabolism: role in cerebral hemorrhage. J Cereb Blood Flow Metab 23: 629–652

16. Wan S, Hua Y, Keep RF, Hoff JT, Xi G (2006) Deferoxamine reduces CSF free iron levels following intracerebral hemorrhage. Acta Neurochir Suppl 96: 199–202

17. Wu J, Hua Y, Keep RF, Nakamura T, Hoff JT, Xi G (2003) Iron and iron-handling proteins in the brain after intracerebral hemorrhage. Stroke 34: 2964–2969

18. Xi G, Keep RF, Hua Y, Xiang J, Hoff JT (1999) Attenuation of thrombin-induced brain edema by cerebral thrombin preconditioning. Stroke 30: 1247–1255

19. Xi G, Keep RF, Hoff JT (2006) Mechanisms of brain injury after intracerebral haemorrhage. Lancet Neurol 5: 53–63

20. Ying W, Chen Y, Alano CC, Swanson RA (2002) Tricarboxylic acid cycle substrates prevent PARP-mediated death of neurons and astrocytes. J Cereb Blood Flow Metab 22: 774–779

21. Yip S, Ip JK, Sastry BR (1996) Electrophysiological actions of hemoglobin on rat hippocampal CA1 pyramidal neurons. Brain Res 713: 134–142

22. Zazulia AR, Diringer MN, Derdeyn CP, Powers WJ (1999) Progression of mass effect after intracerebral hemorrhage. Stroke 30: 1167–1173

Acta Neurochir Suppl (2008) 105: 29–32
© Springer-Verlag 2008
Printed in Austria

Induction of autophagy in rat hippocampus and cultured neurons by iron

Y. He, Y. Hua, S. Song, W. Liu, R. F. Keep, G. Xi

Department of Neurosurgery, University of Michigan Medical School, Ann Arbor, MI, USA

Summary

Autophagy occurs in the brain after intracerebral hemorrhage (ICH). Iron is an important factor causing neuronal death and brain atrophy after ICH. In this study, we examined whether iron can induce autophagy in the hippocampus and in cultured neurons.

For in vivo studies, rats received an infusion of either saline or ferrous iron into the right hippocampus and were killed 1, 3, or 7 days later for Western blot analysis of microtubule-associated protein light chain-3 (LC3). For in vitro studies, primary cultured cortex neurons from rat embryos were exposed to ferrous iron. Cells were used for Western blot analysis of LC3 and monodansylcadaverine (MDC) staining 24 h later.

Intrahippocampal injection of ferrous iron resulted in an increased conversion of LC3-I to LC3-II. Exposure of primary cultured neurons to ferrous iron also induced an enhanced conversion of LC3-I to LC3-II. MDC labeling showed an accumulation of MDC in cultured neurons exposed to ferrous iron.

These results indicate that autophagy is induced by iron in neurons and that iron-induced autophagy may contribute to brain injury after ICH.

Keywords: Autophagy; cerebral hemorrhage; iron; microtubule-associated protein light chain-3.

Introduction

Autophagy plays an important role in cellular homeostasis and is involved in a number of diseases [1, 8–10]. Recently we have demonstrated that autophagy occurs in the brain after intracerebral hemorrhage (ICH) [4].

Our previous studies have shown that iron overload occurs in the brain after ICH and contributes to ICH-induced brain edema, brain atrophy, and prolonged neurological deficits [5, 11, 13, 15]. Recent studies demonstrate iron can also induce neuronal death in hippocampus [5, 13, 15]. Iron-induced brain injury may be through many pathways including the formation of free radicals and oxidative damage [12, 14]. There is evidence showing that oxidative stress can induce autophagic cell death [3].

In this study, therefore, we investigated whether iron can induce autophagy in neurons. Two markers for autophagy, microtubule-associated protein light chain-3 (LC3) and fluorescent dye monodansylcadaverine (MDC), were used. LC3 is a marker for autophagosomes. LC3 has 2 forms: type I is cytosolic and type II is membrane-bound. During autophagy, LC3-II is increased by conversion from LC3-I [7]. MDC is a specific marker for autophagic vacuoles [2].

Materials and methods

Animal preparation and intracerebral injection

The University of Michigan Committee on the Use and Care of Animals approved the protocols for these studies. Male Sprague-Dawley rats weighing 275 to 350 g (Charles River Laboratories, Portage, MI) were used. Rats were anesthetized with pentobarbital (40 mg/kg, i.p.). A polyethylene catheter (PE-50) was then inserted into the right femoral artery to monitor arterial blood pressure and blood gases. Rectal temperature was maintained at 37.5 °C using a feedback-controlled heating pad. The animals were positioned in a stereotactic frame (Kopf Instruments, Tujunga, CA) and a cranial burr hole (1 mm) was drilled. Saline or ferrous chloride was infused into the right hippocampus through a Hamilton syringe at a rate of 1 μL/min using a microinfusion pump (Harvard Apparatus Inc., South Natick, MA). The coordinates were 3.8 mm posterior and 3.5 mm lateral to the bregma, and a depth of 3.2 mm. After intrahippocampal injection, the needle was removed and the skin incision closed with suture. The rats received an intrahippocampal 10-μL injection of either 1 mmol/L ferrous chloride or saline and were killed 1, 3, or 7 days later for Western blot analysis.

Neuronal culture and treatments

Primary neuronal cultures were obtained from embryonic day-17 Sprague-Dawley rats (Charles River Laboratories). Cultures were prepared according to a previously described procedure with some modifications [6]. Briefly, cerebral cortices were dissected, stripped of

Correspondence: Guohua Xi, MD, Department of Neurosurgery, University of Michigan Medical School, 109 Zina Pitcher Place, Room R5018, BSRB, Ann Arbor, MI 48109-2200, USA. e-mail: guohuaxi@umich.edu

meninges, and dissociated by a combination of 0.5% trypsin digestion and mechanical trituration. The dissociated cell suspensions were seeded into poly-L-lysine pre-coated 6- or 24-well plates. The cells were grown in neurobasal medium with 2% B27, 0.5 mM glutamine and 1% antibiotic-antimycotic and maintained in a humidified incubator at 37 °C with 5% CO_2. Half of the cultured media was changed every 3–4 days. Neurons were used for experiments after 7 days.

The cultured neurons were treated with serum-free medium (vehicle control) or 250 μM ferrous chloride. Sodium pyrithione was also added to the medium at a concentration of 20 μM to transport ferrous iron into the cells. Neurons were washed twice with phosphate-buffered saline (PBS; pH 7.4) 30 min after treatment, and then placed in serum-free medium for up to 24 h.

Western blot analysis

For in vivo studies, rats were anesthetized with pentobarbital (60 mg/kg, i.p.) and underwent intracardiac perfusion with 0.1 M PBS. Brain tissues from the ipsilateral hippocampus were dissected and frozen in liquid nitrogen. For in vitro studies, culture medium was removed and plates were washed 3 times with chilled PBS. The cells were quickly scraped and collected by centrifugation at 4 °C, then stored at −80 °C.

Western blot analysis was performed as described previously [16]. Brain and cell samples were sonicated with Western blot lysis buffer. Protein concentration was determined using Bio-Rad protein assay kit (Bio-Rad Laboratories, Hercules, CA). Equal amounts of protein from each sample was separated by sodium dodecyl sulfate-polyacrymide gel electrophoresis and transferred to a hybond-C pure nitrocellulose membrane (Amersham Biosciences, Piscataway, NJ). The membranes were blocked in Carnation nonfat milk and probed with the primary and secondary antibodies. The primary antibody was rabbit anti-MAPLC3 (Abgent Inc., San Diego, CA; 1:700 dilution). The second antibody was goat anti-rabbit IgG (Bio-Rad Laboratories; 1:2500 dilution). The antigen-antibody complexes were visualized with a chemiluminescence system and exposed to Kodak X-OMAT film. Relative densities of bands were analyzed with NIH Image program, Version 1.61 (National Institutes of Health, Bethesda, MD).

MDC labeling

Neurons treated with either vehicle control or 250 μM $FeCl_2$ were incubated with 0.05 mM MDC in PBS for 30 min at 37 °C. The neurons were washed 3 times with PBS and immediately imaged using a fluorescence microscope (Olympus IX51, Olympus America Inc., Melville, NY).

Statistical analysis

All data in this study are presented as mean ± SD. Data were analyzed using Student *t*-test and analysis of variance (ANOVA). Statistical significance was set at $p < 0.05$.

Results

Physiological variables including mean arterial blood pressure, blood pH, PaO_2, $PaCO_2$, hematocrit, and blood glucose level were controlled within normal ranges.

Using Western blot analysis, a time course study of LC3 showed that the ratio of LC3-II to LC3-I in the ipsilateral hippocampus was significantly increased at day 3 and remained at high levels at day 7 after intra-hippocampal injection of ferrous iron (Fig. 1A). The

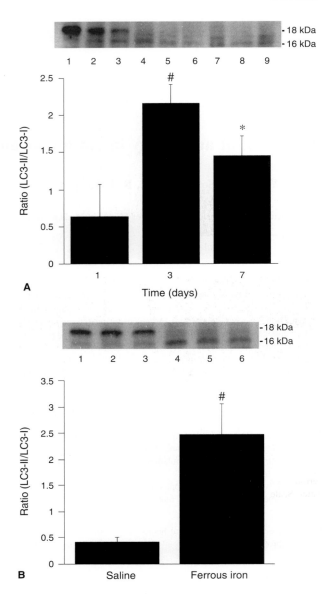

Fig. 1. Ferrous iron induces conversion of LC3-I to LC3-II. (A) Western blot analysis showing LC3-I (18 kDa) and LC3-II (16 kDa) levels in ipsilateral hippocampus at 1 (*1–3*), 3 (*4–6*), and 7 (*7–9*) days after injection of ferrous iron. Values are mean ± SD, $n = 3$. $^{\#}p < 0.01$; $^{*}p < 0.05$ versus day 1. (B) Western blot analysis showing the levels of LC3-I and LC3-II in ipsilateral hippocampus 3 days after injection of saline (*1–3*) or ferrous iron (*4–6*). Values are mean ± SD, $n = 3$. $^{\#}p < 0.01$

ratio of LC3-II to LC3-I in the ipsilateral hippocampus at day 3 after ferrous iron injection was markedly higher than that in the ipsilateral hippocampus after saline injection (2.48 ± 0.57 versus 0.42 ± 0.08; $p < 0.01$; Fig. 1B).

To test whether autophagy also happens after ferrous iron treatment in cultured neurons, cells were exposed to ferrous iron or control medium. Western blotting showed that cells treated with ferrous iron had a higher

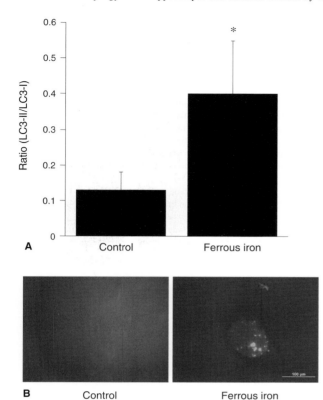

A Control   Ferrous iron

B Control   Ferrous iron

Fig. 2. Ferrous iron induces conversion of LC3-I to LC3-II and accumulation of MDC in cultured neurons. (A) Western blot analysis showing LC3-I (18 kDa) and LC3-II (16 kDa) levels in control neurons and ferrous iron-treated neurons. Values are mean $\pm$ SD, $n = 3$. $^{*}p < 0.05$ versus control. (B) MDC staining of control neurons and ferrous iron-treated neurons. Note the MDC-labeled vacuoles in the latter. Scale bar $= 100\,\mu m$

ratio of LC3-II to LC3-I compared with vehicle control (0.40 ± 0.15 versus 0.13 ± 0.05; $p < 0.01$; Fig. 2A). MDC labeling showed an increase in the number of vacuoles and their size in cells treated with ferrous iron (Fig. 2B).

Discussion

Autophagy is a dynamic process involving bulk degradation of portions of the cytoplasm and intracellular organelles in eukaryotic cells via the lysosomal system. It plays an important role in cellular homeostasis and is involved in a number of human diseases, including cancer, neurodegeneration, and brain ischemia [1, 8–10]. Our recent studies demonstrate that autophagy occurs in the brain after ICH [4].

After ICH, iron concentrations in the brain can reach very high levels and brain non-heme iron is not cleared from the brain within 4 weeks [15]. Iron overload in the brain can cause free radical formation and oxidative damage [12, 14]. There is evidence suggesting that

oxidative stress can induce autophagic cell death [3]. Therefore, iron may be an important trigger for ICH-induced autophagic cell death.

LC3 has been used as a marker of autophagy. LC3 has 2 forms: type I is cytosolic and type II is membrane-bound. During autophagy, LC3 type II is increased by conversion from LC3 type I. The ratio of LC3-II to LC3-I is correlated with the extent of autophagosome formation [7]. In the present study, we found that the ratio of LC3 II to LC3 I in the ipsilateral hippocampus was significantly increased at day 3 and remained at high levels at day 7 after intracerebral injection of ferrous iron. Exposure of primary cultured neurons to ferrous iron also induced an enhanced conversion of LC3-I to LC3-II. These results suggest that iron can induce autophagic cell death in neurons.

MDC is a selective marker for autophagic vacuoles [2]. In the present study, primary cultured neurons exposed to ferrous showed the accumulation of MDC-labeled vacuoles, again indicating that iron induced the occurrence of autophagy.

In summary, intrahippocampal infusion of ferrous iron caused an increased conversion of LC3-I to LC3-II. Exposure of primary cultured neurons to ferrous iron also resulted in an enhanced conversion of LC3-I to LC3-II and the accumulation of MDC, suggesting that autophagy may be involved in iron-induced neuronal death.

Acknowledgments

This study was supported by grants NS-017760, NS-039866 and NS-047245 from the National Institutes of Health (NIH) and 0755717Z from American Heart Association (AHA). The content is solely the responsibility of the authors and does not necessarily represent the official views of the NIH or AHA.

References

1. Adhami F, Liao G, Morozov YM, Schloemer A, Schmithorst VJ, Lorenz JN, Dunn RS, Vorhees CV, Wills-Karp M, Degen JL, Davis RJ, Mizushima N, Rakic P, Dardzinski BJ, Holland SK, Sharp FR, Kuan CY (2006) Cerebral ischemia-hypoxia induces intravascular coagulation and autophagy. Am J Pathol 169: 566–583
2. Biederbick A, Kern HF, Elsässer HP (1995) Monodansylcadaverine (MDC) is a specific in vivo marker for autophagic vacuoles. Eur J Cell Biol 66: 3–14
3. Chen Y, McMillan-Ward E, Kong J, Israels SJ, Gibson SB (2008) Oxidative stress induces autophagic cell death independent of apoptosis in transformed and cancer cells. Cell Death Differ 15: 171–182
4. He Y, Wan S, Hua Y, Keep RF, Xi G (2008) Autophagy after experimental intracerebral hemorrhage. J Cereb Blood Flow Metab 28: 897–905

5. Hua Y, Nakamura T, Keep RF, Wu J, Schallert T, Hoff JT, Xi G (2006) Long-term effects of experimental intracerebral hemorrhage: the role of iron. J Neurosurg 104: 305–312

6. Jiang Y, Wu J, Hua Y, Keep RF, Xiang J, Hoff JT, Xi G (2002) Thrombin-receptor activation and thrombin-induced brain tolerance. J Cereb Blood Flow Metab 22: 404–410

7. Kabeya Y, Mizushima N, Ueno T, Yamamoto A, Kirisako T, Noda T, Kominami E, Ohsumi Y, Yoshimori T (2000) LC3, a mammalian homologue of yeast Apg8p, is localized in autophagosome membranes after processing. EMBO J 19: 5720–5728

8. Klionsky DJ, Emr SD (2000) Autophagy as a regulated pathway of cellular degradation. Science 290: 1717–1721

9. Komatsu M, Waguri S, Chiba T, Murata S, Iwata J, Tanida I, Ueno T, Koike M, Uchiyama Y, Kominami E, Tanaka K (2006) Loss of autophagy in the central nervous system causes neurodegeneration in mice. Nature 441: 880–884

10. Kondo Y, Kanzawa T, Sawaya R, Kondo S (2005) The role of autophagy in cancer development and response to therapy. Nat Rev Cancer 5: 726–734

11. Nakamura T, Keep RF, Hua Y, Schallert T, Hoff JT, Xi G (2004) Deferoxamine-induced attenuation of brain edema and neurological deficits in a rat model of intracerebral hemorrhage. J Neurosurg 100: 672–678

12. Siesjö BK, Agardh CD, Bengtsson F (1989) Free radicals and brain damage. Cerebrovasc Brain Metab Rev 1: 165–211

13. Song S, Hua Y, Keep RF, Hoff JT, Xi G (2007) A new hippocampal model for examining intracerebral hemorrhage-related neuronal death: effects of deferoxamine on hemoglobin-induced neuronal death. Stroke 38: 2861–2863

14. Wagner KR, Sharp FR, Ardizzone TD, Lu A, Clark JF (2003) Heme and iron metabolism: role in cerebral hemorrhage. J Cereb Blood Flow Metab 23: 629–652

15. Wu J, Hua Y, Keep RF, Nakamura T, Hoff JT, Xi G (2003) Iron and iron-handling proteins in the brain after intracerebral hemorrhage. Stroke 34: 2964–2969

16. Xi G, Keep RF, Hua Y, Xiang J, Hoff JT (1999) Attenuation of thrombin-induced brain edema by cerebral thrombin preconditioning. Stroke 30: 1247–1255

Acta Neurochir Suppl (2008) 105: 33–35
© Springer-Verlag 2008
Printed in Austria

Effects of superoxide dismutase and catalase derivates on intracerebral hemorrhage-induced brain injury in rats

E. Titova[5], R. P. Ostrowski[1], J. Rowe[1], W. Chen[1], J. H. Zhang[1,2,3], J. Tang[1,4]

[1] Department of Physiology and Pharmacology, Loma Linda University, Loma Linda, CA, USA
[2] Department of Neurosurgery, Loma Linda University, Loma Linda, CA, USA
[3] Department of Anesthesiology, Loma Linda University, Loma Linda, CA, USA
[4] Department of Physiology, Chongqing Medical University, Chongqing, China
[5] Department of Anesthesiology, Krasnoyarsk State Medical University, Krasnoyarsk, Russia

Summary

The use of exogenous superoxide dismutase (SOD) and catalase (CAT) has been previously evaluated against various reactive oxygen species-mediated brain injuries, especially those associated with ischemia/reperfusion. In this study, we investigated effects of these enzymatic antioxidants on intracerebral hemorrhage (ICH)-induced brain injury.

A total of 65 male Sprague-Dawley rats (300–380 g) were divided into a sham group, an untreated ICH group, 3 groups of ICH rats treated with lecithinized SOD (PC-SOD) at doses of 0.1, 0.3, and 1 mg/kg, and a group treated with polyethylene glycol conjugated CAT (PEG-CAT) at a dose of 10,000 U/kg. An additional group of ICH rats received a combination of PC-SOD (1 mg/kg) and PEG-CAT (10,000 U/kg). ICH was induced by collagenase injection. All drugs were administered intravenously immediately after ICH induction. Brain injury was evaluated by scoring neurological function and measuring brain edema at 24 h after ICH induction.

Our results demonstrated that ICH caused significant neurological deficit associated with remarkable brain edema. Treatment with PC-SOD, PEG-CAT, or PC-SOD in combination with PEG-CAT did not reduce brain edema or neurological deficit after ICH. We conclude that intravenously administered PC-SOD and/or PEG-CAT do not reduce brain injury in the collagenase-induced ICH rat model.

Keywords: Lecithinized superoxide dismutase; polyethylene glycol conjugated catalase; intracerebral hemorrhage; rats.

Introduction

Reactive oxygen species (ROS) are considered a major mediator of intracerebral hemorrhage (ICH)-induced brain injury [1]. Therapeutic effects of exogenous superoxide dismutase (SOD) (catalyzes dismutation of superoxide to hydrogen peroxide) and catalase (CAT) (decomposes hydrogen peroxide) have been examined in experimental focal cerebral ischemia, and spinal cord and traumatic brain injury models [5, 10–12]. *In vitro* studies have confirmed the suppressing effect of CAT on hydroxyl radical production in Hb-driven oxidative reactions [9]. However, the role of free radical elimination in an animal model of ICH has yet to be investigated. The main goal of this study was to analyze effects of exogenous antioxidant enzymes (SOD and CAT) in a rat model of ICH.

In our study we used lecithinized SOD (PC-SOD) which was a Cu, Zn-SOD conjugated with 4 covalently bound molecules of lecithin [14]. Lecithinization of SOD results in its extended half-life in blood, enhanced tissue affinity and pharmacological activity, and improves passage of SOD to the brain. Polyethylene glycol conjugated CAT (PEG-CAT) was used either alone or together with PC-SOD.

Materials and methods

Experimental groups

A total of 65 male Sprague-Dawley rats (300–380 g) were divided into a sham group, an ICH untreated group, 3 ICH groups treated with lecithinized SOD (PC-SOD) at doses of 0.1, 0.3, and 1 mg/kg, and a group treated with PEG-CAT at a dose of 10,000 U/kg. An additional group of ICH rats received a combination of PC-SOD (1 mg/kg) and PEG-CAT (10,000 U/kg). ICH was induced by collagenase injection as previously described [8, 13].

All drugs were administered intravenously immediately after ICH induction. Brain injury was evaluated by investigating neurological function and measuring brain edema at 24 h after ICH induction.

Animal preparation

All procedures for this study were approved by the Animal Care and Use Committee at Loma Linda University and complied with the Guide for

Correspondence: Jiping Tang, MD, Department of Physiology and Pharmacology, Loma Linda University Medical Center, 11041 Campus Street, Risley Hall Room 133, Loma Linda, CA 92354. e-mail: jtang@llu.edu

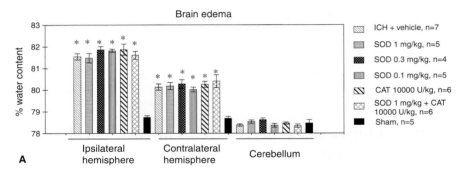

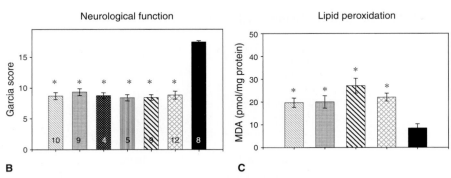

Fig. 1. Effects of PC-SOD and CAT in ICH. (A, B) Collagenase injection increased brain edema and impaired neurological function in ICH animals, but there was no significant difference among groups with ICH ($^*p < 0.05$ vs. sham, ANOVA). (B) Numbers in the bar indicate number of animals used in each group. (C) Lipid peroxidation was significantly increased in ICH animals ($^*p < 0.05$ vs. sham, ANOVA). However, neither SOD, CAT, nor SOD + CAT reduced lipid peroxidation. ICH untreated ($n = 8$); ICH + SOD 1 mg/kg ($n = 4$); ICH + CAT 10,000 U/kg ($n = 6$); ICH + SOD 1 mg/kg + CAT 10,000 U/kg ($n = 6$); Sham ($n = 3$)

the Care and Use of Laboratory Animals. Animals were housed under 12:12 h light/dark cycle, with access to water and food *ad libitum*.

Anesthesia was induced in an induction chamber with 4% isoflurane and maintained with 2–3% isoflurane in a 30% oxygen/70% air mixture using Fluovac Isoflurane/Halothane Scavenger (Stoelting Co., Wood Dale, IL) *via* mask in spontaneously breathing animals. Rectal temperature was maintained at $37 \pm 0.5\,°C$. The right femoral artery was cannulated with a PE-50 polyethylene canula to monitor physiological variables (blood pressure, arterial blood gases, and serum glucose level) before ICH induction, during collagenase injection, and after surgery.

The right femoral vein was cannulated with a PE-10 polyethylene canula for drug administration. PC-SOD was dissolved in distilled water (1 mg/mL) following manufacturer's recommendations (LTT Bio-Pharma, Japan). PEG-CAT (Sigma-Aldrich, St. Louis, MO) was dissolved in normal saline (16,000 U/mL). To avoid any interactions between drugs in the combined treatment group, PC-SOD was used first with subsequent PEG-CAT injection. The ICH with vehicle treatment group (untreated) was injected with the same volume of distilled water.

All animals were sacrificed 24 h after surgery under deep anesthesia with isoflurane inhalation and subsequent decapitation. Brain was collected immediately to measure brain water content. For biochemical studies, rats were deeply anesthetized with isoflurane inhalation and perfused through the left heart ventricle with ice-cold phosphate-buffered saline (PBS). Brains were collected and stored at $-80\,°C$ until analysis.

Neurological deficits

Twenty-four hours after surgery, each rat was graded neurologically for focal deficits in a blinded fashion using an 18-point neurological scoring system developed by Garcia *et al.* [3].

Brain water content and lipid peroxidation

Brain water content was measured and calculated using the previously described wet weight (WW)/dry weight (DW) formula, as follows: $[(WW - DW)/WW] \times 100$ [7].

The level of lipid peroxidation products (malondialdehyde, MDA) was measured using an LPO-586 kit (Oxis Research, Portland, OR) in brain samples 24 h after ICH, as described previously [6].

Results

Neurological deficit was detected in all animals with ICH. There was no statistical difference between treated and untreated groups, however (Fig. 1B).

Brain water content was markedly increased in all hemorrhagic groups of animals compared with sham ($p < 0.05$, ANOVA). We failed to find statistically significant difference between treated and untreated groups (Fig. 1A).

Lipid peroxidation significantly increased in rats with ICH when compared with sham-operated rats ($p < 0.005$, *t*-test). Intergroup comparison did not show any significant difference. Interestingly, however, there is a tendency toward an increase in the level of lipid peroxidation products in the CAT-treated brain samples ($p = 0.066$) (Fig. 1C).

Discussion

Oxidative stress largely contributes to ICH-induced injury due to the impact of hemoglobin degradation products. Moreover, decreased plasma SOD and reduced total superoxide scavenger activities have been found in patients' plasma within 24 h after onset of hemorrhagic stroke [2].

Therefore, we used treatment with exogenous SOD, aiming to target superoxide-derived free radical cascades while scavenger activities are impaired. It was proven ineffective, which may raise a question of the dosage used in our study. A dose similar to ours was effective in transient focal cerebral ischemia [14]; however, more aggravated oxidative stress in ICH might surpass the antioxidant effect of our dose of PC-SOD.

It has been postulated that induction of CAT can protect brain cells from oxidative damage after ICH [15]. Surprisingly, we found a trend toward an increased level of lipid peroxidation products in brains of CAT-treated animals compared with vehicle-treated ones. It is therefore possible that heme included in high-dose CAT contributed to aggravation of oxidative stress, which overwhelmed effects of CAT H_2O_2-decomposing function. The injurious effect might be mediated by products of interaction between CAT heme and superoxide radical [4], as CAT did not seem to cause aggravation of injury when given in combination with SOD.

The use of a solely collagenase model of ICH is a limitation of this study. Although there is no evidence of direct interaction between collagenase and antioxidant enzymes, it is still conceivable that in the blood injection model, results of the same treatment would be different. In the collagenase model, acute tissue necrosis with release of intracellular proteolytic enzymes might largely contribute to the final extent of early brain injury [8].

We conclude that, at the dosage used in our study, neither PC-SOD nor PEG-CAT offered protection against ICH-induced brain injury. CAT treatment alone resulted in a tendency toward exacerbation of brain damage, the effect at least partly mediated by superoxide. Although treatment with antioxidant enzymes in ICH may be further investigated using different dosages and different hemorrhage models, the results of our study may favor pursuing other therapeutic directions including iron chelation and/or augmented hematoma resolution.

Acknowledgment

This work was supported by a grant from National Institutes of Health (NS052492) to Jiping Tang.

References

1. Aronowski J, Hall CE (2005) New horizons for primary intracerebral hemorrhage treatment: experience from preclinical studies. Neurol Res 27: 268–279
2. Aygul R, Demircan B, Erdem F, Ulvi H, Yildirim A, Demirbas F (2005) Plasma values of oxidants and antioxidants in acute brain hemorrhage: role of free radicals in the development of brain injury. Biol Trace Elem Res 108: 43–52
3. Garcia JH, Wagner S, Liu KF, Hu XJ (1995) Neurological deficit and extent of neuronal necrosis attributable to middle cerebral artery occlusion in rats. Statistical validation. Stroke 26: 627–635
4. Lardot C, Broeckaert F, Lison D, Buchet JP, Lauwerys R (1996) Exogenous catalase may potentiate oxidant-mediated lung injury in the female Sprague-Dawley rat. J Toxicol Environ Health 47: 509–522
5. Liu TH, Beckman JS, Freeman BA, Hogan EL, Hsu CY (1989) Polyethylene glycol-conjugated superoxide dismutase and catalase reduce ischemic brain injury. Am J Physiol 256: H589–H593
6. Lo W, Bravo T, Jadhav V, Titova E, Zhang JH, Tang J (2007) NADPH oxidase inhibition improves neurological outcomes in surgically-induced brain injury. Neurosci Lett 414: 228–232
7. Qin Z, Song S, Xi G, Silbergleit R, Keep RF, Hoff JT, Hua Y (2007) Preconditioning with hyperbaric oxygen attenuates brain edema after experimental intracerebral hemorrhage. Neurosurg Focus 22: E13
8. Rosenberg GA, Mun-Bryce S, Wesley M, Kornfeld M (1990) Collagenase-induced intracerebral hemorrhage in rats. Stroke 21: 801–807
9. Sadrzadeh SM, Graf E, Panter SS, Hallaway PE, Eaton JW (1984) Hemoglobin. A biologic fenton reagent. J Biol Chem 259: 14354–14356
10. Sugawara T, Lewén A, Gasche Y, Yu F, Chan PH (2002) Overexpression of SOD1 protects vulnerable motor neurons after spinal cord injury by attenuating mitochondrial cytochrome c release. FASEB J 16: 1997–1999
11. Sugawara T, Noshita N, Lewén A, Gasche Y, Ferrand-Drake M, Fujimura M, Morita-Fujimura Y, Chan PH (2002) Overexpression of copper/zinc superoxide dismutase in transgenic rats protects vulnerable neurons against ischemic damage by blocking the mitochondrial pathway of caspase activation. J Neurosci 22: 209–217
12. Takenaga M, Ohta Y, Tokura Y, Hamaguchi A, Nakamura M, Okano H, Igarashi R (2006) Lecithinized superoxide dismutase (PC-SOD) improved spinal cord injury-induced motor dysfunction through suppression of oxidative stress and enhancement of neurotrophic factor production. J Control Release 110: 283–289
13. Titova E, Ostrowski RP, Sowers LC, Zhang JH, Tang J (2007) Effects of apocynin and ethanol on intracerebral haemorrhage-induced brain injury in rats. Clin Exp Pharmacol P 34: 845–850
14. Tsubokawa T, Jadhav V, Solaroglu I, Shiokawa Y, Konishi Y, Zhang JH (2007) Lecithinized superoxide dismutase improves outcomes and attenuates focal cerebral ischemic injury via antiapoptotic mechanisms in rats. Stroke 38: 1057–1062
15. Zhao X, Sun G, Zhang J, Strong R, Song W, Gonzales N, Grotta JC, Aronowski J (2007) Hematoma resolution as a target for intracerebral hemorrhage treatment: role for peroxisome proliferator-activated receptor gamma in microglia/macrophages. Ann Neurol 61: 352–362

Acta Neurochir Suppl (2008) 105: 37–40
© Springer-Verlag 2008
Printed in Austria

Metallothionein and brain injury after intracerebral hemorrhage

S. Yamashita, M. Okauchi, Y. Hua, W. Liu, R. F. Keep, G. Xi

Department of Neurosurgery, University of Michigan Medical School, Ann Arbor, MI, USA

Summary

Metallothioneins (MTs) are metal-binding proteins that can be upregulated in the brain after injury and are associated with neuroprotection. A recent genomics study has shown that brain MT-1 and MT-2 mRNA levels are upregulated following intracerebral hemorrhage (ICH) in rats. Our study examines whether brain MT-1 and MT-2 protein levels are increased after ICH. We also investigated the effect of exogenous MT-1 in perihematomal edema formation *in vivo* and iron-induced cell death *in vitro*. We found that MT-1/-2 immunoreactivity in ipsilateral basal ganglia was significantly increased after ICH and exogenous MT-1 attenuated perihematomal edema formation. In addition, MT-1 also reduced cell death induced by iron in cultured astrocytes. These results suggest a role for MT in ICH-induced brain injury, and MT could be a therapeutic target for ICH.

Keywords: Astrocytes; cerebral hemorrhage; iron; metallothionein.

Introduction

Metallothioneins (MTs) are zinc-binding proteins that may be neuroprotective [12]. Four isoforms of MT (1–4) have been found. Within the brain, MT-1 and MT-2 (MT-1/-2) comprise approximately two-thirds of total brain MT [2]. In central nervous system (CNS), they are mainly expressed in astrocytes [1]. Previously, MT proteins had unexpected roles within the cellular response to brain injury. For example, MT-1 is considered to be a rapidly acting cellular defense protein and is induced in the brain by exposure to a variety of stresses [1]. Intracerebral hemorrhage (ICH) upregulates many genes in the brain including MT-1 and MT-2 [6].

Iron has an important role in ICH-induced brain injury [5, 14]. After erythrocyte lysis, iron concentrations in the brain reach very high levels. We found a 3-fold increase in brain non-heme iron after ICH in rats, and this level remains high for at least 1 month [13]. Our recent study found that ferrous iron in low concentrations (e.g., 0.2 mM) can also induce brain damage [15]. Deferoxamine, an iron chelator, reduces brain damage after ICH [9].

In this study, we examine whether ICH induces MT upregulation in the brain, and whether exogenous MT-1 attenuates perihematomal brain edema and iron-induced cell death.

Materials and methods

Experimental groups

There were 3 sets of experiments in this study. In the first set, male Sprague-Dawley rats received a 100-μL intracaudate injection of autologous whole blood. Sham animals had needle insertion only. The rats were killed 1, 3, or 7 days later, and brains were sampled for Western blot analysis and immunohistochemistry. The antibody used detects both MT-1 and MT-2.

In the second set of experiments, rats received a 100-μL intracaudate infusion of blood with 10 μL MT-1 (0.1 or 0.2 nmol) or saline. The rats were euthanized 3 days later for brain water content measurement.

In the last set, cultured primary astrocytes were treated with MT-1 (5, 10, 50, and 100 nM) or vehicle for 1 h. The astrocytes were then exposed to ferrous chloride (500 μM). Culture medium was collected for lactate dehydrogenase (LDH) measurement 48 h following treatment.

Animal preparation and intracerebral infusion

Animal protocols were approved by the University of Michigan Committee on the Use and Care of Animals. Male Sprague-Dawley rats (Charles River Laboratories, Portage, MI), each weighing 300–350 g, were used in the *in vivo* study. Rats were allowed free access to food and water. Rats were anesthetized with pentobarbital (40 mg/kg i.p.) and the right femoral artery was catheterized to monitor arterial blood pressure and to sample blood for intracerebral infusion. Blood pH, PaO_2, $PaCO_2$, hematocrit, and glucose levels were monitored. Rectal temperature was maintained at 37.5 °C using a feedback-controlled heating pad. The rats were positioned in a stereotactic frame (David Kopf Instruments, Tujunga, CA) and a 1-mm cranial burr hole was drilled near the right

Correspondence: Guohua Xi, MD, Department of Neurosurgery, University of Michigan Medical School, 109 Zina Pitcher Place, R5018 Biomedical Science Research Building, Ann Arbor, MI 48109-2200, USA. e-mail: guohuaxi@umich.edu

coronal suture 3.5 mm lateral to the midline. A 26-gauge needle was inserted stereotaxically into right basal ganglia (coordinates: 0.2 mm anterior, 5.5 mm ventral, and 3.5 mm lateral to bregma). The animals received injections of autologous whole blood at a rate of 10 μL/min. Sham rats received needle insertion in the right caudate. The needle was removed and the skin incision was closed with suture after infusion.

Brain water content measurement

Rats were anesthetized intraperitoneally (60 mg/kg) and decapitated 72 h after intracerebral blood injection. Brains were removed and a 4-mm coronal brain slice was cut from the frontal pole (approximately 3 mm thick). The brain slice was divided into ipsilateral and contralateral cortex, and ipsilateral and contralateral basal ganglia. The cerebellum served as control. Brain samples were weighed on an electronic analytical balance (model AE 100; Mettler Instrument, Hightstown, NJ) to obtain the wet weight (WW). Brain samples were then dried in a gravity oven at 100 °C for 24 h to obtain the dry weight (DW). Brain water content was determined as follows: (WW – DW)/WW.

Immunohistochemistry

Rats were anesthetized and underwent intracardiac perfusion with 4% paraformaldehyde in 0.1 mol/L phosphate-buffered saline (pH 7.4). The brains were removed and kept in 4% paraformaldehyde for 6 h, then immersed in 25% sucrose for 3–4 days at 4 °C. Brains were then placed in optimal cutting temperature embedding compound and sectioned on a cryostat (18 μm). For immunofluorescent single-labeling, anti-MT-1/-2 antibody (E9 monoclonal mouse anti-horse MT; Dako Cytomation, Carpinteria, CA) was incubated overnight at 4 °C. Rhodamine conjugated rabbit anti-mouse (1:50) secondary antibody was incubated with sections for 2 h at room temperature. The single-labeled cells were analyzed using a fluorescence microscope.

Cell preparation and treatment

Astrocyte culture method was modified from that used by McCarthy and deVellis [8]. Cell cultures were established in T75 Falcon flasks from cerebral cortex of 1- to 3-day-old Sprague-Dawley rats. Cerebra were dissected and placed in medium for astrocytes (DMEM plus 10% FBS, 1% glutamine, and 2% antibiotic-antimycotic). Meninges and blood vessels were removed. The medium was removed and the cerebra dissociated with a blade. Tissues were then suspended in modified Hank's Balanced Solution (500 mL HBSS, Gibco +25 mM HEPES,

Gibco + 5 mL antibiotic-antimycotic; Gibco BRL, Carlsbad, CA). After centrifugation, cell pellets were digested in 0.5% trypsin at 37 °C for 20 min, then re-suspended in Buffer T (23.5 mL of modified HBSS + 200 U DNase + 0.5 mL 3.8% $MgSO_4$) and astrocyte medium (half) + HBSS (half) and centrifuged. Pellets were re-suspended in astrocyte medium and the cells plated into T75 Falcon flasks coated with poly-L-lysine at a density of 10,000,000 cells and cultured at 37 °C in an atmosphere of 5% CO_2 in air. The medium was changed after 3 to 4 days and twice per week thereafter. After cells reached confluence (approximately 7 days), astrocyte cultures were deprived of microglia by shaking the flask at 200 RPM for 1.5 h on a gyratory shaker at 4 °C. The cells were re-plated on poly-L-lysine coated 24-well plates (500,000 cells/well) for LDH measurements.

Measurement of LDH activity

Cell medium was collected and centrifuged. LDH activity in cell culture media was measured using a commercially available kit (Roche Pharmaceuticals, Germany) according to manufacturer's instructions.

Statistical analysis

All data in this study are presented as mean ± standard deviation. Data were analyzed using Student *t*-test or one-way analysis of variance (ANOVA). Significance levels were set at $p < 0.05$.

Results

MT-1/-2 immunoreactivity was very low in normal brain tissue, but immunoreactivity was significantly increased in ipsilateral basal ganglia after ICH. MT-1/-2 positive cells were found in ipsilateral basal ganglia after ICH and most of those positive cells appeared to be glia-like (Fig. 1). Western blot analysis showed a marked increase in MT-1/-2 content at day 1 after ICH, and it was still detectable at day 7. At day 3 after ICH, MT-1/-2 levels in the ipsilateral basal ganglia were 3327 ± 1523 vs. 338 ± 270 pixels in sham control, $p < 0.01$.

Exogenous MT-1 attenuated edema formation following ICH *in vivo*. ICH-induced brain edema at day 3 was

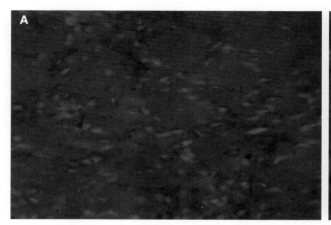 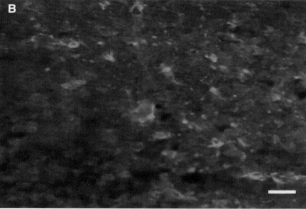

Fig. 1. Immunoreactivity of MT-1/-2 in (A) contralateral or (B) ipsilateral basal ganglia 3 days after ICH. Scale bar = 25 μm

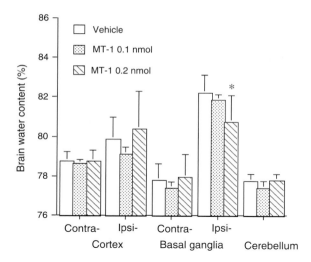

Fig. 2. Brain water content in basal ganglia 3 days after ICH. Rats were treated with or without MT-1 (0.1 or 0.2 nmol). Values are mean ± SD; $n = 5–6$; $^*p < 0.05$ vs. vehicle-treated group

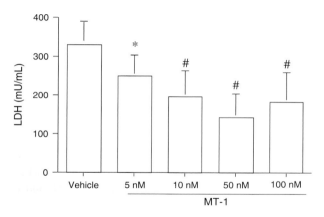

Fig. 3. LDH levels in cultured astrocyte medium 48 h after exposure to ferrous iron. Astrocytes were pretreated (30 min earlier) with vehicle or MT-1. Values are mean ± SD; $^*p < 0.05$, $^\#p < 0.01$ vs. vehicle

reduced by co-injection of MT-1 at dose of 0.2 nmol ($80.7 \pm 1.4\%$ vs. $82.2 \pm 0.9\%$ in vehicle-treated group; $p < 0.05$; Fig. 2) but not at dose of 0.1 nmol ($81.9 \pm 0.1\%$ vs. $82.2 \pm 0.9\%$ in vehicle-treated group; $p > 0.05$; Fig. 2).

MT-1 also protected against iron-induced cell death in cultured astrocytes. LDH release induced by ferrous chloride was significantly reduced by MT-1 pretreatment at all doses (e.g., MT-1 at dose of 50 nM: 141 ± 62 vs. 313 ± 71 mU/mL in vehicle-treated group; $p < 0.05$; Fig. 3).

Discussion

In this study, we found that MT-1/-2 protein levels increase in the brain after ICH. Exogenous MT-1 attenuated perihematomal edema *in vivo* and reduced astrocyte

death *in vitro*. These results suggest a neuroprotective effect for MT in ICH.

Astrocytes are the most abundant cells in the CNS and have roles in both neuroprotection and neurogeneration. In the normal brain, MTs are mainly expressed in astrocytes [1]. An increase in MT expression has been reported in a rat model of ICH [6]. In the current study, we found that ICH results in an increase of MT-1/-2 in the brain, and most MT-1/-2 positive cells are glia. Previous studies show that overexpression of MT protein is helpful for protecting from brain damage, and MT-1/-2 knock-out models are vulnerable to brain damage [12]. Although it is not clear whether MT upregulation in glia after ICH is neuroprotective, a weaker astrocytic reaction to the hematoma has been associated with more severe brain swelling and neurological deficits in aged rats [4].

Iron overload in the brain after ICH contributes to brain damage [5, 14]. MT-1 injection diminishes ICH-induced brain edema and MT-1 reduces iron-induced astrocyte death, indicating that MT-1 may decrease iron toxicity following ICH. This evidence also suggests that both endogenous and exogenous MT proteins may be neuroprotective. While the mechanisms for brain protection by MTs are still unclear, MT can act as a free radical scavenger and as an antioxidant by modulating inflammatory response to injury and by having anti-apoptotic effects [12]. It should be noted that free radicals, oxidative stress, inflammation, and apoptosis all contribute to brain injury after ICH [7, 10, 11, 14]. MTs also contain high levels of sulfur, which can bind transition metals. However, while intracellular copper and zinc are normally bound to MT, MTs are not thought to be a major chelator of iron, which is primarily bound to ferritin [3].

In conclusion, our results indicate that MTs may be protective in ICH by reducing iron toxicity.

Acknowledgments

This study was supported by grants NS-017760, NS-039866, and NS-047245 from the National Institutes of Health (NIH), and 0755717Z and 0840016N from American Heart Association (AHA). The content is solely the responsibility of the authors and does not necessarily represent the official views of the NIH or AHA.

References

1. Chung RS, Hidalgo J, West AK (2008) New insight into the molecular pathways of metallothionein-mediated neuroprotection and regeneration. J Neurochem 104: 14–20
2. Erickson JC, Sewell AK, Jensen LT, Winge DR, Palmiter RD (1994) Enhanced neurotrophic activity in Alzheimer's disease cortex is not

associated with down-regulation of metallothionein-III (GIF). Brain Res 649: 297–304

3. Formigari A, Irato P, Santon A (2007) Zinc, antioxidant systems and metallothionein in metal mediated-apoptosis: biochemical and cytochemical aspects. Comp Biochem Physiol C Toxicol Pharmacol 146: 443–459

4. Gong Y, Hua Y, Keep RF, Hoff JT, Xi G (2004) Intracerebral hemorrhage: effects of aging on brain edema and neurological deficits. Stroke 35: 2571–2575

5. Hua Y, Keep RF, Hoff JT, Xi G (2007) Brain injury after intracerebral hemorrhage: the role of thrombin and iron. Stroke 38: 759–762

6. Lu A, Tang Y, Ran R, Ardizzone TL, Wagner KR, Sharp FR (2006) Brain genomics of intracerebral hemorrhage. J Cereb Blood Flow Metab 26: 230–252

7. Matsushita K, Meng W, Wang X, Asahi M, Asahi K, Moskowitz MA, Lo EH (2000) Evidence for apoptosis after intercerebral hemorrhage in rat striatum. J Cereb Blood Flow Metab 20: 396–404

8. McCarthy KD, de Vellis J (1980) Preparation of separate astroglial and oligodendroglial cell cultures from rat cerebral tissue. J Cell Biol 85: 890–902

9. Nakamura T, Keep RF, Hua Y, Schallert T, Hoff JT, Xi G (2004) Deferoxamine-induced attenuation of brain edema and neurological deficits in a rat model of intracerebral hemorrhage. J Neurosurg 100: 672–678

10. Nakamura T, Keep RF, Hua Y, Hoff JT, Xi G (2005) Oxidative DNA injury after experimental intracerebral hemorrhage. Brain Res 1039: 30–36

11. Peeling J, Yan HJ, Chen SG, Campbell M, Del Bigio MR (1998) Protective effects of free radical inhibitors in intracerebral hemorrhage in rat. Brain Res 795: 63–70

12. Penkowa M (2006) Metallothioneins are multipurpose neuroprotectants during brain pathology. FEBS J 273: 1857–1870

13. Wu J, Hua Y, Keep RF, Nakamura T, Hoff JT, Xi G (2003) Iron and iron-handling proteins in the brain after intracerebral hemorrhage. Stroke 34: 2964–2969

14. Xi G, Keep RF, Hoff JT (2006) Mechanisms of brain injury after intracerebral hemorrhage. Lancet Neurol 5: 53–63

15. Yang S, Hua Y, Nakamura T, Keep RF, Xi G (2006) Up-regulation of brain ceruloplasmin in thrombin preconditioning. Acta Neurochir Suppl 96: 203–206

Experimental intracerebral hemorrhage – inflammation and thrombin

Acta Neurochir Suppl (2008) 105: 43–46
© Springer-Verlag 2008
Printed in Austria

Intracerebral hemorrhage injury mechanisms: glutamate neurotoxicity, thrombin, and Src

F. Sharp, D.-Z. Liu, X. Zhan, B. P. Ander

Department of Neurology, MIND Institute, University of California at Davis Medical Center, Sacramento, CA, USA

Summary

The mechanisms accounting for variable increases in blood flow and seizures following intracerebral hemorrhage (ICH) are unknown. Local cerebral glucose utilization (LCGU) studies performed to address this issue demonstrate increased LCGU within hours around an ICH that is blocked by NMDA and AMPA glutamate receptor antagonists. Local injections of NMDA or AMPA increased LCGU whereas glutamate did not, suggesting an ICH effect on glutamate uptake or glutamate receptors. To address these possibilities, we performed genomic studies of brain following ICH. Among the many regulated genes, an Src family member, Lyn, increased expression over 20-fold. This was important, since Src is known to phosphorylate NMDA receptors and augment their function, and thrombin is known to activate PARs that activate Src. This prompted us to study the Src antagonist, PP2. PP2 decreased LCGU and cell death around ICH and improved behavioral function following ICH. This data leads us to suggest our hypothesis, that ICH, possibly via thrombin activation of protease-activated receptors, activates Src that phosphorylates NMDA receptors and other proteins that mediate injury after ICH.

Keywords: Intracerebral hemorrhage; thrombin; Src; glutamate; excitatory amino acids.

Introduction

Experimental studies of intracerebral hemorrhage (ICH) are in relative infancy compared to experimental ischemic stroke. This has occurred in part because most clinicians have assumed the major morbidity and mortality were due to mass effect. Although probably true to a large extent, particularly for early mortality, experimental studies of ICH are beginning to show that various aspects of hemorrhage can be manipulated and perhaps improved. A good example of this is a series of studies by Xi and colleagues, showing that thrombin appears to be the major mediator of acute edema following ICH in

experimental models [19, 20]. These proof-of-principle studies could lead to treatment of early edema due to ICH.

Our group has been particularly interested in the role of heme oxygenase 1 and 2 in metabolizing the heme and iron released from hemoglobin following subarachnoid hemorrhage (SAH) and ICH [9, 14, 15]. Indeed, either ICH or SAH induce HO-1 in microglia throughout the involved hemisphere(s), presumably in response to extracellular heme taken up into the microglia [13, 14].

In addition to the heme and iron load following ICH, a number of studies have described both local decreases and local increases in cerebral blood flow at the margins of ICH [10]. Although local decreases of blood flow seemed to make sense on the basis of mass effect, the explanation for increases in blood flow following ICH was less clear and not always appreciated [11]. The role of decreased blood flow has been debated throughout the literature, but the consensus now seems to be that although flow decreases around ICH, it does not decrease to levels that appear to produce ischemia in most cases [12].

Based on scattered reports of increases of glutamate in brain and cerebrospinal fluid following SAH and ICH, we explored the possibility that local increases in blood flow were related to glutamate release. To do this, we examined local cerebral glucose utilization (LCGU) following experimental ICH.

Glucose metabolism and glutamate receptors following ICH

Adult male Sprague-Dawley rats were anesthetized and lysed blood or saline (50 μL) was injected into one striatum. Anesthesia was discontinued, and the rats were allowed to recover 1 to 72 h. [14C]-2-deoxyglucose

Correspondence: Frank R. Sharp, MD, Department of Neurology and the MIND Institute, UCD Medical Center, 2805 50th Street – Room 2416, Sacramento, CA 95817, USA. e-mail: frank.sharp@ucdmc.ucdavis.edu

(intraperitoneally) was then injected and subjects sacrificed 30 min later. To examine the mechanisms of changes in glucose utilization, animals were pretreated with the NMDA antagonist MK-801 (1 mg/kg) or the AMPA glutamate receptor antagonist NBQX (30 mg/kg), or saline vehicle [1].

The results showed that [14C]-2-deoxyglucose uptake decreased in the region of ICH, but increased in the perihematomal region, peaking at about 3 h after the lysed blood injection. Saline injections did not affect striatal glucose utilization. Pretreatment with either MK-801 or NBQX blocked the increased [14C]-2-deoxyglucose uptake produced by the ICH.

To examine possible mechanisms of increased [14C]-2-deoxyglucose uptake, we showed that glutamate injections alone had no effect on striatal glucose metabolism. This confirmed that glutamate release *per se* was not sufficient to increase glucose metabolism. In contrast, NMDA and AMPA injections increased [14C]-2-deoxyglucose uptake [1]. The data imply that glutamate activation of NMDA or AMPA receptors increases glucose metabolism in perihematomal brain early after ICH, but that either the glutamate uptake or glutamate receptors must be changed following ICH to account for ICH-induced, glutamate receptor-dependent increases in glucose metabolism [1].

Genomic studies of brain following ICH

We next performed genomic studies of brain following ICH to look for genes that might account for altered glutamate uptake or altered glutamate receptors following ICH [7]. Gene expression was assessed using Affymetrix microarrays (Affymetrix, Santa Clara, CA) in the striatum and the overlying cortex 24 h after infusions of blood into the striatum of adult rats [7]. Three hundred and sixty-nine of 8,740 transcripts were regulated with ICH as compared with saline-injected controls, with 104 regulated genes shared by the striatum and cortex. Real-time reverse transcriptase-polymerase chain reaction (RT-PCR) confirmed up regulation of IL-1-beta, Lipcortin 1 (annexin), and metallothionein 1, 2, and down regulation of potassium voltage-gated channel, shaker-related subfamily, beta member 2 (Kcnab2). Pathways analyses showed that many metabolism and signal transduction-related genes decreased in striatum but increased in adjacent cortex. In contrast, most enzyme, cytokine, chemokine, and immune response genes were up regulated in both striatum and in the cortex after ICH, likely in response to foreign blood proteins. Many

growth factor pathways and the phosphatidylinositol 3-kinase (PI3K)/Akt pathway were down regulated. Activation of immune systems and down regulation of trophic and survival pathways could contribute to cell death and edema following ICH. ICH-related down regulation of GABA-related genes and potassium channels might contribute to perihematomal cellular excitability and increased risk of post-ICH seizures [7].

Of relevance to increased glucose metabolism following ICH, we found that Lyn expression increased over 20-fold in perihematomal brain [7]. Lyn is an Src family kinase (SFK) that is related to Src, the first described protooncogene. Src and SFKs are known to phosphorylate the NR2A subunit of the NMDA receptor and increase calcium flux through the receptor and increase glutamate excitotoxicity [8]. This was also of interest since thrombin is known to activate protease-activated receptors (PARs) that in turn phosphorylate and activate Src [16]. Thus, we postulated that ICH would activate thrombin that caused PARs to phosphorylate Src that would, in turn, phosphorylate the NR2A subunit of the NMDA receptor to exacerbate glutamate-mediated injury following ICH. To test this idea, we performed the following preliminary studies.

Src mediates glutamate neurotoxicity following ICH

Src is a 60 kDa protein that is the prototypical member of a family of non-receptor tyrosine kinases (reviewed in [3]). Src is myristoylated on the amino terminus, thus allowing it to associate with the inner surface of the plasma membrane. Structurally, Src contains Src homology SH3 and SH2 domains and the catalytic domain in the amino-terminal region. The carboxy-terminus contains a non-catalytic regulatory sequence that has a proline rich segment and a terminal tyrosine residue. The SH2 domain binds the phosphorylated form of the carboxy-terminal tyrosine and the SH3 domain reinforces this interaction by binding the proline-rich region in the regulatory domain. These intramolecular interactions inactivate Src, thus regulating its function through its phosphorylation. Therefore, the phosphorylation of the C-terminal tyrosine should give an indication of the activity of Src under different conditions. In stroke it has recently been shown that the Src kinase inhibitor PP2 decreases infarct volumes and improves neurological outcomes following middle cerebral artery occlusion [5].

The physiological function of Src in the central nervous system is not well understood. However, Src activity can potentially contribute to glutamate excitotoxicity and edema formation. Src is activated by thrombin in cells of the central nervous system [16, 17]. Src directly phosphorylates the NR2A subunit of the NMDA receptor to potentiate its function and increase the risk of neurons to excitotoxic insults [6]. Src could also contribute to edema in ICH by inducing the translation of HIF-1alpha or by activating a variety of metalloproteinases (MMPs) and by interacting with tight junction proteins.

As noted above, NMDA receptors are potentiated by thrombin receptor activation that causes Src-mediated phosphorylation of NR2A subunits [6]. NMDA receptors are directly linked to Src via a recently-identified adapter protein to produce NMDA (NR2a)-NADH dehydrogenase subunit 2 – Src complexes [4]. Finally, Src kinases appear to be important in glutamate release from synaptic vesicles, since the Src kinase inhibitor PP2 can block glutamate release [18].

Based on this background information, we have begun to test the hypothesis that ICH activates Src kinases that phosphorylate other molecules to produce cell injury and behavioral deficits after ICH (Fig. 1) [2]. ICH was produced by direct injection of autologous blood (50 μL) into striatum of anesthetized adult Sprague Dawley rats. Src kinase activity, glucose hypermetabolic areas around the ICH, TUNEL-stained cells, and apomorphine-induced rotational behaviors were assessed in animals with ICH pretreated with the Src kinase inhibitor, PP1, or with vehicle [2]. PP1 completely blocked local regions of increased glucose metabolism in the perihematomal brain that appeared to be identical to those

produced by MK-801 or NBQX. PP1 blocked increases in Src kinase activity (5-fold) at 3 h after ICH and decreased the numbers of TUNEL-stained cells surrounding the ICH at 24 h. PP1 also marked reduced apomorphine-induced (1 mg/kg) rotation at 24 h after ICH [2]. Thus, PP1 produced improvement on all of the measures that the glutamate receptor antagonists also improved. The data are consistent with the hypothesis that ICH, possibly via thrombin activation of protease-activated receptors, activates Src that phosphorylates NMDA receptors and other proteins that mediate injury after ICH [2].

Future directions

Future studies will need to determine if thrombin activation of PARs causes phosphorylation and activation of Src or Src family members. In addition, does PAR activation of Src activate NMDA receptors as proposed above? Other potential actions of Src in experimental ICH also need to be explored in order to test whether other thrombin-mediated injuries to brain are mediated by Src. Several of these studies are underway.

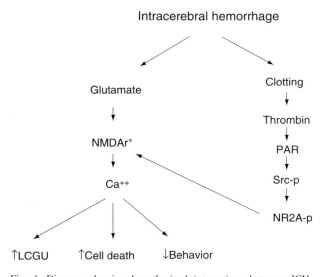

Fig. 1. Diagram showing hypothesized interactions between ICH, thrombin, Src, and NMDA glutamate receptors. *PAR* Protease activated receptor; *NR2A* subunit of NMDA receptor; *LCGU* local cerebral glucose utilization in brain adjacent to ICH

References

1. Ardizzone TD, Lu A, Wagner KR, Tang Y, Ran R, Sharp FR (2004) Glutamate receptor blockade attenuates glucose hypermetabolism in perihematomal brain after experimental intracerebral hemorrhage in rat. Stroke 35: 2587–2591
2. Ardizzone TD, Zhan X, Ander BP, Sharp FR (2007) Src kinase inhibition improves acute outcomes after experimental intracerebral hemorrhage. Stroke 38: 1621–1625
3. Fukami Y, Nagao T, Iwasaki T, Sato K (2002) Inhibition and activation of c-Src: the head and tail of a coin. Pharmacol Ther 93: 263–270
4. Gingrich JR, Pelkey KA, Fam SR, Huang Y, Petralia RS, Wenthold RJ, Salter MW (2004) Unique domain anchoring of Src to synaptic NMDA receptors via the mitochondrial protein NADH dehydrogenase subunit 2. Proc Natl Acad Sci USA 101: 6237–6242
5. Lennmyr F, Ericsson A, Gerwins P, Akterin S, Ahlström H, Terént A (2004) Src family kinase-inhibitor PP2 reduces focal ischemic brain injury. Acta Neurol Scand 110: 175–179
6. Liu Y, Zhang G, Gao C, Hou X (2001) NMDA receptor activation results in tyrosine phosphorylation of NMDA receptor subunit 2A(NR2A) and interaction of Pyk2 and Src with NR2A after transient cerebral ischemia and reperfusion. Brain Res 909: 51–58
7. Lu A, Tang Y, Ran R, Ardizzone TL, Wagner KR, Sharp FR (2006) Brain genomics of intracerebral hemorrhage. J Cereb Blood Flow Metab 26: 230–252
8. Manzerra P, Behrens MM, Canzoniero LM, Wang XQ, Heidinger V, Ichinose T, Yu SP, Choi DW (2001) Zinc induces a Src family kinase-mediated up-regulation of NMDA receptor activity and excitotoxicity. Proc Natl Acad Sci USA 98: 11055–11061
9. Matz PG, Weinstein PR, Sharp FR (1997) Heme oxygenase-1 and heat shock protein 70 induction in glia and neurons throughout rat brain after experimental intracerebral hemorrhage. Neurosurgery 40: 152–162

10. Miyazawa N, Mitsuka S, Asahara T, Uchida M, Fukamachi A, Fukasawa I, Sasaki H, Nukui H (1998) Clinical features of relative focal hyperfusion in patients with intracerebral hemorrhage detected by contrast-enhanced xenon CT. Am J Neuroradiol 19: 1741–1746

11. Ogasawara K, Koshu K, Yoshimoto T, Ogawa A (1999) Transient hyperemia immediately after rapid decompression of chronic subdural hematoma. Neurosurgery 45: 484–489

12. Qureshi AI, Wilson DA, Hanley DF, Traystman RJ (1999) No evidence for an ischemic penumbra in massive experimental intracerebral hemorrhage. Neurology 52: 266–272

13. Sharp FR, Massa SM, Swanson RA (1999) Heat-shock protein protection. Trends Neurosci 22: 97–99

14. Turner CP, Bergeron M, Matz P, Zegna A, Noble LJ, Panter SS, Sharp FR (1998) Heme oxygenase-1 is induced in glia throughout brain by subarachnoid hemoglobin. J Cereb Blood Flow Metab 18: 257–273

15. Turner CP, Panter SS, Sharp FR (1999) Anti-oxidants prevent focal rat brain injury as assessed by induction of heat shock proteins (HSP70, HO-1/HSP32, HSP47) following subarachnoid injections of lysed blood. Brain Res Mol Brain Res 65: 87–102

16. Wang H, Reiser G (2003) Thrombin signaling in the brain: the role of protease-activated receptors. Biol Chem 384: 193–202

17. Wang H, Reiser G (2003) The role of the Ca^{2+}-sensitive tyrosine kinase Pyk2 and Src in thrombin signalling in rat astrocytes. J Neurochem 84: 1349–1357

18. Wang SJ (2003) A role for Src kinase in the regulation of glutamate release from rat cerebrocortical nerve terminals. Neuroreport 14: 1519–1522

19. Xi G, Keep RF, Hoff JT (1998) Erythrocytes and delayed brain edema formation following intracerebral hemorrhage in rats. J Neurosurg 89: 991–996

20. Xi G, Keep RF, Hoff JT (2006) Mechanisms of brain injury after intracerebral haemorrhage. Lancet Neurol 5: 53–63

Acta Neurochir Suppl (2008) 105: 47–50
© Springer-Verlag 2008
Printed in Austria

Increase in brain thrombin activity after experimental intracerebral hemorrhage

Y. Gong[1,2], G. Xi[1], H. Hu[1], Y. Gu[1,2], F. Huang[2], R. F. Keep[1], Y. Hua[1]

[1] Department of Neurosurgery, University of Michigan Medical School, Ann Arbor, MI, USA
[2] Department of Neurosurgery, Huashan Hospital, Fudan University, Shanghai, China

Summary

Thrombin has been shown to play a major role in brain injury after intracerebral hemorrhage (ICH). In this study, we measured thrombin activity in the perihematomal zone and examined the role of thrombin in ICH-induced brain tissue loss.

There were 2 experiments in this study. In the first part, adult male Sprague-Dawley rats received 100 μL of either autologous whole blood or saline. The rats were killed at 1 h or 24 h later for thrombin activity measurement. Thrombin activity was measured using the thrombin-specific chromogenic substrate, S2238. In the second part, rats received a 50-μL intracaudate injection of either thrombin or saline, and the rats were killed at days 1, 3, or 28 for determination of neuronal death and brain tissue loss.

We found that brain thrombin activity was elevated in ipsilateral basal ganglia 1 h after ICH. Intracerebral injection of thrombin rather than saline caused significant neuronal death at days 1 and 3, and resulted in significant brain tissue loss at day 28. These results suggest that thrombin inhibition in the acute phase may reduce ICH-induced brain damage.

Keywords: Cerebral hemorrhage; thrombin activity; neuronal death.

Introduction

Intracerebral hemorrhage (ICH) is a subtype of stroke with high morbidity and mortality, accounting for approximately 15% of all deaths from stroke [8]. Many factors affect outcomes in ICH patients. Experimental investigations have indicated that thrombin formation and iron toxicity play a major role in ICH-induced injury [24].

Thrombin is a serine protease and an essential component in the coagulation cascade. It is produced in the brain immediately after an ICH to stop the hemorrhage. Thrombin at low concentrations is neuroprotective [22].

However, direct infusion of large doses of thrombin into brain causes inflammatory cell infiltration and brain edema formation [22, 24]. We have demonstrated that thrombin is responsible for early brain edema formation following ICH and that such edema results partly from a direct opening of the blood–brain barrier [13]. Because thrombin can be harmful at high concentrations and protective at low concentrations, it is important to know what concentrations of thrombin may occur in the brain after ICH.

In this study, we measured thrombin activity around the hematoma. We also examined whether or not thrombin causes neuronal death and brain tissue loss.

Materials and methods

Animal preparation and intracerebral injection

Our animal protocol was approved by the University of Michigan Committee on the Use and Care of Animals. Male Sprague-Dawley rats weighing 300–400 g were used in this study. The animals were anesthetized with pentobarbital (40 mg/kg, i.p.). Aseptic precautions were taken for all surgical procedures. The right femoral artery was catheterized for continuous blood pressure monitoring and for blood sampling during surgery. Arterial blood was obtained for analysis of pH, PaO_2, $PaCO_2$, hematocrit, and blood glucose. Core body temperature was maintained at 37.5 °C using a feedback-controlled heating pad. The rats were positioned in a stereotactic frame and a 1-mm cranial burr hole was drilled in the right coronal suture 4.0 mm lateral to the midline. Autologous whole blood, thrombin, or saline were infused into the right caudate nucleus through a 26-gauge needle (coordinates: 0.2 mm anterior, 5.5 mm ventral, and 4.0 mm lateral to the bregma) at a rate of 10 μL per minute using a microinfusion pump. The needle was removed and the skin incision closed with suture.

Experimental groups

There were 2 parts to this study. In the first part, rats received a 100-μL intracaudate injection of either autologous whole blood or saline. The

Correspondence: Ya Hua, M.D., Department of Neurosurgery, University of Michigan Medical School, 109 Zina Pitcher Place, R5018 Biomedical Science Research Building, Ann Arbor, MI 48109-2200, USA. e-mail: yahua@umich.edu

rats were killed 1 h or 24 h later for thrombin activity measurement. In the second part, rats received a 50-µL injection of either thrombin (5 U) or saline into right caudate and the rats were killed at day 1, 3, or 28 for determination of neuronal death and brain tissue loss.

Thrombin activity measurement

For thrombin activity measurements, rat brains were perfused transcardially with saline. Brain samples were homogenized and thrombin activities were measured using the thrombin-specific chromogenic substrate, S2238 (Chromogenix, Milano, Italy) [4]. The final concentration of S2238 was 0.3 mmol/L in phosphate-buffered saline, and absorption at 405 nm of supernatant was measured 1 h later.

Morphometric analyses

The rat brains were removed and kept in 4% paraformaldehyde for 4–6 h, then immersed in 25% sucrose for 3–4 days at 4 °C. Brains were embedded in optimal cutting temperature compound (Sakura Finetek USA, Inc., Torrance, CA) and 18-µm-thick sections were taken on a cryostat. Coronal sections from 1 mm posterior to the blood injection site were stained with hematoxylin and eosin. The caudate, cortex, and lateral ventricle were outlined on a computer and the outlined areas were measured using NIH Image software, version 1.62 (National Institutes of Health, Bethesda, MD). All measurements were repeated 3 times and the average value was recorded [6].

Fluoro-Jade staining

Brain sections were kept 15 min in 0.06% potassium permanganate (KMnO4) and rinsed in distilled water. Sections were stained by gently shaking for 30 min in working solution of Fluoro-Jade composed of 10 mL 0.01% Fluoro-Jade in distilled water and 90 mL 0.1% acetic acid, then rinsed in distilled water 3 times. After drying with a blower, slides were quickly dipped into xylol and covered for microscopic examination [16].

Statistical analysis

All data in this study are presented as mean ± SD. Data were analyzed using Student *t*-test. Statistical significance was set at $p < 0.05$.

Results

One hour after ICH, thrombin activity was elevated in ipsilateral basal ganglia (3.3 ± 1.4 vs. 0.1 ± 0.2 U/g in

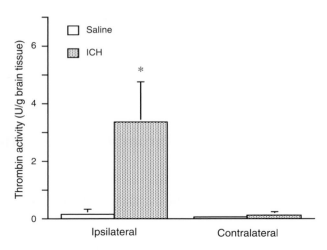

Fig. 1. Thrombin activity in ipsilateral and contralateral basal ganglia 1 h after ICH or saline injection into the ipsilateral basal ganglia. Values are mean ± SD; $n = 6$; *$p < 0.05$ vs. saline

saline control, $p < 0.01$, Fig. 1). Twenty-four hours after ICH, the level of thrombin activity in ipsilateral basal ganglia was still higher (2.4 ± 1.0 vs. 0.3 ± 0.2 U/g in contralateral side, $p < 0.01$). Intracerebral saline injection did not increase thrombin activity in the brain. One hour after saline injection, thrombin activity in ipsilateral basal ganglia and contralateral basal ganglia were the same (0.1 ± 0.2 and 0.1 ± 0.1 U/g, respectively).

Fluoro-Jade can be effectively utilized to stain degenerating neuronal cells in the central nervous system of mammals. There were many Fluoro-Jade-positive cells in ipsilateral basal ganglia at day 1 and day 3 after 5-U thrombin injection. Only a few Fluoro-Jade-positive cells were detected in ipsilateral basal ganglia after saline injection (Fig. 2).

Thrombin caused a significant loss of brain tissue. At 28 days after thrombin injection, marked brain tissue loss occurred in ipsilateral basal ganglia (6.2 ± 1.4 mm^2 vs. 0.7 ± 0.4 mm^2 in saline control, $p < 0.01$). In addi-

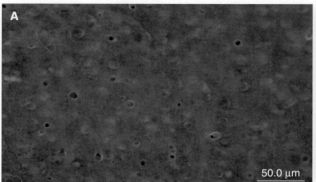
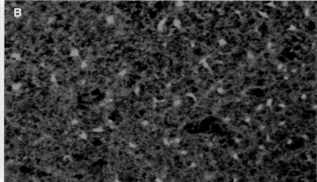

Fig. 2. Fluoro-Jade-positive cells in ipsilateral basal ganglia 24 h after injection of (A) saline or (B) 5 U thrombin. Scale bar = 50 µm

tion, lateral ventricle sizes were larger in thrombin-injected rats ($4.0 \pm 3.3 \, mm^2$ vs. $0.3 \pm 0.2 \, mm^2$ in saline control, $p < 0.05$).

Discussion

Our results show a significant increase in thrombin activity in the brain shortly after ICH. The concentration of prothrombin in plasma is high enough (1-$5 \, \mu M$) to produce a substantial amount of thrombin in brain parenchyma after hemorrhage. The brain as well as blood may be a site of thrombin production. In vitro studies have shown that prothrombin mRNA is expressed in the cells of the nervous system [1]. These results suggest that thrombin may be formed and cause brain injury, even if the blood–brain barrier is intact.

Thrombin is a serine protease and an essential component in the coagulation cascade. It is produced in the brain immediately after intracerebral hemorrhage, brain trauma, or blood–brain barrier breakdown following many kinds of brain injury [3]. Direct infusion of large doses of thrombin into brain causes inflammatory cell infiltration, mesenchymal cell proliferation, scar formation, brain edema formation, and seizures [9–13, 15, 20, 21]. Thrombin in high concentrations also kills neurons and astrocytes in vitro [7, 18, 19]. Our previous studies have demonstrated that thrombin is responsible for early brain edema formation following ICH [11].

Clinical and experimental data have shown that brain atrophy occurs after ICH [2, 5, 17, 23]. Our recent study showed that iron has a role in ICH-induced brain atrophy [6]. In the present study, we found that thrombin causes neuronal death and also can result in brain tissue loss.

It is very important to determine thrombin activity in the brain after ICH, because high concentrations of thrombin are detrimental and low concentrations of thrombin are protective. In addition, thrombin also contributes to brain recovery following ICH [25]. Our findings in this study indicate that thrombin is harmful in acute phase, at least the first 24 h, after ICH. The concentration of thrombin in ipsilateral basal ganglia 1 h after ICH was about $3.3 \, U/g$. Previously, we found that direct intracaudate injection of 5 U of thrombin causes marked brain damage, whereas 1 U is neuroprotective [22]. It should be noted, though, that the neurotoxicity of thrombin may be enhanced by the presence of other factors after an ICH, such as iron [14].

In summary, thrombin activity is increased in the brain after ICH, which results in neuronal death and brain tissue loss. The measured thrombin levels were 5-fold higher than we previously found in cerebral ischemia [4]. Limiting thrombin activation in the acute phase of ICH may reduce brain damage.

Acknowledgments

This study was supported by grants NS-017760, NS-039866, and NS-047245 from the National Institutes of Health (NIH), and 0755717Z and 0840016N from American Heart Association (AHA). The content is solely the responsibility of the authors and does not necessarily represent the official views of the NIH or AHA.

References

1. Dihanich M, Kaser M, Reinhard E, Cunningham D, Monard D (1991) Prothrombin mRNA is expressed by cells of the nervous system. Neuron 6: 575–581
2. Felberg RA, Grotta JC, Shirzadi AL, Strong R, Narayana P, Hill-Felberg SJ, Aronowski J (2002) Cell death in experimental intracerebral hemorrhage: the "black hole" model of hemorrhagic damage. Ann Neurol 51: 517–524
3. Gingrich MB, Traynelis SF (2000) Serine proteases and brain damage – is there a link? Trends Neurosci 23: 399–407
4. Hua Y, Wu J, Keep RF, Hoff JT, Xi G (2003) Thrombin exacerbates brain edema in focal cerebral ischemia. Acta Neurochir Suppl 86: 163–166
5. Hua Y, Wu J, Kitaoka T, Keep RF, Schallert T, Zhu W, Hoff JT, Xi G (2003) Iron overload, brain atrophy, calcification and long-term neurological deficits after experimental intracerebral hemorrhage. J Cereb Blood Flow Metab 23 (Suppl 1): 233 (Abstract)
6. Hua Y, Nakamura T, Keep RF, Wu J, Schallert T, Hoff JT, Xi G (2006) Long-term effects of experimental intracerebral hemorrhage: the role of iron. J Neurosurg 104: 305–312
7. Jiang Y, Wu J, Hua Y, Keep RF, Xiang J, Hoff JT, Xi G (2002) Thrombin-receptor activation and thrombin-induced brain tolerance. J Cereb Blood Flow Metab 22: 404–410
8. Kase CS, Caplan LR (1994) Intracerebral hemorrhage. Butterworth-Heinemann, Boston
9. Lee KR, Betz AL, Keep RF, Chenevert TL, Kim S, Hoff JT (1995) Intracerebral infusion of thrombin as a cause of brain edema. J Neurosurg 83: 1045–1050
10. Lee KR, Betz AL, Kim S, Keep RF, Hoff JT (1996) The role of the coagulation cascade in brain edema formation after intracerebral hemorrhage. Acta Neurochir (Wien) 138: 396–401
11. Lee KR, Colon GP, Betz AL, Keep RF, Kim S, Hoff JT (1996) Edema from intracerebral hemorrhage: the role of thrombin. J Neurosurg 84: 91–96
12. Lee KR, Drury I, Vitarbo E, Hoff JT (1997) Seizures induced by intracerebral injection of thrombin: a model of intracerebral hemorrhage. J Neurosurg 87: 73–78
13. Lee KR, Kawai N, Kim S, Sagher O, Hoff JT (1997) Mechanisms of edema formation after intracerebral hemorrhage: effects of thrombin on cerebral blood flow, blood–brain barrier permeability, and cell survival in a rat model. J Neurosurg 86: 272–278
14. Nakamura T, Xi G, Park JW, Hua Y, Hoff JT, Keep RF (2005) Holo-transferrin and thrombin can interact to cause brain damage. Stroke 36: 348–352
15. Nishino A, Suzuki M, Ohtani H, Motohashi O, Umezawa K, Nagura H, Yoshimoto T (1993) Thrombin may contribute to the pathophysiology of central nervous system injury. J Neurotrauma 10: 167–179
16. Schmued LC, Albertson C, Slikker W Jr (1997) Fluoro-Jade: a novel fluorochrome for the sensitive and reliable histochemical localization of neuronal degeneration. Brain Res 751: 37–46

17. Skriver EB, Olsen TS (1986) Tissue damage at computed tomography following resolution of intracerebral hematomas. Acta Radiol Diagn (Stockh) 27: 495–500

18. Striggow F, Riek M, Breder J, Henrich-Noack P, Reymann KG, Reiser G (2000) The protease thrombin is an endogenous mediator of hippocampal neuroprotection against ischemia at low concentrations but causes degeneration at high concentrations. Proc Natl Acad Sci USA 97: 2264–2269

19. Vaughan PJ, Pike CJ, Cotman CW, Cunningham DD (1995) Thrombin receptor activation protects neurons and astrocytes from cell death produced by environmental insults. J Neurosci 15: 5389–5401

20. Xi G, Keep RF, Hoff JT (1998) Erythrocytes and delayed brain edema formation following intracerebral hemorrhage in rats. J Neurosurg 89: 991–996

21. Xi G, Wagner KR, Keep RF, Hua Y, de Courten-Myers GM, Broderick JP, Brott TG, Hoff JT (1998) The role of blood clot formation on early edema development after experimental intracerebral hemorrhage. Stroke 29: 2580–2586

22. Xi G, Reiser G, Keep RF (2003) The role of thrombin and thrombin receptors in ischemic, hemorrhagic and traumatic brain injury: deleterious or protective? J Neurochem 84: 3–9

23. Xi G, Fewel ME, Hua Y, Thompson BG Jr, Hoff JT, Keep RF (2004) Intracerebral hemorrhage: pathophysiology and therapy. Neurocrit Care 1: 5–18

24. Xi G, Keep RF, Hoff JT (2006) Mechanisms of brain injury after intracerebral hemorrhage. Lancet Neurol 5: 53–63

25. Yang S, Song S, Hua Y, Nakamura T, Keep RF, Xi G (2008) Effects of thrombin on neurogenesis after intracerebral hemorrhage. Stroke (in press)

Acta Neurochir Suppl (2008) 105: 51–53
© Springer-Verlag 2008
Printed in Austria

Microglial activation and intracerebral hemorrhage

Z. Gao[1], J. Wang[1], R. Thiex[1], A. D. Rogove[1], F. L. Heppner[2], S. E. Tsirka[1]

[1] Department of Pharmacological Sciences, Stony Brook University, Stony Brook, New York, USA
[2] Institute of Neuropathology, Charité – Universitätsmedizin Berlin, Berlin, Germany

Summary

Introduction. Microglia activate upon injury, migrate to the injury site, proliferate locally, undergo morphological and gene expression changes, and phagocytose injured and dying cells. Cytokines and proteases secreted by these cells contribute to the injury and edema formed. We studied the injury outcome after local elimination/paralysis of microglia.

Methods. Adult male mice were subjected to intracerebral hemorrhage (ICH) by intra-caudate injection of either collagenase or autologous blood. Mice survived for different periods of time, and were subsequently evaluated for neurological deficits, size of the hematoma, and microglia activation. Mice expressing an fms-GFP transgene or the CD11b-HSVTK transgene were also used. For elimination of monocytes/macrophages, CD11b-HSVTK mice were treated with ganciclovir prior to hemorrhage. Modifiers of microglial activation were also used.

Results. Induction of ICH resulted in robust microglia activation and recruitment of macrophages. Inactivation of these cells, genetically or pharmacologically, pointed to a critical role of the time of such inactivation, indicating that their role is distinct at different time points following injury. Edema formation is decreased when microglia activation is inhibited, and neurological outcomes are improved.

Conclusions. Microglia, as immunomodulatory cells, have the ability to modify the final presentation of ICH.

Keywords: Microglia; intracerebral hemorrhage; edema; tissue plasminogen activator.

Introduction

Intracerebral hemorrhage (ICH) comprises 15 to 20% of all strokes that take place annually in the United States, and occurs when a small artery or an arteriole ruptures spontaneously in the brain. During ICH, a series of cellular events take place. As blood extravasated from arteries accumulates in the brain, it exerts pressure on surrounding tissue and triggers formation of edema

Correspondence: Stella E. Tsirka, Ph.D., Department of Pharmacological Sciences, Stony Brook University, Stony Brook, NY 11794-8651, USA. e-mail: stella@pharm.stonybrook.edu

and reactivity of the neighboring cells. Among the events that follow an ICH, activation of immune-competent microglia cells is a key process [11]. The assumed function of microglia in this context is that they migrate to the site of hemorrhage where they secrete cytokines, proteases, and other factors. Activated microglia are also able to phagocytose neuronal and cellular debris. The accumulation of activated microglia is thought to contribute to the neuronal death observed in several acute adverse settings (e.g., stroke, infection) and in chronic neurodegenerative pathologies (e.g., Alzheimer's disease, amyotrophic lateral sclerosis, multiple sclerosis) [6, 7].

Although awareness of the presence and functions of microglia is rapidly increasing, the roles attributed to these cells and their contributions to injury remain controversial. Some reports indicate a direct or indirect neurotoxic role for microglia in different injury settings, whereas others emphasize their ability to act as antigen-presenting cells and thus contain and minimize infections in the CNS. Moreover, the fact that they can also secrete anti-inflammatory cytokines points to neuroprotective properties [3, 4].

Many reports exist in the literature targeting the presence and reactivity of inflammatory cells in the brain, primarily microglia but also infiltrating leukocytes. That approach seemed beneficial, as it improved neurological score of animals and decreased hemorrhage volume [11]. Anti-inflammatory agents, such as minocycline, neutralize cytokine antibodies and scavengers of reactive oxygen species, and have shown to be beneficial in animal models of ICH (little information is available for human samples). An effective, rational approach to treating small-volume ICH is to remove the hematoma that has formed [9]. The removal is accomplished with infusion of tissue plasminogen activator (tPA), a secreted serine protease that catalyzes the formation of plasmin, another serine protease with a broad specificity towards several extracellular matrix proteins and specifically fibrin [2, 8]. Such approach has, however, been shown to result in the generation of edema, which compromises treatment outcome [10]. Extensive microglia activation and blood cell infiltration accompanies tPA-mediated liquefaction of the hematoma.

In this report, we summarize the work we have performed in an effort to characterize the relationship between inflammation (microglia) and outcome of ICH in a mouse model of collagenase-induced ICH.

Materials and methods

Induction of intracerebral hemorrhage

We used the collagenase injection model to induce hemorrhage, as previously described [12–14]. Briefly, mice were anesthetized with Avertin, and 0.075 units of bacterial collagenase were injected stereotactically (1.0 mm posterior and 3.0 mm lateral of bregma, 4.0 mm in depth) unilaterally into the caudate putamen of adult mice. At different time points after collagenase injection, the mice were euthanized and their brains were analyzed histologically using cresyl violet/Luxol fast blue histological stain to determine neuronal survival, hemorrhage volume, and edema formation.

Immunohistochemistry

Microglia were visualized using Iba-1 and F4/80, markers that recognize surface antigens on cells of monocytic origin (monocytes/macrophages/microglia). Astrocytes were visualized using an antibody to glial fibrillary acidic protein.

Intracerebral infusion

The mice were anesthetized as described above and a micro-osmotic pump (Durect Corp., Cupertino, CA) containing normal saline (control animals) or the infusion compound (macrophage/microglial inhibitory factor [MIF] or ganciclovir [GCV]) was inserted subcutaneously through a midline incision toward the back of the animal. A brain infusion cannula connected to the pump was positioned at coordinates mentioned above. The pump was secured in place on the skull with dental cement. The infusion rate was 0.5 µL/h. After installing the pump, the midline incision was closed with sutures. The pump was allowed to infuse the designated solution for 2 days, and then collagenase was injected as described above. The mice are sacrificed at various time points, and their brains were examined for neuronal survival, hemorrhage volume, edema formation, and microglial activation.

Neurological deficit

MIF- or GCV-treated and control mice were scored blindly for neurological deficits using a 28-point neurological scoring system on day 1 after ICH. The tests included body symmetry, gait, climbing, circling behavior, front limb symmetry, compulsory circling, and whisker response. Each point graded from 0 to 4. Maximum deficit score was 28 [1].

Results and discussion

We used 2 models for inhibition of microglia activation. In the first method, we infused the tripeptide MIF into the brain at the same midline and dorsoventral coordinates as the collagenase injection [13, 14]. The infusion was started either before (one day prior) or 2 h after collagenase injection and continued for 24 or 72 h. In both cases, the presence of MIF attenuated the ICH injury volume and improved neurological outcome in the animals. It also reduced the extent of edema formed and the numbers of immune cells (resident or infiltrating). Neuronal death decreased and so did the oxidative state of the tissue. Overall, the use of MIF was beneficial to the animals.

The monocytic/inflammatory reaction was attenuated in a second model of ICH: we subjected the CD11b-HSVTK transgenic animals to collagenase-induced ICH [5]. These are animals that express thymidine kinase (TK) of herpes simplex virus (HSV) under the control of the CD11b promoter. Since CD11b-HSVTK is expressed in cells of monocytic origin, all microglia, monocytes, and macrophages express the transgene. When these animals are treated with GCV, the HSVTK protein is inhibited and the cells that express TK are eliminated, as they are unable to replicate further. Therefore, the GCV-treated CD11b-HSVTK gene can practically be devoid of microglia/monocytes/macrophages. We delivered GCV locally into the brain parenchyma, induced ICH, and evaluated the extent of injury and microglial activation at several time points. We found that, although at early time points the extent of ICH was similar, the injury volume was smaller in GCV-treated animals. Moreover, hematoma was eliminated faster in GCV-treated animals compared to control mice.

Although our results are still preliminary, they indicate that microglia and their activation status can modulate the severity and clearance of ICH. Activation of microglia can exacerbate ICH outcome both at early and later time points. It is possible that proinflammatory cytokines, secreted by activated microglia, affect ICH outcome. Therefore, one can imagine that an effective ICH treatment approach may result from combinations of previous methods, namely, the seemingly indispensable liquefaction of hematoma, aspiration of the majority of the liquefied blood volume, and immediate delivery of scavenger of reactive oxygen species or a microglia activation inhibitor. Such combinatorial treatment may allow for decreasing pressure of the ICH on surrounding tissue, while neutralizing the action of tPA on microglia and other inflammatory, blood-derived cells.

References

1. Clark WM, Lessov NS, Dixon MP, Eckenstein F (1997) Monofilament intraluminal middle cerebral artery occlusion in the mouse. Neurol Res 19: 641–648

2. Gravanis I, Tsirka SE (2008) Tissue-type plasminogen activator as a therapeutic target in stroke. Expert Opin Ther Targets 12: 159–170

3. Hailer NP (2008) Immunosuppression after traumatic or ischemic CNS damage: it is neuroprotective and illuminates the role of microglial cells. Prog Neurobiol 84: 211–233

4. Hanisch UK, Kettenmann H (2007) Microglia: active sensor and versatile effector cells in the normal and pathologic brain. Nat Neurosci 10: 1387–1394

5. Heppner FL, Greter M, Marino D, Falsig J, Raivich G, Hövelmeyer N, Waisman A, Rülicke T, Prinz M, Priller J, Becher B, Aguzzi A (2005) Experimental autoimmune encephalomyelitis repressed by microglial paralysis. Nat Med 11: 146–152

6. Kreutzberg GW (1995) Microglia, the first line of defense in brain pathologies. Arzneimittelforschung 45: 357–360

7. Kreutzberg GW (1996) Microglia: a sensor for pathological events in the CNS. Trends Neurosci 19: 312–318

8. Sheehan JJ, Tsirka SE (2005) Fibrin-modifying serine proteases thrombin, tPA, and plasmin in ischemic stroke: a review. Glia 50: 340–350

9. Thiex R, Küker W, Müller HD, Rohde I, Schröder JM, Gilsbach JM, Rohde V (2003) The long-term effect of recombinant tissue-plasminogen-activator (rt-PA) on edema formation in a large-animal model of intracerebral hemorrhage. Neurol Res 25: 254–262

10. Thiex R, Mayfrank L, Rohde V, Gilsbach JM, Tsirka SA (2004) The role of endogenous versus exogenous tPA on edema formation in murine ICH. Exp Neurol 189: 25–32

11. Wang J, Doré S (2007) Inflammation after intracerebral hemorrhage. J Cereb Blood Flow Metab 27: 894–908

12. Wang J, Tsirka SE (2005) Neuroprotection by inhibition of matrix metalloproteinases in a mouse model of intracerebral haemorrhage. Brain 128: 1622–1633

13. Wang J, Tsirka SE (2005) Tuftsin fragment 1–3 is beneficial when delivered after the induction of intracerebral hemorrhage. Stroke 36: 613–618

14. Wang J, Rogove AD, Tsirka AE, Tsirka SE (2003) Protective role of tuftsin fragment 1–3 in an animal model of intracerebral hemorrhage. Ann Neurol 54: 655–664

Acta Neurochir Suppl (2008) 105: 55–58
© Springer-Verlag 2008
Printed in Austria

Concomitant intracerebral infusion of tissue plasminogen activator and thrombin leads to brain injury

T. O'Lynnger, Y. He, H. Hu, Y. Hua, K. M. Muraszko, G. Xi

Department of Neurosurgery, University of Michigan Medical School, Ann Arbor, MI, USA

Summary

Low doses of thrombin are neuroprotective while high doses are neurotoxic and lead to brain injury. However, evidence suggests that low doses of thrombin cause brain injury when infused concomitantly with tissue plasminogen activator (tPA), which is used clinically to facilitate evacuation of intracerebral hematomas. In this study, we examined the effects of intracerebral infusion of tPA and thrombin, individually and in combination.

Rats were infused in the right basal ganglia with 50 µL saline solutions containing thrombin, tPA, or thrombin + tPA. In the first experiment, rats were used for blood–brain barrier (BBB) permeability measurements at 24 h after infusion. In the second experiment, animals were euthanized 3 days after infusion, and brain sections were stained with Fluoro-Jade to measure neuronal cell death. Behavioral tests were carried out before and after surgery.

Infusion of thrombin + tPA markedly increased Evans blue tissue content in ipsilateral brain samples ($p < 0.05$). Fluoro-Jade-stained sections from thrombin + tPA group demonstrated significantly higher cell death counts ($p < 0.01$). Significant neurological deficit was revealed in thrombin + tPA group in forelimb-placing and corner-turn tests ($p < 0.01$).

This study shows that tPA potentiates the neurotoxic effects of thrombin and leads to increased BBB permeability, neuronal cell death, and neurological deficit. Our results suggest that using tPA to lyse intracerebral hematomas has potential to produce neuronal cell death and disruption of BBB.

Keywords: Blood–brain barrier permeability; tissue plasminogen activator; thrombin.

Introduction

Tissue plasminogen activator (tPA) has been used to lyse intracerebral hematomas to facilitate their removal [9, 16]. Its function is to activate the fibrinolytic substance, plasmin, which breaks down blood clots. Thrombin is a

serine protease that is responsible for forming blood clots. While it has been shown that thrombin at low doses is neuroprotective [13, 15], it has also been demonstrated that thrombin causes brain injury at sufficiently high doses and contributes to brain injury after intracerebral hemorrhage (ICH) [5, 12]. However, evidence suggests that low doses of thrombin cause brain injury when infused concomitantly with tPA [1].

This is significant because the use of tPA to lyse intracerebral hematomas in humans could cause increased blood–brain barrier (BBB) permeability and neuronal injury, further exacerbating the brain injury caused by ICH. This particularly applies to the stereotactic injection of tPA directly into the coagulum, which is used in certain neurosurgical procedures in humans [4]. In this study, we examined the effects of intracerebral infusion of tPA and thrombin, individually and in combination. We hypothesized that tPA potentiates BBB disruption, cell death, and neurological deficit induced by thrombin.

Materials and methods

Animal preparation and intracerebral infusion

Animal protocols were approved by the University of Michigan Committee on the Use and Care of Animals. Male Sprague-Dawley rats (Charles River Laboratories, Portage, MI), each weighing 250–300 g, were used for all experiments. Animals were allowed free access to food and water before and after surgery. Rats anesthetized with pentobarbital (50 mg/kg, i.p.) were placed in a stereotactic frame, and the scalp was incised along the sagittal midline using a sterile technique. A 1-mm cranial burr-hole was drilled on the right coronal suture 4.0 mm lateral to the bregma. A 26-gauge needle was inserted into the right caudate with stereotactic guidance (coordinates: 0.1 mm anterior, 5.5 mm ventral, and 4.0 mm lateral to bregma). Animals were divided into 3 groups, and each group was infused with either 1 U thrombin, 2 µg tPA, or 1 U thrombin + 2 µg tPA dissolved in 50 µL saline. Solutions were infused into the brain at a rate of 10 µL/min using an infusion pump (Harvard

Correspondence: Guohua Xi, MD, Department of Neurosurgery, University of Michigan Medical School, R5018 Biomedical Science Research Building, 109 Zina Pitcher Place, Ann Arbor, MI 48109-2200, USA. e-mail: guohuaxi@umich.edu

Apparatus Inc., Holliston, MA), and after infusion the needle was left in place for 2 min. The needle was then withdrawn, the burr-hole filled with bone wax, and the scalp incision closed with 2–3 sutures [1, 2]. The rats were sacrificed either 24 or 72 h after intracerebral infusion so that measurements of BBB permeability or cell death, respectively, could be made [2, 10, 11, 14].

In animals with a 72-h recovery period, behavioral testing was carried out the day before surgery and the day of sacrifice to measure any neurological deficit present [3].

Measurement of BBB permeability

BBB permeability was investigated by measuring the extravasation of Evans blue in each of the 3 groups ($n = 6$ each) [6]. Evans blue dye (2% in saline, 4 mL/kg) was injected intravenously 24 h after intracerebral infusion. Two hours after Evans blue injection, the chest wall was opened under lethal anesthesia and the animals were perfused with 0.1 mol/L phosphate-buffered saline (PBS) through the left ventricle until colorless perfusion fluid was obtained from the right atrium. After decapitation, the brain was removed and dissected into left and right hemispheres, which were then weighed. Brain samples were placed in 3 mL 50% trichloroacetic acid solution, and then homogenized and centrifuged (4000 rpm for 60 min). The supernatant was measured at 610 nm for absorbance using a spectrophotometer (Ultrospec 3; Pharmacia LKB Biotechnology, Uppsala, Sweden). The tissue content of Evans blue was quantified from a linear standard curve and was expressed as micrograms per gram of brain tissue.

Measurement of cell death

To measure cell death, brain sections were prepared according to standard protocols for histopathological study [6]. The same 3 groups were once again established ($n = 4$ each), and 3 days after intracerebral infusion, animals were perfused intracardially under lethal anesthesia with 4% paraformaldehyde in 0.1 mol/L PBS (pH 7.4). Brains were placed in 4% paraformaldehyde overnight and then immersed in 30% sucrose for 3 days and stored at 4 °C. The brains were embedded in a mixture of 30% sucrose and optimal cutting temperature compound, and 18-μm-thick coronal frozen sections were made on a cryostat. For each group, 2 slices of the basal ganglia were taken from each brain. The slices were analyzed using the Fluoro-Jade staining technique described by Schmued et al. [8]. Briefly, tissue sections were immersed in 100% alcohol for 3 min, 70% alcohol for 1 min, then deionized H$_2$O for 1 min before being stained with 0.06% potassium permanganate for 15 min. After washing again in deionized water for 1 min, tissue sections were immersed in 0.001% Fluoro-Jade staining solution for 30 min, and then washed 3 times in deionized water for 1 min each time. After drying under a fan for 30 min, sections were placed into 100% xylene for 6 min and then given a coverslip with DPX. This technique is useful for detecting neuronal cell death because it causes dead neurons to fluoresce bright green while leaving healthy neurons and glial cells unstained. Using a camera mounted to a fluorescent microscope, 3 pictures of different areas in the basal ganglia were taken at 400× for each slide and cell counts were made. Fluorescing dead neurons in the area of the basal ganglia were photographed if present; otherwise, pictures were taken in unstained regions throughout the basal ganglia. For each brain slice, the mean number of degenerating neurons was calculated by adding up the number of fluorescing cells in all 3 pictures and then taking the average.

Measurement of neurological deficit

Forelimb-placing test, forelimb-use asymmetry test, and corner-turn test were preformed in order to assess neurological deficit, as described in our previous studies [3]. For the behavioral tests, all animal behavior was

tested the day before surgery and 3 days after surgery, and scored by experimenters blind to both neurological and treatment conditions. Three groups were established ($n = 8$ each) based on infusion of thrombin, tPA, or thrombin + tPA, as described previously.

Statistical analysis

All data were reported as mean ± SD. Student t-test was used to analyze data for statistical significance. Values of $p < 0.05$ were considered significant.

Results

BBB permeability

Two hours after intravenous injection of Evans blue, the thrombin + tPA group showed a significant increase in Evans blue content of the ipsilateral hemisphere as compared with the thrombin and tPA groups, demonstrating disruption of the BBB and increased permeability (4.9 ± 2.0 vs 2.5 ± 0.7 with thrombin, and $2.4 \pm 0.8\,\mu g/g$ with tPA, $p < 0.05$; Fig. 1). There was no significant difference in the amount of extravasated Evans blue in the contralateral hemisphere among any of the 3 groups. The net Evans blue content, which was calculated by taking the difference between the ipsilateral and contralateral measurements, was substantially higher in the thrombin + tPA group as compared with the other 2 groups (2.9 ± 1.7 vs 1.2 ± 0.6 with thrombin, $p = 0.06$, and $1.0 \pm 0.3\,\mu g/g$ with tPA, $p < 0.05$; Fig. 1). While the net Evans blue content in the thrombin + tPA group was not significantly greater than the thrombin group statistically, this may be due to inadequate perfusion resulting in the presence of excess dye liquid in the contralateral hemisphere. Nevertheless, there was still a marked in-

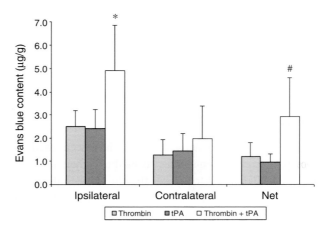

Fig. 1. Evans blue content in the brain 24 h after intracerebral injection of thrombin, tPA, and thrombin + tPA. Values are mean ± SD, $n = 6$. *$p < 0.05$ vs thrombin and tPA; #$p = 0.06$ vs thrombin and $p < 0.05$ vs tPA

crease in net Evans blue extravasation that almost met the requirements for statistical significance.

Cell death

The Fluoro-Jade stain revealed a marked increase in the mean number of dead neurons per section in the thrombin + tPA group as compared with the other groups that received infusions of either thrombin or tPA alone (39.5 ± 26.8 vs 1.1 ± 2.1 with thrombin and 2.5 ± 5.2 with tPA, $p < 0.01$; Fig. 2). A sharp contrast can be seen in the number of bright green cells in each image between the first 2 groups and the thrombin + tPA group as few, if any, neurons fluoresce in the thrombin and tPA groups, while the entire field of view is filled with stained, degenerating neurons in the thrombin + tPA group.

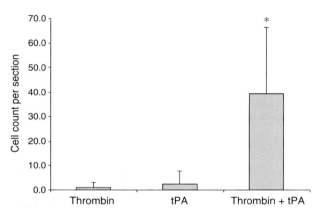

Fig. 2. Dead neuronal cell count on Fluoro-Jade-stained brain sections. Values are mean $\pm$ SD, $n = 4$. $^{*}p < 0.01$ vs thrombin and tPA

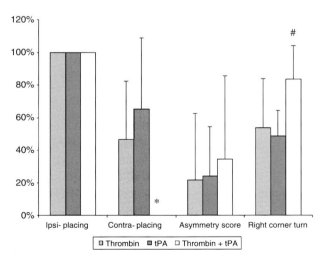

Fig. 3. Results of postoperative behavioral tests after 3 days of recovery. Values are mean $\pm$ SD, $n = 8$. $^{*}p < 0.01$ vs thrombin and tPA; $^{\#}p < 0.05$ vs thrombin and $p < 0.01$ vs tPA

Neurological deficit

As compared with the thrombin and tPA groups, there was a significantly greater deficit in the thrombin + tPA group in both the contralateral forelimb-placing test ($0.0 \pm 0.0\%$ vs $46.3 \pm 36.2\%$ with thrombin and $65.0 \pm 43.8\%$ with tPA, $p < 0.01$; Fig. 3) and the right corner-turn test ($83.8 \pm 20.7\%$ vs $53.8 \pm 30.2\%$ with thrombin, $p < 0.04$, and $48.8 \pm 15.5\%$ with tPA, $p < 0.01$; Fig. 3). None of the animals in the thrombin + tPA group was able to respond to contralateral vibrissae contact, indicating neurological injury in the ipsilateral side. Similarly, this group exhibited a significantly higher percentage of right corner turns, which further evidences the neurological damage to the ipsilateral side. While the mean asymmetry score was higher for the thrombin + tPA group as compared with the other 2 groups, the large variation led to a difference that was not significant.

Discussion

The results of this study suggest that administering tPA with a low dose of thrombin potentiates the neurotoxic effects induced by thrombin, resulting in increased BBB permeability, neuronal cell death, and neurological deficit. While tPA and low doses of thrombin do not result in significant disruption of the BBB or neuronal cell death when administered separately, when given in combination they produce a marked increase in BBB permeability and neuronal injury, in addition to a neurological deficit.

It has been shown that thrombin in high doses kills neurons and astrocytes *in vitro* [16]. As evidenced in this study, a low dose of thrombin can become equally deleterious after potentiation with tPA. Disruption in the BBB may be due to the death of astrocytes and other glial cells in the brain rather than the death of neurons, as the linkage between neuronal cell death and increased BBB permeability is unclear. The neurological deficit may be associated with the death of both glial cells and neurons in the basal ganglia.

Our results suggest that using tPA to lyse intracerebral hematomas has the potential to produce neuronal cell death and disruption of the BBB. The clinical usage of tPA to treat ICH is widespread. Certain neurosurgical protocols call for direct stereotactic puncture of the intracerebral hematoma and injection of tPA [7], and a parallel can be drawn between this direct infusion into the coagulum and the procedures used in this study. Thus, further research into the clinical usage of tPA to lyse intracerebral hematomas is warranted in order to investigate the potentially neurotoxic effects that tPA may have on the brain.

Acknowledgments

This study was supported by grants NS-017760, NS-39866, NS-047245, and NS-052510 from the National Institutes of Health, and Grant-in-Aid 075571Z from American Heart Association.

References

1. Figueroa BE, Keep RF, Betz AL, Hoff JT (1998) Plasminogen activators potentiate thrombin-induced brain injury. Stroke 29: 1202–1208
2. Gong C, Boulis N, Qian J, Turner DE, Hoff JT, Keep RF (2001) Intracerebral hemorrhage-induced neuronal death. Neurosurgery 48: 875–883
3. Hua Y, Schallert T, Keep RF, Wu J, Hoff JT, Xi G (2002) Behavioral tests after intracerebral hemorrhage in the rat. Stroke 33: 2478–2484
4. Kaufman HH (1993) Treatment of deep spontaneous intracerebral hematomas: a review. Stroke 24: I101–I108
5. Lee KR, Colon GP, Betz AL, Keep RF, Kim S, Hoff JT (1996) Edema from intracerebral hemorrhage: the role of thrombin. J Neurosurg 84: 91–96
6. Qin Z, Karabiyikoglu M, Hua Y, Silbergleit R, He Y, Keep RF, Xi G (2007) Hyperbaric oxygen-induced attenuation of hemorrhagic transformation after experimental focal transient cerebral ischemia. Stroke 38: 1362–1367
7. Schaller C, Rohde V, Meyer B, Hassler W (1995) Stereotactic puncture and lysis of spontaneous intracerebral hemorrhage using recombinant tissue-plasminogen activator. Neurosurgery 36: 328–335
8. Schmued LC, Albertson C, Slikker W Jr (1997) Fluoro-Jade: a novel fluorochrome for the sensitive and reliable histochemical localization of neuronal degeneration. Brain Res 751: 37–46
9. Wagner KR, Xi G, Hua Y, Zuccarello M, de Courten-Myers GM, Broderick JP, Brott TG (1999) Ultra-early clot aspiration after lysis with tissue plasminogen activator in a porcine model of intracerebral hemorrhage: edema reduction and blood–brain barrier protection. J Neurosurg 90: 491–498
10. Wu J, Hua Y, Keep RF, Schallert T, Hoff JT, Xi G (2002) Oxidative brain injury from extravasated erythrocytes after intracerebral hemorrhage. Brain Res 953: 45–52
11. Xi G, Keep RF, Hoff JT (1998) Erythrocytes and delayed brain edema formation following intracerebral hemorrhage in rats. J Neurosurg 89: 991–996
12. Xi G, Wagner KR, Keep RF, Hua Y, de Courten-Myers GM, Broderick JP, Brott TG, Hoff JT (1998) Role of blood clot formation on early edema development after experimental intracerebral hemorrhage. Stroke 29: 2580–2586
13. Xi G, Keep RF, Hua Y, Xiang J, Hoff JT (1999) Attenuation of thrombin-induced brain edema by cerebral thrombin preconditioning. Stroke 30: 1247–1255
14. Xi G, Hua Y, Bhasin RR, Ennis SR, Keep RF, Hoff JT (2001) Mechanisms of edema formation after intracerebral hemorrhage: effects of extravasated red blood cells on blood flow and blood–brain barrier integrity. Stroke 32: 2932–2938
15. Xi G, Reiser G, Keep RF (2003) The role of thrombin and thrombin receptors in ischemic, hemorrhagic and traumatic brain injury: deleterious or protective? J Neurochem 84: 3–9
16. Xi G, Keep RF, Hoff J (2006) Mechanisms of brain injury after intracerebral hemorrhage. Lancet Neurol 5: 53–63

Acta Neurochir Suppl (2008) 105: 59–65
© Springer-Verlag 2008
Printed in Austria

Microglial activation and brain injury after intracerebral hemorrhage

J. Wu[1,2], **S. Yang**[1,2], **G. Xi**[2], **S. Song**[1,2], **G. Fu**[1], **R. F. Keep**[2], **Y. Hua**[2]

[1] Medical School, Zhejiang University, Hangzhou, China
[2] Department of Neurosurgery, University of Michigan Medical School, Ann Arbor, MI, USA

Summary

Microglial activation and thrombin formation contribute to brain injury after intracerebral hemorrhage (ICH). Tumor necrosis factor-alpha (TNF-α) and interleukin-1 beta (IL-1β) are 2 major proinflammatory cytokines. In this study, we investigated whether thrombin stimulates TNF-α and IL-1β secretion in vitro, and whether microglial inhibition reduces ICH-induced brain injury in vivo.

There were 2 parts to this study. In the first part, cultured rat microglial cells were treated with vehicle, thrombin (5 and 10 U/mL), or thrombin plus tuftsin (0.05 µg/mL), an inhibitor of microglia activation. Levels of TNF-α and IL-1β in culture medium were measured by ELISA at 4, 8, and 24 h after thrombin treatment. In the second part of the study, rats received an intracerebral infusion of 100 µL autologous whole blood with or without 25 µg of tuftsin 1–3 fragment. Rats were killed at day 1 or day 3 for immunohistochemistry and brain water content measurement.

We found that thrombin receptors were expressed in cultured microglia cells, and TNF-α and IL-1β levels in the culture medium were increased after thrombin treatment. Tuftsin reduced thrombin-induced upregulation of TNF-α and IL-1β. In vivo, microglia were activated after ICH, and intracerebral injection of tuftsin reduced brain edema in the ipsilateral basal ganglia (81.1 ± 0.7% vs. 82.7 ± 1.3% in vehicle-treated group; $p < 0.05$) after ICH.

These results suggest a critical role of microglia activation in ICH-related brain injury.

Keywords: Cerebral hemorrhage; interleukin-1β; microglia; thrombin; tumor necrosis factor-α.

Introduction

Microglia are cells within the brain that are activated in response to injury. Depending upon specific conditions, they can have neurotrophic or neurotoxic actions [24]. In normal brain, microglia are in a quiescent state, but in the event of injury they become highly phagocytic and are involved in clearing debris from the damaged site [24]. Activated microglia are associated with ischemic and hemorrhagic brain injury including intracerebral hemorrhage (ICH), and there is evidence that microglia contribute to ICH-induced brain damage [9, 36, 37]. The activation of microglia that occurs after ICH is marked by changes in cellular morphology, size, and number.

Thrombin is a serine protease and an essential component in the coagulation cascade. It is produced immediately in the brain after ICH. Thrombin in high concentrations kills neurons and astrocytes in vitro [13, 25, 28], and we have demonstrated that thrombin is responsible for early brain damage following ICH in vivo [10, 15, 31, 32].

Some of the normal cellular effects of thrombin are receptor mediated. Three protease-activated receptors (PARs), PAR-1, PAR-3, and PAR-4, are thrombin receptors [2–4]. Expression of thrombin receptor mRNA is found in neurons and astrocytes [20, 30]. Recent studies indicate that PARs mediate some of the pathological effects of thrombin and are involved in central nervous system pathophysiology [21, 35]. Thrombin can activate microglia, and activated microglia release proinflammatory cytokines such as tumor necrosis factor-alpha (TNF-α) and interleukin-1 beta (IL-1β), which are harmful to the brain [19]. It has been reported that a tripeptide tuftsin fragment 1–3, Thr-Lys-Pro, also called macrophage/microglial inhibitory factor [1], significantly reduces brain injury and improves functional outcomes in an ICH model in mice [29].

In this study, we examined whether or not thrombin can stimulate TNF-α and IL-1β secretion in cultured microglial cells and whether or not microglial inhibition with tuftsin fragment 1–3 can reduce perihematomal edema in rats.

Correspondence: Ya Hua, M.D., Department of Neurosurgery, University of Michigan Medical School, 109 Zina Pitcher Place, R5018 Biomedical Science Research Building, Ann Arbor, MI 48109-2200, USA. e-mail: yahua@umich.edu

Materials and methods

Experiments in vitro

Microglia culture

Cultures of microglia were established based on the differential adherence of cells harvested from neonatal (day 1–3) Sprague-Dawley rat cortex. The methods used were a modification of those used by McCarthy and deVellis [18]. Mixed cell cultures were initially established in T75 Falcon flasks. Cerebra were dissected and placed in a medium for astrocytes (DMEM plus 10% FBS, 1% glutamine and 2% Antibiotic-Antimycotic; GIBCO, Carlsbad, CA). Meninges and blood vessels were removed. The medium was then removed and cerebra were minced with a blade. Tissues were suspended in modified Hanks' Balanced Salt Solution (HBSS) (500 mL HBSS + 25 mM HEPES + 5 mL Antibiotic-Antimycotic; GIBCO). After centrifugation, the cell pellet was digested in 0.5% trypsin at 37 °C for 20 min, then re-suspended in Buffer T (23.5 mL modified HBSS + 200 U DNase I [Invitrogen, Carlsbad, CA] + 0.5 mL 3.8% MgSO$_4$ [Sigma-Aldrich Co., St. Louis, MO]). The cells were then re-centrifuged and re-suspended in astrocyte medium and HBSS (1:1 ratio). After centrifugation, the pellet was re-suspended in astrocyte medium, and the cells plated into T75 Falcon flasks coated with poly-L-lysine at a density of 1×10^6/mL. The cells were cultured at 37 °C in an atmosphere of 5% CO$_2$ in air. The medium was changed after 3–4 days. After 7–10 days, the flask was shaken at 200 rpm for 1 h on a gyratory shaker at 4 °C. The supernatant cells were plated on uncoated T25 flasks and incubated for 30 min at 37 °C. The cells were then washed with Tris-buffered saline containing 1 nM EDTA (Sigma-Aldrich Co.) and the supernatant discarded. The remaining microglia cells were fed with microglia culture medium (10% FBS, 2% AA, 1% glutamine and M-CSF 10 ng/mL [Sigma-Aldrich Co.] in DMEM). The purity of the cultured microglial cells was confirmed by OX-42 staining.

Experimental groups

There were 2 groups of experiments. In the first, cultured microglia were collected for immunocytochemistry. In the second, microglia were treated with different doses of human thrombin (5 and 10 U/mL; Sigma-Aldrich Co.) or thrombin (10 U/mL) ± tuftsin (0.05 µg/mL; Sigma-Aldrich Co.). Culture medium was collected for IL-1β and TNF-α measurements.

Immunocytochemistry

Microglia were seeded on 8-chamber glass slides at a density of 1×10^4/well. Five days later, cultures were washed with phosphate-buffered saline (PBS), fixed with 4% paraformaldehyde for 20 min followed by washing with PBS. Slides were incubated overnight at 4 °C with the primary antibodies for either mouse anti-rat OX-42 (Serotec Inc., Raleigh, NC), rabbit anti-human PAR-1, rabbit anti-human PAR-3, or goat anti-mouse PAR-4 (Santa Cruz Biotechnology Inc., Santa Cruz, CA) at a concentration of 1:400. They were then incubated with avidin-biotinylated horseradish peroxidase (Vector Laboratories, Burlingame, CA) second antibodies and diamino-benzidine hydrogen peroxide (Stable DAB; Research Genetics Inc., Huntsville, AL) for 90 min each at room temperature. After dehydration, sections were cover-slipped for microphotography. Normal IgG (from the same species as the primary antibody) or omission of the primary antibody was used as a negative control.

Measurements of IL-1β and TNF-α

Cells were seeded at a density of 1×10^5 in 24-well plates. After 24 h in growth media, the cells were cultured in serum-free media for 18 h prior to treatment with thrombin at doses of 0, 5, and 10 U/mL. Microglia-conditioned medium from each well was collected at 4, 8, and 24 h, and the concentrations of IL-1β and TNF-α were quantified by ELISA (R & D Systems, Inc., Minneapolis, MN). The final IL-1β and TNF-α concentration from each well was standardized by protein concentration.

Experiments in vivo

Animal preparation and intracerebral injection

The University of Michigan Committee on the Use and Care of Animals approved the protocols for these animal studies, which used male Sprague-Dawley rats aged 3 to 4 months (Charles River Laboratories, Wilmington, MA). Septic precautions were used for all surgical procedures, and body temperature was maintained at 37.5 °C using a feedback-controlled heating pad. Rats were anesthetized with pentobarbital (50 mg/kg, i.p.) and the right femoral artery was catheterized for continuous blood pressure monitoring and blood sampling. Blood from the catheter was used to determine pH, PaO$_2$, PaCO$_2$, hematocrit, and glucose. It was also the source for the intracerebral blood infusion. The animals were positioned in a stereotactic frame (David Kopf Instruments, Tujunga, CA). Blood or thrombin was injected into the right caudate nucleus through a 26-gauge needle at a rate of 10 µL per minute using a microinfusion pump (Harvard Apparatus Inc., Holliston, MA). The coordinates were 0.2 mm anterior to bregma, 5.5 mm ventral, and 4.0 mm lateral to midline. After intracerebral infusion, the needle was removed and the skin incision closed with suture.

Experimental groups

Rats had intracerebral injection of 5 U of thrombin in 50 µL saline, or 100 µL of blood with or without 25 µg tuftsin. Rats were killed at days 1 and 3 and the brains used for brain water content, sodium ion measurements, and immunohistochemistry.

Immunohistochemistry

Rats were anesthetized with pentobarbital (60 mg/kg, i.p.) and perfused with 4% paraformaldehyde in 0.1 M PBS (pH 7.4). Brains were removed, kept in 4% paraformaldehyde for 6 h, and then immersed in 25% sucrose for 3 to 4 days at 4 °C. The brains were then embedded in O.C.T compound (Sakura Finetek U.S.A. Inc., Torrance, CA) and sectioned on a cryostat (18 µm thick) for immunohistochemistry, as previously described [34]. Briefly, sections were incubated overnight at 4 °C with the primary antibody mouse anti-rat OX-42 (Serotec Inc.) at a concentration of 1:400. They were then incubated with avidin-biotinylated horseradish peroxidase (Vector Laboratories) second antibody and diamino-benzidine hydrogen peroxide (Stable DAB; Research Genetics Inc.) for 90 min each at room temperature. After dehydration, sections were cover-slipped for microphotography. Normal IgG (from the same species as the primary antibody) or omission of the primary antibody was used as a negative control.

Brain water and ion content measurements

Rats received an injection of 100 µL blood with 5 µL saline or 25 µg tuftsin (in 5 µL saline) into right basal ganglia. Rats were killed under deep pentobarbital anesthesia at day 3. The brains were removed immediately and a 4-mm thick coronal section was taken 3 mm from the frontal pole. The brain sample was then divided into cortex or basal ganglia (ipsilateral or contralateral). Tissue samples were weighed to obtain the wet weight (WW). The tissue was then dried in a gravity oven at 100 °C for more than 24 h to determine the dry weight (DW). Tissue water content (%) was calculated as ([WW − DW]/WW) × 100.

Dehydrated brain samples were digested in 1 mL of 1 N nitric acid for 1 week. Sodium and potassium ion contents in this solution were measured by flame photometry and expressed in micro-equivalents per gram of dehydrated brain tissue (μEq/gm DW).

Statistical analysis

All data in this study are presented as mean ± standard deviation. Data were analyzed using Student *t*-test or ANOVA with a Scheffe's post-hoc multiple comparison test. Significance levels were set at $p < 0.05$.

Results

Experiments in vitro

Thrombin receptor expression in cultured rat microglia

Purity of microglial cultures was determined by immunocytochemistry. Most cultured cells were OX-42 (a marker of microglia)-positive (Fig. 1A) and glial fibrillary acidic protein (a marker of astrocytes)-negative (Fig. 1B). Immunoreactivity of thrombin receptors PAR-1, PAR-3, and PAR-4 were detected in the cultured microglia. PAR-1 immunoreactivity and PAR-4 immunoreactivity were present in large numbers of cultured

microglia (Fig. 2A and C). However, PAR-3 immunoreactivity was found in some microglia (Fig. 2B).

Thrombin-induced secretion of IL-1β and TNF-α

Cultured microglia released IL-1β and TNF-α into the culture medium. Thrombin treatment (5 or 10 U/mL) increased IL-1β and TNF-α secretion at 4, 8, and 24 h in a dose-dependent manner (Fig. 3A and B). Co-treatment of thrombin (10 U/mL) for 24 h with tuftsin (0.05 μg/mL) significantly reduced levels of IL-1β (a 35% decrease compared with the vehicle-treated group; $p < 0.05$) and TNF-α (a 22% decrease compared with the vehicle-treated group; $p < 0.05$) in the culture medium.

Experiments in vivo

All physiologic variables were measured immediately before intracerebral injections. Mean arterial blood pressure (MABP), pH, arterial oxygen and carbon dioxide tensions (PO_2 and PCO_2), hematocrit, and blood glucose were controlled within normal range (MABP, 80–120 mmHg; PO_2, 80–120 mmHg; PCO_2,

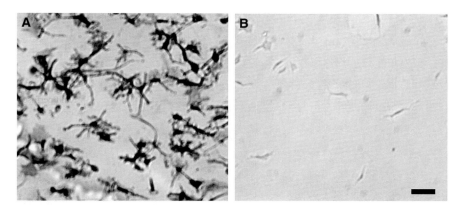

Fig. 1. (A) OX-42 and (B) GFAP immunostaining in cultured rat microglia. Scale bar = 20 μm

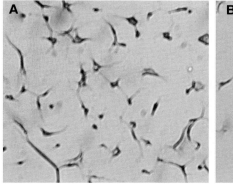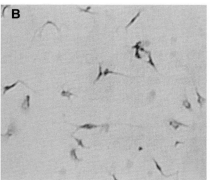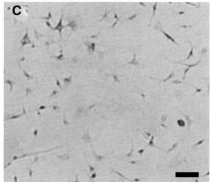

Fig. 2. Immunocytochemistry of cultured rat microglia. (A) PAR-1, (B) PAR-3, and (C) PAR-4. Scale bar = 20 μm

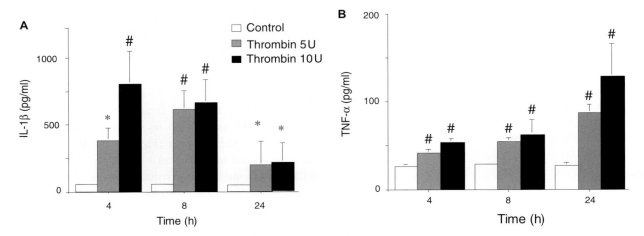

Fig. 3. IL-1β and TNF-α levels in microglia culture medium after different durations of thrombin treatment. (A) Cultured microglia treated with either vehicle or thrombin (5 and 10 U/mL). Values are mean $\pm$ SD, *$p < 0.05$ and #$p < 0.01$ vs. control (ANOVA test + Scheffe's post hoc test). (B) Cultured microglia treated with either vehicle or thrombin (5 and 10 U/mL). Values are mean $\pm$ SD, #$p < 0.05$ vs. control

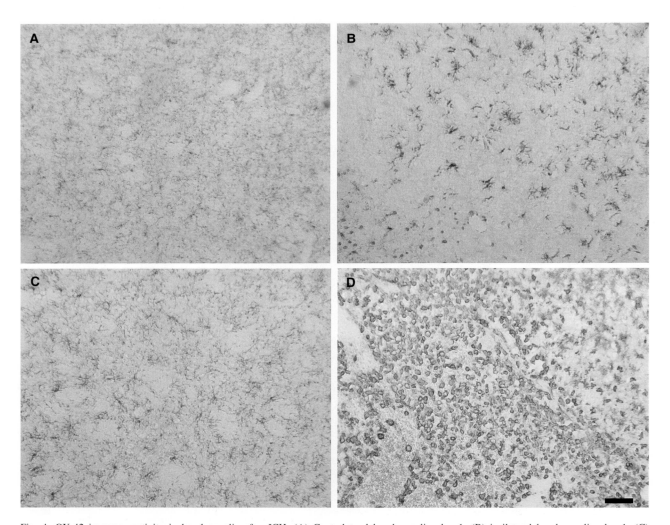

Fig. 4. OX-42 immunoreactivity in basal ganglia after ICH. (A) Contralateral basal ganglia, day 1; (B) ipsilateral basal ganglia, day 1; (C) contralateral basal ganglia, day 3; (D) ipsilateral basal ganglia, day 3. Scale bar = 50 μm

35–45 mmHg; hematocrit, 38–43%; blood glucose, 80–120 mg/dL).

Microglia activation after intracerebral blood and thrombin infusion

Immunohistochemistry showed microglia activation after ICH. Reactive and phagocytic microglia were found around the hematoma at day 1 and day 3 after ICH. On the first day after ICH, microglial cells were significantly activated and the activated microglial cells were enlarged and bushy (Fig. 4B). Three days later, many microglia around the hematoma were phagocytic (Fig. 4D). Activated and phagocytic microglial cells were also found in the ipsilateral caudate after 5-U thrombin injection at 1 and 3 days, respectively (data not shown).

Attenuation of ICH-induced brain edema by tuftsin

To test the role of microglia activation in brain edema formation after ICH, rats received an injection of 100 μL autologous whole blood with 5 μL saline ± 25 μg tuftsin

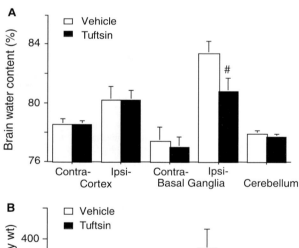

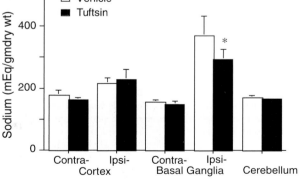

Fig. 5. (A) Brain water and (B) sodium content 3 days after ICH. Rats received an injection of either blood + vehicle or blood + tuftsin into the right basal ganglia. Values are mean ± SD, $n = 5$. $^{*}p < 0.05$, $^{\#}p < 0.01$ vs. vehicle; Student t-test

into the right basal ganglia. Brain water content was measured 3 days later. We found that tuftsin treatment reduced brain edema in the ipsilateral basal ganglia ($80.8 \pm 0.9\%$ vs. $83.4 \pm 0.8\%$ in the saline-treated group; $p < 0.01$; Fig. 5A). Tuftsin treatment did not affect brain water content in the cerebellum. Reduction of perihematomal edema was associated with a reduction in brain sodium levels (294 ± 31 vs. $368 \pm 64\,\mu Eq/gm$ DW in the saline-treated group; $p < 0.05$).

Discussion

In this study, we demonstrated that microglia are activated after ICH, that thrombin can stimulate microglia to secrete IL-1β and TNF-α, and that microglia inhibition with tuftsin reduces ICH-mediated perihematomal brain edema. These results suggest an important role of thrombin-activated microglia in brain injury following ICH, and that this injury may transpire by way of proinflammatory cytokines.

Thrombin is produced immediately in the brain after an ICH. Thrombin is necessary to stop the bleeding and it can also have direct neuroprotective actions at very low concentrations [25, 28, 33]. However, at high concentrations, thrombin can also activate potentially harmful pathways. *In vivo*, thrombin contributes to ICH-related injury, including brain edema formation and neuronal death [35, 36]. We have shown that thrombin-induced edema occurs in part from a direct opening in the blood-brain barrier [16]. *In vitro*, thrombin induces apoptosis in cultured neurons and astrocytes [6], potentiates N-methyl-D-aspartate (NMDA) receptor function [7], and activates rodent microglia [19, 26, 27]. Our current study focused on the effects of the latter, examining which thrombin receptors are present on microglia, the effects of thrombin on the secretion of proinflammatory cytokines by microglia, the extent of microglia activation after ICH, and the results of microglia inhibition on ICH-induced brain injury.

Whether thrombin activates microglia through thrombin receptors is a concept that has not been well-studied. Three PARs, including PAR-1, PAR-3, and PAR-4, are thrombin receptors. It has been reported that PARs are expressed in microglia [19, 26, 27]. We showed that PAR-1 and PAR-4 are the 2 major thrombin receptors in microglia. PAR-1 and PAR-4 are linked to a wide variety of intracellular signaling cascades [3]. Recent studies indicate that many of the effects of thrombin are PAR-mediated [35]. For example, Suo *et al.* [26, 27]

found that PAR-4, but not PAR-1, mediates thrombin-induced TNF-α production in microglia.

Activated microglia secrete many toxic materials such as free radicals [14]. Here, we found that rat microglia can secrete IL-1β and TNF-α upon exposure to thrombin. TNF-α is a major proinflammatory cytokine. TNF-α levels in the brain are increased after intracerebral injection of thrombin, and ICH [11] and ICH-induced brain edema was less in TNF-α knockout mice compared with wild-type mice [12]. It appears that TNF-α is involved in ICH- and thrombin-induced brain injury. Similarly, IL-1β is also a proinflammatory cytokine. Although it is important in initiating tissue repair, it can also induce prolonged inflammation and it is associated with certain pathologies in humans. IL-1β has multiple potentially harmful effects on the brain, including neurotoxicity, opening of the blood-brain barrier, and inducting apoptosis and neutrophil infiltration. Our previous study showed attenuation of ICH and thrombin-induced brain edema by overexpression of IL-1β receptor antagonist in the brain [17]. In all, these results and those in our current study suggest that thrombin-induced production of these proinflammatory cytokines by microglia may have an important role in ICH-induced brain injury.

Activation of microglia around the hematoma occurs after ICH [8, 9, and this study]. We found that microglia activation is associated with brain edema formation following ICH since tuftsin fragment 1–3, an inhibitor of microglia activation [1], results in less perihematomal edema. We have previously found that microglial activation enhances brain injury in aged rats after ICH [9]. In addition, microglial inhibition decreases injury volume and improves neurobehavioral deficits in a collagenase-induced ICH model in mice [29]. Recently, minocycline, a second-generation tetracycline-based molecule, has been reported to provide neuroprotection by inhibiting microglia [22]. We believe, therefore, that tuftsin reduces ICH-induced brain edema through microglia inhibition. However, it should be noted that although microglial activation is a brain injury marker for many central nervous system diseases [5, 23], it has neurotrophic actions [24]. The precise role of microglial activation in ICH-induced brain injury may depend upon the timing and degree of microglial activation.

In summary, thrombin formation after ICH activates microglia and activated microglia secrete IL-1β and TNF-α. Clarification of the role of microglia activation in ICH-induced brain injury should help in development of new therapies to limit hemorrhagic brain damage.

Acknowledgments

This study was supported by grants NS-017760, NS-039866, and NS-047245 from the National Institutes of Health (NIH), 0755717Z from American Heart Association (AHA), and NSFC30600195 from National Natural Science Foundation of China (NSFC). The content is solely the responsibility of the authors and does not necessarily represent the official views of the NIH, AHA, or NSFC.

References

1. Auriault C, Joseph M, Tartar A, Capron A (1983) Characterization and synthesis of a macrophage inhibitory peptide from the second constant domain of human immunoglobulin G. FEBS Lett 153: 11–15
2. Coughlin SR (1999) How the protease thrombin talks to cells. Proc Natl Acad Sci USA 96: 11023–11027
3. Coughlin SR (2000) Thrombin signalling and protease-activated receptors. Nature 407: 258–264
4. Déry O, Corvera CU, Steinhoff M, Bunnett NW (1998) Proteinase-activated receptors: novel mechanisms of signaling by serine proteases. Am J Physiol 274: C1429–C1452
5. Dirnagl U, Iadecola C, Moskowitz MA (1999) Pathobiology of ischaemic stroke: an integrated view. Trends Neurosci 22: 391–397
6. Donovan FM, Pike CJ, Cotman CW, Cunningham DD (1997) Thrombin induces apoptosis in cultured neurons and astrocytes via a pathway requiring tyrosine kinase and RhoA activities. J Neurosci 17: 5316–5326
7. Gingrich MB, Junge CE, Lyuboslavsky P, Traynelis SF (2000) Potentiation of NMDA receptor function by the serine protease thrombin. J Neurosci 20: 4582–4595
8. Gong C, Hoff JT, Keep RF (2000) Acute inflammatory reaction following experimental intracerebral hemorrhage. Brain Res 871: 57–65
9. Gong Y, Hua Y, Keep RF, Hoff JT, Xi G (2004) Intracerebral hemorrhage: effects of aging on brain edema and neurological deficits. Stroke 35: 2571–2575
10. Hua Y, Schallert T, Keep RF, Wu J, Hoff JT, Xi G (2002) Behavioral tests after intracerebral hemorrhage in the rat. Stroke 33: 2478–2484
11. Hua Y, Wu J, Keep RF, Nakamura T, Hoff JT, Xi G (2006) Tumor necrosis factor-alpha increases in the brain following intracerebral hemorrhage and thrombin stimulation. Neurosurgery 58: 542–550
12. Hua Y, Keep RF, Hoff JT, Xi G (2007) Brain injury after intracerebral hemorrhage: the role of thrombin and iron. Stroke 38(2 Suppl): 759–762
13. Jiang Y, Wu J, Hua Y, Keep RF, Xiang J, Hoff JT, Xi G (2002) Thrombin-receptor activation and thrombin-induced brain tolerance. J Cereb Blood Flow Metab 22: 404–410
14. Klegeris A, McGeer PL (2000) Interaction of various intracellular signaling mechanisms involved in mononuclear phagocyte toxicity toward neuronal cells. J Leukoc Biol 67: 127–133
15. Lee KR, Colon GP, Betz AL, Keep RF, Kim S, Hoff JT (1996) Edema from intracerebral hemorrhage: the role of thrombin. J Neurosurg 84: 91–96
16. Lee KR, Kawai N, Kim S, Sagher O, Hoff JT (1997) Mechanisms of edema formation after intracerebral hemorrhage: effects of thrombin on cerebral blood flow, blood–brain barrier permeability, and cell survival in a rat model. J Neurosurg 86: 272–278
17. Masada T, Hua Y, Xi G, Yang GY, Hoff JT, Keep RF (2001) Attenuation of intracerebral hemorrhage and thrombin-induced brain edema by overexpression of interleukin-1 receptor antagonist. J Neurosurg 95: 680–686

18. McCarthy KD, de Vellis J (1980) Preparation of separate astroglial and oligodendroglial cell cultures from rat cerebral tissue. J Cell Biol 85: 890–902

19. Möller T, Hanisch UK, Ransom BR (2000) Thrombin-induced activation of cultured rodent microglia. J Neurochem 75: 1539–1547

20. Niclou S, Suidan HS, Brown-Luedi M, Monard D (1994) Expression of the thrombin receptor mRNA in rat brain. Cell Mol Biol (Noisy-le-grand) 40: 421–428

21. Noorbakhsh F, Vergnolle N, Hollenberg MD, Power C (2003) Proteinase-activated receptors in the nervous system. Nat Rev Neurosci 4: 981–990

22. Power C, Henry S, Del Bigio MR, Larsen PH, Corbett D, Imai Y, Yong VW, Peeling J (2003) Intracerebral hemorrhage induces macrophage activation and matrix metalloproteinases. Ann Neurol 53: 731–742

23. Schwartz M (2003) Macrophages and microglia in central nervous system injury: are they helpful or harmful? J Cereb Blood Flow Metab 23: 385–394

24. Streit WJ, Walter SA, Pennell NA (1999) Reactive microgliosis. Prog Neurobiol 57: 563–581

25. Striggow F, Riek M, Breder J, Henrich-Noack P, Reymann KG, Reiser G (2000) The protease thrombin is an endogenous mediator of hippocampal neuroprotection against ischemia at low concentrations but causes degeneration at high concentrations. Proc Natl Acad Sci USA 97: 2264–2269

26. Suo Z, Wu M, Ameenuddin S, Anderson HE, Zoloty JE, Citron BA, Andrade-Gordon P, Festoff BW (2002) Participation of protease-activated receptor-1 in thrombin-induced microglial activation. J Neurochem 80: 655–666

27. Suo Z, Wu M, Citron BA, Gao C, Festoff BW (2003) Persistent protease-activated receptor 4 signaling mediates thrombin-induced microglial activation. J Biol Chem 278: 31177–31183

28. Vaughan PJ, Pike CJ, Cotman CW, Cunningham DD (1995) Thrombin receptor activation protects neurons and astrocytes from cell death produced by environmental insults. J Neurosci 15: 5389–5401

29. Wang J, Rogove AD, Tsirka AE, Tsirka SE (2003) Protective role of tuftsin fragment 1–3 in an animal model of intracerebral hemorrhage. Ann Neurol 54: 655–664

30. Weinstein JR, Gold SJ, Cunningham DD, Gall CM (1995) Cellular localization of thrombin receptor mRNA in rat brain: expression by mesencephalic dopaminergic neurons and codistribution with pro-thrombin mRNA. J Neurosci 15: 2906–2919

31. Xi G, Keep RF, Hoff JT (1998) Erythrocytes and delayed brain edema formation following intracerebral hemorrhage in rats. J Neurosurg 89: 991–996

32. Xi G, Wagner KR, Keep RF, Hua Y, de Courten-Myers GM, Broderick JP, Brott TG, Hoff JT (1998) Role of blood clot formation on early edema development after experimental intracerebral hemorrhage. Stroke 29: 2580–2586

33. Xi G, Keep RF, Hua Y, Xiang JM, Hoff JT (1999) Attenuation of thrombin-induced brain edema by cerebral thrombin preconditioning. Stroke 30: 1247–1255

34. Xi G, Keep RF, Hua Y, Hoff JT (2000) Thrombin preconditioning, heat shock proteins and thrombin-induced brain edema. Acta Neurochir Suppl 76: 511–515

35. Xi G, Reiser G, Keep RF (2003) The role of thrombin and thrombin receptors in ischemic, hemorrhagic and traumatic brain injury: deleterious or protective? J Neurochem 84: 3–9

36. Xi G, Keep RF, Hoff JT (2006) Mechanisms of brain injury after intracerebral hemorrhage. Lancet Neurol 5: 53–63

37. Yang S, Nakamura T, Hua Y, Keep RF, Younger JG, He Y, Hoff JT, Xi G (2006) The role of complement C3 in intracerebral hemorrhage-induced brain injury. J Cereb Blood Flow Metab 26: 1490–1495

Acta Neurochir Suppl (2008) 105: 67–70
© Springer-Verlag 2008
Printed in Austria

Effects of aging on complement activation and neutrophil infiltration after intracerebral hemorrhage

Y. Gong[1,2], G. Xi[1], S. Wan[1], Y. Gu[1,2], R. F. Keep[1], Y. Hua[1]

[1] Department of Neurosurgery, University of Michigan Medical School, Ann Arbor, MI, USA
[2] Department of Neurosurgery, Huashan Hospital, Fudan University, Shanghai, China

Summary

Intracerebral hemorrhage (ICH)-induced brain edema and neurological deficits are greater in aged rats than in young rats. Complement activation and neutrophil infiltration contribute to brain injury after ICH. In this study, we investigated the effects of aging on activation of the complement cascade and neutrophil influx following ICH.

Male Sprague-Dawley rats (3 or 18 months old) received an infusion of 100 μL autologous blood into right caudate. Rats were killed at 1, 3, 7, and 28 days after ICH and the brains were sampled for immunohistochemistry and Western blot analysis. Levels of complement factor C9 and clusterin were used as markers for complement activation, and myeloperoxidase (MPO) staining was performed to detect neutrophil infiltration. Western blot analysis showed that complement C9 and clusterin levels in ipsilateral basal ganglia after ICH were higher in aged rats than in young rats ($p < 0.05$). Immunohistochemistry showed there were more C9- and clusterin-positive cells around the hematoma in aged rats. However, MPO-positive cells in ipsilateral basal ganglia were fewer in aged rats ($p < 0.05$) after ICH.

Our results suggest that ICH causes more severe complement activation and less neutrophil infiltration in aged rats. Clarification of the mechanisms of brain injury after ICH in the aging brain should help develop new therapeutic strategies for ICH.

Keywords: Aging; cerebral hemorrhage; complement; myeloperoxidase.

Introduction

Age is an important factor affecting brain injury in intracerebral hemorrhage (ICH) in both animals and humans [2, 5, 13]. In ICH patients, age is a key predictor of functional outcome [2]. Our recent studies found that ICH causes more severe brain injury in aged rats compared to young ones [5].

Correspondence: Ya Hua, MD, Department of Neurosurgery, University of Michigan Medical School, 109 Zina Pitcher Place, R5018 Biomedical Science Research Building, Ann Arbor, MI 48109-2200, USA. e-mail: yahua@umich.edu

The complement system is involved in various immune reactions, including cell lysis and the inflammatory response [1, 8]. The complement cascade is activated in brain parenchyma after ICH. Inhibition of the complement cascade attenuates ICH-induced brain damage in rats [6]. Recently, we found that complement C3 deficient mice had less brain edema and less microglial activation around the hematoma compared to complement C3 sufficient mice [15].

Inflammation exacerbates hemorrhagic brain injury. An inflammatory response in the tissue surrounding brain occurs soon after ICH and peaks several days later in humans and in animals [3, 4, 7, 14]. Neutrophil infiltration develops within 2 days in rats and activated microglia persist for a month [5, 7].

In the present study, we examined the role of age in complement cascade activation and neutrophil infiltration after ICH.

Materials and methods

Animal preparation and intracerebral infusion

Animal use protocols were approved by the University of Michigan Committee on the Use and Care of Animals. Male Sprague-Dawley rats (Charles River Laboratories, Wilmington, MA) 3 months or 18 months old were used in this study. These age groups are henceforth called young and aged rats, respectively. Animals were anesthetized with pentobarbital (40 mg/kg, i.p.). The right femoral artery was catheterized for continuous blood pressure monitoring and blood sampling. Blood was obtained from the catheter for analysis of blood pH, PaO_2, $PaCO_2$, hematocrit, and blood glucose. Core temperature was maintained at 37 °C with use of a feedback-controlled heating pad. Rats were positioned in a stereotactic frame, and a cranial burr hole (1 mm) was drilled in the right coronal suture 3.5 mm lateral to the midline. All rats received a 100-μL injection of autologous whole blood into the right caudate nucleus at a rate of 10 μL per minute through a 26-gauge needle (coordinates 0.2 mm anterior, 5.5 mm ventral, and 3.5 mm lateral to bregma) using a microinfusion pump. The needle was removed, and the skin incision was closed with suture after infusion.

Immunohistochemistry

Rats were anesthetized with pentobarbital (60 mg/kg, i.p.) and perfused with 4% paraformaldehyde in 0.1 M phosphate-buffered saline (pH 7.4). Brains were removed and kept in 4% paraformaldehyde for 4 to 6 h, then immersed in 25% sucrose for 3 to 4 days at 4 °C. Brains were embedded in O.C.T compound (Sakura Finetek USA Inc., Torrance, CA) and sectioned on a cryostat (18 μm thick).

Immunohistochemistry was performed using avidin-biotin complex technique as previously described [11]. The primary antibodies were rabbit anti-rat C9 (1:800 dilution; a gift from Dr. P. Morgan, University of Wales), rabbit anti-rat clusterin (1:400 dilution; a gift from Dr. M. Griswold, Washington State University), rabbit anti-human myeloperoxidase (MPO; 1:200 dilution; DAKO, Dakopatts, Denmark). Normal rabbit IgG and the absence of primary antibody were used for negative controls.

Western blot analysis

Animals were anesthetized and decapitated at different time points. Animals were perfused transcardially with saline. The brain was then removed and a 4-mm coronal brain slice was cut from the frontal pole (approximately 3 mm thick). The brain slice was divided into ipsilateral and contralateral cortex, and ipsilateral and contralateral basal ganglia. Brain tissues were immersed in 0.5 mL Western sample buffer (62.5 mM

Tris–HCl, pH 6.8, 2.3% sodium dodecyl sulfate, 10% glycerol, and 5% β-mercaptoethanol) and then sonicated for 10 sec. Sample solution (10 μL) was taken for protein assay (Bio-Rad Laboratories, Hercules, CA), while the rest was frozen at −20 °C for Western blot. Western blot analysis was performed as described previously [11]. Briefly, 50 μg

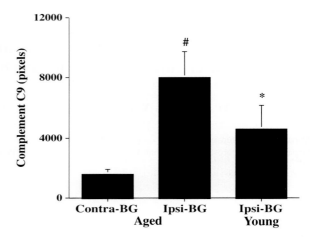

Fig. 1. Complement C9 protein levels in ipsilateral (*Ipsi-*) and contralateral (*Contra-*) basal ganglia (BG) 1 day after ICH in aged and young rats. Values are mean ± SD; #$p < 0.01$ and *$p < 0.05$ vs. contralateral basal ganglia (*Contra-BG*)

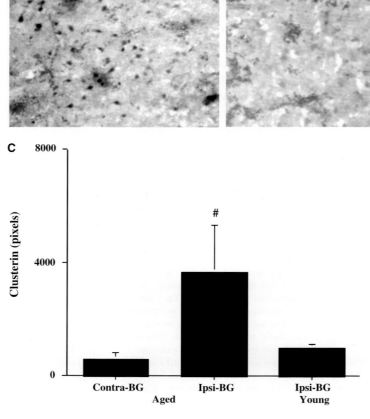

Fig. 2. Immunoreactivity of clusterin in ipsilateral basal ganglia of (A) aged or (B) young rats 1 day after ICH. Scale bar = 50 μm. (C) Clusterin protein levels in contralateral (*Contra-*) and ipsilateral (*Ipsi-*) basal ganglia (BG) in aged and young rats 1 day after ICH. Values are mean ± SD; #$p < 0.01$ vs. the other groups

protein was run on polyacrylamide gels with a 4% stacking gel (SDS-PAGE) after 5 min boiling at 95 °C. The protein was transferred to a hybond-C pure nitrocellulose membrane (Amersham Biosciences, Piscataway, NJ). The membranes were blocked in 5% Carnation non-fat dry milk in TBST (150 mM NaCl, 100 mM Tris-base, 0.1% Tween 20, pH 7.6) buffer for 1 h at 37 °C. After washing in TBST buffer 3 times, membranes were probed with primary antibody for 90 min at room temperature. After washing the membranes with TBST buffer 3 times, the membranes were immuno-probed again with the second antibody for 1 h at room temperature. Finally, membranes were washed 3 times in TBST buffer and the antigen-antibody complexes visualized with the ECL chemiluminescence system (Amersham Biosciences) and exposed to Kodak X-OMAT film. The relative densities of the protein bands were analyzed with NIH Image software, version 1.61 (National Institutes of Health, Bethesda, MD).

Statistical analysis

Student *t*-test and ANOVA test were used. Values are mean ± SD. Statistical significance was set at $p < 0.05$.

Results

Time-course showed that complement C9 protein levels (Western blotting) were significantly increased in ipsilateral basal ganglia and peaked 1 day after intracerebral injection of 100 μL autologous whole blood in both young and aged rats. Complement C9 content then decreased with time and was very low by day 28. Compared to young rats, aged rats had higher levels of complement C9 in ipsilateral basal ganglia 1 day after ICH (8006 ± 1726 vs. 4578 ± 1597 pixels in young rats, $p < 0.05$; Fig. 1).

By Western blot analysis, clusterin was markedly increased 1 day after ICH in both aged and young rats. There were more clusterin-positive cells in the ipsilateral caudate in aged rats compared to young rats (Fig. 2A, B). Protein levels of brain clusterin in aged rats were significantly higher than in young rats (3646 ± 1656 vs. 1009 ± 134 pixels; $p < 0.05$; Fig. 2C) 1 day after ICH.

Neutrophil infiltration occurred in the brain after ICH. There were more MPO-positive cells in ipsilateral basal

ganglia at day 3 than at day 1 after ICH. At day 3, the numbers of MPO-positive cells were lower in aged rats (35 ± 6 vs. 97 ± 53 cells/mm^2; $p < 0.05$, Fig. 3).

Discussion

Our previous studies have indicated that complement is activated in the brain after ICH, contributing to perihematomal edema formation, and complement inhibition and depletion attenuate ICH-induced brain edema formation [6, 12]. The complement system is involved in various immune reactions, including cell lysis and the inflammatory response [8]. Membrane attack complex (MAC) formation may be involved in lysis of erythrocytes in the clot. We have demonstrated that complement depletion reduces ICH-induced brain edema and is associated with inhibition of the inflammatory response and MAC-mediated erythrocytes lysis [12]. MAC insertion may also occur in neurons, glia, and endothelial cells, causing neuronal death and blood-brain barrier leakage. MAC-induced cell lysis plays a major role in aged rats after ICH. In the present study, complement activation was greater in aged rats compared to young rats after ICH. We found that ICH-induced brain injury in aged rats was more severe than that found in young rats [5]. The extensive activation of complement cascade in aged rats may contribute to severe ICH-induced brain injury in aged rats.

We hypothesized that neutrophil infiltration would also be enhanced after ICH in aged rats. However, in this study, there was less neutrophil infiltration in aged rats after ICH compared to young rats. Inflammation and phagocytosis are involved in hematoma resolution [16], but they may also be involved in brain injury. There is evidence that microglia activation and neutrophil infiltration contribute to brain injury after ICH [9, 10, 13]. In rat models of ICH, neutrophil infiltration develops within 2 days and activated microglial cells persist for at least a month [5, 7]. There were more activated microglial cells in aged rats than in young rats [5]. The role of neutrophils in aged brain after ICH should be studied further.

In summary, ICH results in greater complement activation and less neutrophil infiltration around the hematoma in aged rats. Complement inhibition may be a new therapeutic target for ICH.

Acknowledgment

This study was supported by grants NS-017760, NS-039866, and NS-047245 from the National Institutes of Health (NIH), and 0755717Z and

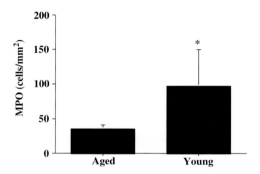

Fig. 3. MPO-positive cells in ipsilateral basal ganglia of aged and young rats 3 days after ICH. Values are mean ± SD; *$p < 0.05$ vs. aged rats

0840016N from American Heart Association (AHA). The content is solely the responsibility of the authors and does not necessarily represent the official views of the NIH or AHA.

References

1. Cole DS, Morgan BP (2003) Beyond lysis: how complement influences cell fate. Clin Sci (London) 104: 455–466
2. Daverat P, Castel JP, Dartigues JF, Orgogozo JM (1991) Death and functional outcome after spontaneous intracerebral hemorrhage. A prospective study of 166 cases using multivariate analysis. Stroke 22: 1–6
3. Enzmann DR, Britt RH, Lyons BE, Buxton JL, Wilson DA (1981) Natural history of experimental intracerebral hemorrhage: sonography, computed tomography and neuropathology. Am J Neuroradiol 2: 517–526
4. Gong C, Hoff JT, Keep RF (2000) Acute inflammatory reaction following experimental intracerebral hemorrhage in rat. Brain Res 871: 57–65
5. Gong Y, Hua Y, Keep RF, Hoff JT, Xi G (2004) Intracerebral hemorrhage: effects of aging on brain edema and neurological deficits. Stroke 35: 2571–2575
6. Hua Y, Xi G, Keep RF, Hoff JT (2000) Complement activation in the brain after experimental intracerebral hemorrhage. J Neurosurg 92: 1016–1022
7. Jenkins A, Maxwell WL, Graham DI (1989) Experimental intracerebral hematoma in the rat: sequential light microscopical changes. Neuropathol Appl Neurobiol 15: 477–486
8. Morgan BP, Gasque P, Singhrao S, Piddlesden SJ (1997) The role of complement in disorders of the nervous system. Immunopharmacology 38: 43–50
9. Wang J, Rogove AD, Tsirka AE, Tsirka SE (2003) Protective role of tuftsin fragment 1–3 in an animal model of intracerebral hemorrhage. Ann Neurol 54: 655–664
10. Wang J, Tsirka SE (2005) Tuftsin fragment 1–3 is beneficial when delivered after the induction of intracerebral hemorrhage. Stroke 36: 613–618
11. Xi G, Keep RF, Hua Y, Xiang J, Hoff JT (1999) Attenuation of thrombin-induced brain edema by cerebral thrombin preconditioning. Stroke 30: 1247–1255
12. Xi G, Hua Y, Keep RF, Younger JG, Hoff JT (2001) Systemic complement depletion diminishes perihematomal brain edema in rats. Stroke 32: 162–167
13. Xi G, Keep RF, Hoff JT (2006) Mechanisms of brain injury after intracerebral haemorrhage. Lancet Neurol 5: 53–63
14. Xue M, Del Bigio MR (2000) Intracerebral injection of autologous whole blood in rats: time course of inflammation and cell death. Neurosci Lett 283: 230–232
15. Yang S, Nakamura T, Hua Y, Keep RF, Younger JG, He Y, Hoff JT, Xi G (2006) The role of complement C3 in intracerebral hemorrhage-induced brain injury. J Cereb Blood Flow Metab 26: 1490–1495
16. Zhao X, Sun G, Zhang J, Strong R, Song W, Gonzales N, Grotta JC, Aronowski J (2007) Hematoma resolution as a target for intracerebral hemorrhage treatment: role for peroxisome proliferator-activated receptor gamma in microglia/macrophages. Ann Neurol 61: 352–362

Experimental intracerebral hemorrhage – other mechanisms

Acta Neurochir Suppl (2008) 105: 73–77
© Springer-Verlag 2008
Printed in Austria

Blood–brain barrier function in intracerebral hemorrhage

R. F. Keep[1,2], **J. Xiang**[1], **S. R. Ennis**[1], **A. Andjelkovic**[1,3], **Y. Hua**[1], **G. Xi**[1], **J. T. Hoff**[1,*]

[1] Department of Neurosurgery, University of Michigan Medical School, Ann Arbor, MI, USA
[2] Department of Molecular and Integrative Physiology, University of Michigan Medical School, Ann Arbor, MI, USA
[3] Department of Pathology, University of Michigan Medical School, Ann Arbor, MI, USA

Summary

In this paper, we review current knowledge on blood–brain barrier (BBB) dysfunction following intracerebral hemorrhage (ICH). BBB disruption is a hallmark of ICH-induced brain injury. Such disruption contributes to edema formation, the influx of leukocytes, and the entry of potentially neuroactive agents into the perihematomal brain, all of which may contribute to brain injury. A range of factors have been implicated in inducing BBB disruption, including inflammatory mediators (e.g., cytokines and chemokines), thrombin, hemoglobin breakdown products, oxidative stress, complement, and matrix metalloproteinases. While there is interaction between some of these mediators, it is probable that prevention of ICH-induced BBB disruption will involve blocking multiple pathways or blocking a common end pathway (e.g., by stabilizing tight junction structure). While the effects of ICH on BBB passive permeability have been extensively examined, effects on other 'barrier' properties (metabolic and transport functions) have been less well-studied. However, recent data suggests that ICH can affect transport and that this may help protect the BBB and the brain. Indeed, it is possible in small bleeds that BBB disruption may be beneficial, and it is only in the presence of larger bleeds that disruption has detrimental effects.

Keywords: Blood–brain barrier; tight junctions; transport; intracerebral hemorrhage.

Introduction

The blood–brain barrier (BBB) is formed by cerebral endothelial cells and their linking tight junctions. It severely curtails the diffusion of compounds between blood and brain, protecting the brain from changes in plasma composition [11, 15]. The BBB also possesses many transport systems that move nutrients from blood to brain or potentially harmful compounds from brain to blood [15]. The BBB is not static and the cells of the neurovascular unit, particularly astrocytes, appear to have a major role in inducing and regulating BBB function [2].

A wide variety of disease states, including ischemic stroke, traumatic brain injury, multiple sclerosis, and brain tumors, result in BBB disruption and the migration of macromolecules from blood to brain [11, 15]. Such disruption also occurs after intracerebral hemorrhage (ICH) in man and animals [17, 36, 40]. BBB disruption can result in vasogenic brain edema, facilitate the migration of leukocytes from blood to brain, and cause an influx of potentially neurotoxic compounds from blood. All of these events may contribute to morbidity and mortality after ICH. Increases in intracranial pressure after ICH can be exacerbated by edema formation, leading to brain herniation and death [39]. Leukocyte entry after ICH may cause secondary brain injury [39], as may an influx of prothrombin and complement [13, 18]. There has, therefore, been great interest in developing therapeutics that can reduce BBB disruption after ICH and other disease states. In this paper, we review current knowledge of normal BBB function, how the BBB is affected by ICH, which mediators may alter BBB function, and potential therapeutic strategies.

Normal BBB function

Cerebral and systemic endothelial cells share some common characteristics, particularly in relation to hemostasis, regulation of blood flow, and regulation of leukocyte transmigration. However, cerebral endothelial cells differ: they are linked by continuous tight junctions, have very low paracellular permeability, limited endocytosis, an absence of fenestrations, the presence of metabolizing enzymes for neuroactive compounds, and high expression of

---

* Dr. Julian T. Hoff died prior to publication of this article.

Correspondence: Richard F. Keep, Ph.D., Department of Neurosurgery, University of Michigan Medical School, Room 5018, BSRB, Ann Arbor, MI 48109-2200, USA. e-mail: rkeep@umich.edu

a wide range of transporters [15]. Thus, the BBB has unique physical, metabolic, and transport barrier properties.

The most prominent feature of the BBB is the very limited passive diffusion of compounds from blood to brain. Thus, large molecular weight compounds in plasma, such as proteins, are virtually excluded from brain. This limited diffusion is due to the tight junctions linking the cerebral endothelial cells, which virtually occlude the paracellular route, and a low level of transcytosis [11, 15]. Considerable progress has been made in understanding tight junction structure during the past decade. Tight junctions are composed of transmembrane proteins that undergo homodimeric interactions with proteins on adjacent endothelial cells to occlude the paracellular pathway [11]. These transmembrane proteins include claudins (particularly claudin 5), occludin, and the junctional adhesion molecules. In addition, a wide range of proteins form a cytoplasmic plaque associated with the tight junction. These plaque proteins (e.g., ZO-1) link the tight junctions to the actin cytoskeleton and, in turn, regulate junction properties [11, 15]. Phosphorylation of transmembrane tight junction proteins and their loss from the plasma membrane occurs in a number of disease states, thereby increasing BBB permeability [8, 11, 32, 33].

Although tight junctions limit paracellular diffusion, lipid-soluble compounds can cross the BBB by diffusing through the plasma membrane [15]. Other compounds can cross the BBB because of specific transporters. BBB transporters may be involved in transporting nutrients into the brain (e.g., GLUT1, LAT1, and the transferrin receptor) or regulating the composition (homeostasis) of the brain extracellular space [15]. With regard to the latter, there are BBB transporters that move waste products from brain to blood, clear potentially toxic agents from the endothelium to blood to prevent their entry into brain, and regulate ion concentrations in the brain interstitial space [15]. It should be noted, however, that some transporters at the cerebral endothelium may be involved in regulating endothelial rather than brain composition.

The entry of some compounds into brain is prevented by metabolism at the BBB. Such metabolism may degrade neuroactive compounds, but it may also facilitate their clearance from brain by converting them into substrates for BBB efflux transporters [15].

BBB disruption during ICH

BBB disruption after ICH has been examined both in man and in animal models. In animals, evidence on disruption has come from studies using intracerebral injection of blood [36, 40] or collagenase [29, 31], the latter inducing hemorrhage due to blood vessel disruption. Both models have disadvantages. The blood injection model only examines blood toxicity and has no disrupted vessel as its cause. The collagenase model does not replicate the normal cause of vessel rupture in man and injects an exogenous molecule that may have multiple effects on the brain. Unfortunately, there are few animal models of spontaneous ICH (e.g., [14]), and the pathophysiological relevance of those genetic models to man are open to debate.

After intracerebral blood injection in rat or pig, there is delayed BBB opening. Thus, after intracaudate blood injection, Yang *et al.* [40] found no BBB disruption at 4 h, but progressive disruption at 12 to 48 h. Similarly, following blood injection into cortical white matter in pigs, there is no disruption early (1 to 8 h) [21, 35], but there is by 24 h [36].

Following collagenase-induced ICH, there is a marked increase in BBB permeability by 30 min, a lower degree of hyperpermeability is then maintained from 5 h to 7 days, with normal permeability being restored by day 14 [29]. The initial BBB hyperpermeability is due to collagenase-induced degradation of the endothelial basement membrane, which causes extravasation of blood and compounds present in blood [29]. It is, however, unclear whether prolonged hyperpermeability (up to day 7) is solely the residual effect of endothelial basement membrane degradation or whether blood-derived factors contribute to the disruption (as indicated by models with blood injection).

In man, there is evidence of both acute and delayed vascular disruption after ICH [9, 17, 24]. There has been interest in the penetration of contrast agents into the brain in the hyperacute phase after ICH, as it may be an indicator of hematoma expansion [9, 24]. Some continued bleeding after the initial ictus occurs in about 14–38% of patients [39], and the extravasation of contrast agent is associated with such hematoma expansion [9, 24]. Since this hyperacute vascular leakage is probably due to continued extravasation at the site of the initial hemorrhage, it should probably not be considered as BBB disruption. There is also, however, delayed BBB disruption [17] after human ICH, and this may be more analogous to the disruption found after intracerebral blood injection in animals.

While most ICH studies have focused on the movement of compounds from blood to brain, there has been interest in examining whether proteins from brain appear in plasma, as they might be useful biomarkers. The appearance of such proteins in plasma would indicate BBB disruption, which would allow movement of proteins released from damaged parenchymal cells into the bloodstream [21]. Delgado *et al.* [7] have found that S100B, a primarily glial protein, appears in plasma after ICH and that plasma levels correlated with ICH volume. Plasma S100B levels were also higher in patients who deteriorated early and had an unfavorable outcome.

The underlying cause of BBB disruption after ICH has not really been examined. In cerebral ischemia, there is much evidence indicating a loss of tight junction proteins from the plasma membrane, resulting in junction disruption [8, 11]. Based on the fact that some of the compounds that can cause tight junction protein redistribution are increased after ICH (e.g., inflammatory mediators), it seems probable that ICH-induced disruption also involves tight junction modification. However, this needs to be directly examined.

There is evidence for increased pinocytosis at the BBB after cerebral ischemia, and this may contribute to increased migration of large molecular-weight compounds [6, 26]. There are, however, questions over its quantitative importance [27], and its role in ICH-induced BBB disruption is unknown.

The BBB functions as more than a physical barrier. There have, however, been very few studies that have examined the effect of ICH on other BBB functions (transport or metabolic). In cerebral ischemia, a number

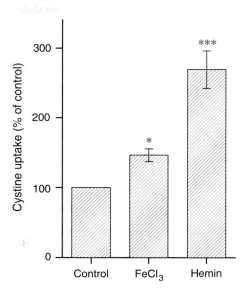

Fig. 1. Effect on L-[^{35}S] cystine uptake (expressed as % of control uptake) when exposing cerebral endothelial cells (bEnd.3) to FeCl$_3$ or hemin (both at 50 μM) for 24 h. Values are means ± SE, $n = 4$. *,***indicate a significant difference from control at the $p < 0.05$ and $p < 0.001$ levels, respectively

of Na-dependent transporters at the BBB are inhibited, probably due to ATP depletion [16]. In contrast, we failed to find a reduction in Na-dependent transport in a rat ICH model, probably reflecting an absence of endothelial energy depletion following ICH [25]. We have, however, found that exposure to heme or Fe can induce a marked increase in cystine uptake in cerebral endothelial cells (Fig. 1). Cystine uptake is rate limiting for glutathione production [12], and this may be a mechanism to protect the BBB from oxidative stress.

Mediators of BBB dysfunction and therapeutic targets

There are currently no agents that prevent ICH-induced BBB disruption in man. Therapeutic strategies may be suggested by 2 types of evidence regarding the mediators of ICH-induced BBB disruption in animals. There are experiments that have directly examined the role of particular mediators using administration of the mediator or an inhibitor, and there are those that have shown increases in the levels of specific compounds after ICH, compounds that can increase BBB permeability in other disease states or conditions (e.g., there are increases in cytokine levels in the brain after ICH, and cytokines can induce BBB disruption [1, 11, 34]).

Matrix metalloproteinases (MMPs) can cause BBB disruption and even hemorrhage by degrading the endothelial basement membrane [29, 31]. There is evidence that MMPs are increased after ICH in man and in animal models [3, 23], and a MMP inhibitor, tissue inhibitor of metalloproteinase-2 (TIMP2) can reduce ICH-induced BBB disruption in rats [30].

A number of compounds that can be produced by blood have the potential to cause BBB disruption. Thus, thrombin can cause BBB disruption, and inhibition of thrombin reduces ICH-edema and BBB disruption [10, 18]. Products released from erythrocytes during lysis can cause marked BBB disruption [5, 38]. This is likely due to the release of hemoglobin and iron with resultant oxidative stress [39].

Inflammation occurs after ICH with an influx of leukocytes, activation of microglia, and production of inflammatory mediators including cytokines and chemokines [19, 34]. Evidence indicates that such inflammation contributes to ICH-induced brain injury [34, 39]. Leukocytes and inflammatory mediators have been shown to participate in BBB disruption in other disease states [1, 8, 11, 32, 33], making it very likely that they also participate in ICH-induced disruption.

Belayev *et al.* [4] have found that intravenous injection of albumin can reduce BBB disruption in a rat ICH model. The mechanisms underlying this protection are as yet uncertain.

Whether ischemia occurs after ICH (in man or animals) and whether ischemia plays a role in ICH-induced brain injury is contentious. Certainly BBB disruption after ICH can occur in animal models where blood flow does not decrease to levels that cause ischemic brain damage [39, 40].

From the above discussion, it seems probable that ICH-induced BBB disruption is induced by multiple factors. An approach that would potentially reduce multiple mediators is clot evacuation. Indeed, Wagner *et al.* [36] found that evacuation did reduce BBB disruption in a pig ICH model, although clot evacuation has yet to be proven beneficial in reducing brain injury in human ICH [22]. Hypothermia and preconditioning stimuli may also be methods of inhibiting multiple pathways. The potential of hypothermia to reduce brain injury, including BBB damage, has received much attention for ischemic stroke and trauma, and there is evidence that general or localized hypothermia is protective in animal models of ICH [20, 37]. Similarly, we have also found that preconditioning with hyperbaric oxygen can protect the BBB after ICH [28].

Another approach may be to target downstream pathways shared by multiple mediators of BBB disruption, e.g., by blocking the pathways that cause tight junction disassembly. BBB disruption involves phosphorylation of tight junction proteins and their removal from the plasma membrane [8, 11, 32, 33], both of which may be amenable to therapeutic intervention.

Conclusion

ICH-induced BBB disruption occurs in man and in animal ICH models. Such disruption may contribute to the morbidity and mortality that occurs after ICH. Multiple potential mediators of ICH-induced BBB disruption have been identified, but whether they can be therapeutically modified in man has yet to be determined. However, in addition to potentially harmful effects, recent evidence indicating that BBB disruption is an orchestrated event involving specific tight junction protein phosphorylation and internalization suggests that under certain circumstances that disruption might have beneficial consequences. For example, with small hematomas, BBB disruption may aid in clot resolution.

Acknowledgments

This work was supported by grants NS-17760, NS-39866, NS-34709, NS-52510 from the National Institutes of Health, and an AHA Scientist Development Award, 0635403N. The content is solely the authors and does not necessarily represent the official views of the NIH or AHA.

References

1. Abbott NJ (2000) Inflammatory mediators and modulation of blood–brain barrier permeability. Cell Mol Neurobiol 20: 131–147
2. Abbott NJ, Rönnbäck L, Hansson E (2006) Astrocyte-endothelial interactions at the blood–brain barrier. Nat Rev Neurosci 7: 41–53
3. Alvarez-Sabin J, Delgado P, Abilleira S, Molina CA, Arenillas J, Ribó M, Santamarina E, Quintana M, Monasterio J, Montaner J (2004) Temporal profile of matrix metalloproteinases and their inhibitors after spontaneous intracerebral hemorrhage: relationship to clinical and radiological outcome. Stroke 35: 1316–1322
4. Belayev L, Saul I, Busto R, Danielyan K, Vigdorchik A, Khoutorova L, Ginsberg MD (2005) Albumin treatment reduces neurological deficit and protects blood–brain barrier integrity after acute intracortical hematoma in the rat. Stroke 36: 326–331
5. Bhasin RR, Xi G, Hua Y, Keep RF, Hoff JT (2002) Experimental intracerebral hemorrhage: effect of lysed erythrocytes on brain edema and blood–brain barrier permeability. Acta Neurochir Suppl 81: 249–251
6. Cipolla MJ, Crete R, Vitullo L, Rix RD (2004) Transcellular transport as a mechanism of blood–brain barrier disruption during stroke. Front Biosci 9: 777–785
7. Delgado P, Alvarez Sabin J, Santamarina E, Molina CA, Quintana M, Rosell A, Montaner J (2006) Plasma S100B level after acute spontaneous intracerebral hemorrhage. Stroke 37: 2837–2839
8. Dimitrijevic OB, Stamatovic SM, Keep RF, Andjelkovic AV (2006) Effects of the chemokine CCL2 on blood–brain barrier permeability during ischemia – reperfusion injury. J Cereb Blood Flow Metab 26: 797–810
9. Goldstein JN, Fazen LE, Snider R, Schwab K, Greenberg SM, Smith EE, Lev MH, Rosand J (2007) Contrast extravasation on CT angiography predicts hematoma expansion in intracerebral hemorrhage. Neurology 68: 889–894
10. Guan JX, Sun SG, Cao XB, Chen ZB, Tong ET (2004) Effect of thrombin on blood–brain barrier permeability and its mechanism. Chin Med J (Engl) 117: 1677–1681
11. Hawkins BT, Davis TP (2005) The blood–brain barrier/neurovascular unit in health and disease. Pharmacol Rev 57: 173–185
12. Hosoya K, Tomi M, Ohtsuki S, Takanaga H, Saeki S, Kanai Y, Endou H, Naito M, Tsuruo T, Terasaki T (2002) Enhancement of L-cystine transport activity and its relation to xCT gene induction at the blood–brain barrier by diethyl maleate treatment. J Pharmacol Exp Ther 302: 225–231
13. Hua Y, Xi G, Keep RF, Hoff JT (2000) Complement activation in the brain after experimental intracerebral hemorrhage. J Neurosurg 92: 1016–1022
14. Iida S, Baumbach GL, Lavoie JL, Faraci FM, Sigmund CD, Heistad DD (2005) Spontaneous stroke in a genetic model of hypertension in mice. Stroke 36: 1253–1258
15. Keep RF (2001) The blood–brain barrier. In: Walz W (ed) The neuronal microenvironment: brain homeostasis in health and disease. Humana Press, Totowa, pp 277–307
16. Keep RF, Kawai N, Stummer W, Fujisawa M, Patel T, Abdelkarim GE, Ennis SR, Betz AL (1999) Sodium-dependent transport at the blood–brain barrier and the effects of cerebral ischemia. In: Paulson OB, Knudsen GM, Moos T (eds) Review of brain barrier systems, Alfred Benzon Symposium 45. Munksgaard Press, Copenhagen, pp 387–395

17. Kidwell CS, Latour LL, Hsia AW, Merino JG, Burgess RE, Copenhaver BR, Castle A, Warach S (2007) Demonstration of blood–brain barrier disruption in humans with primary intracerebral hemorrhage (Abstract #47). Stroke 38: 464

18. Lee KR, Kawai N, Kim S, Sagher O, Hoff JT (1997) Mechanisms of edema formation after intracerebral hemorrhage: effects of thrombin on cerebral blood flow, blood–brain barrier permeability, and cell survival in a rat model. J Neurosurg 86: 272–278

19. Lu A, Tang Y, Ran R, Ardizzone TL, Wagner KR, Sharp FR (2006) Brain genomics of intracerebral hemorrhage. J Cereb Blood Flow Metab 26: 230–252

20. MacLellan CL, Davies LM, Fingas MS, Colbourne F (2006) The influence of hypothermia on outcome after intracerebral hemorrhage in rats. Stroke 37:1266–1270

21. Marchi N, Rasmussen P, Kapural M, Fazio V, Kight K, Mayberg MR, Kanner A, Ayumar B, Albensi B, Cavaglia M, Janigro D (2003) Peripheral markers of brain damage and blood–brain barrier dysfunction. Restor Neurol Neuros 21: 109–121

22. Mendelow AD, Gregson BA, Fernandes HM, Murray GD, Teasdale GM, Hope DT, Karimi A, Shaw MD, Barer DH, STICH investigators (2005) Early surgery versus initial conservative treatment in patients with spontaneous supratentorial intracerebral haematomas in the International Surgical Trial in Intracerebral Haemorrhage (STICH): a randomised trial. Lancet 365: 387–397

23. Mun-Bryce S, Rosenberg GA (1998) Metrix metalloproteinases in cerebrovascular disease. J Cereb Blood Flow Metab 18: 1163–1172

24. Murai Y, Ikeda Y, Teramoto A, Tsuji Y (1998) Magnetic resonance imaging-documented extravasation as an indicator of acute hypertensive intracerebral hemorrhage. J Neurosurg 88: 650–655

25. Patel TR, Fujisawa M, Schielke GP, Hoff JT, Betz AL, Keep RF (1999) Effect of intracerebral and subdural hematomas on energy-dependent transport across the blood–brain barrier. J Neurotraum 16: 1049–1055

26. Petito CK (1979) Early and late mechanisms of increased vascular permeability following experimental cerebral infarction. J Neuropathol Exp Neurol 38: 222–234

27. Preston E, Webster J (2002) Differential passage of [^{14}C]sucrose and [^{3}H]inulin across rat blood–brain barrier after cerebral ischemia. Acta Neuropathol 103: 237–242

28. Qin Z, Song S, Xi G, Silbergleit R, Keep RF, Hoff JT, Hua Y (2007) Preconditioning with hyperbaric oxygen attenuates brain edema after experimental intracerebral hemorrhage. Neurosurg Focus 22: E13

29. Rosenberg GA, Estrada E, Kelley RO, Kornfeld M (1993) Bacterial collagenase disrupts extracellular matrix and opens blood–brain barrier in rat. Neurosci Lett 160: 117–119

30. Rosenberg GA, Kornfeld M, Estrada E, Kelley RO, Liotta LA, Stetler-Stevenson WG (1992) TIMP-2 reduces proteolytic opening of blood–brain barrier by type IV collagenase. Brain Res 576: 203–207

31. Rosenberg GA, Mun-Bryce S, Wesley M, Kornfeld M (1990) Collagenase-induced intracerebral hemorrhage in rats. Stroke 21: 801–807

32. Stamatovic SM, Shakui P, Keep RF, Moore BB, Kunkel SL, Van Rooijen N, Andjelkovic AV (2005) Monocyte chemoattractant protein-1 regulation of blood–brain barrier permeability. J Cereb Blood Flow Metab 25: 593–606

33. Stamatovic SM, Dimitrijevic OB, Keep RF, Andjelkovic AV (2006) Protein kinase C-alpha-RhoA cross-talk in CCL2-induced alterations in brain endothelial permeability. J Biol Chem 281: 8379–8388

34. Wagner KR (2007) Modeling intracerebral hemorrhage: glutamate, nuclear factor-kappa B signaling and cytokines. Stroke 38: 753–758

35. Wagner KR, Xi G, Hua Y, Kleinholz M, de Courten-Myers GM, Myers RE, Broderick JP, Brott TG (1996) Lobar intracerebral hemorrhage model in pigs: rapid edema development in perihematomal white matter. Stroke 27: 490–497

36. Wagner KR, Xi G, Hua Y, Zuccarello M, de Courten-Myers GM, Broderick JP, Brott TG (1999) Ultra-early clot aspiration after lysis with tissue plasminogen activator in a porcine model of intracerebral hemorrhage: edema reduction and blood brain barrier protection. J Neurosurg 90: 491–498

37. Wagner KR, Beiler S, Beiler C, Kirkman J, Casey K, Robinson T, Larnard D, de Courten-Myers GM, Linke MJ, Zuccarello M (2006) Delayed profound local brain hypothermia markedly reduces interleukin-1beta gene expression and vasogenic edema development in a porcine model of intracerebral hemorrhage. Acta Neurochir Suppl 96: 177–182

38. Xi G, Hua Y, Bhasin RR, Ennis SR, Keep RF, Hoff JT (2001) Mechanisms of edema formation after intracerebral hemorrhage: effects of extravasated red blood cells on blood flow and blood–brain barrier integrity. Stroke 32: 2932–2938

39. Xi G, Keep RF, Hoff JT (2006) Mechanisms of brain injury after intracerebral hemorrhage. Lancet Neurol 5: 53–63

40. Yang GY, Betz AL, Chenevert TL, Brunberg JA, Hoff JT (1994) Experimental intracerebral hemorrhage: relationship between brain edema, blood flow, and blood–brain barrier permeability in rats. J Neurosurg 81: 93–102

Acta Neurochir Suppl (2008) 105: 79–83
© Springer-Verlag 2008
Printed in Austria

Treatment of stroke and intracerebral hemorrhage with cellular and pharmacological restorative therapies

M. Chopp, Y. Li

Department of Neurology, Henry Ford Hospital, Detroit, MI, USA

Summary

We describe some of our studies on use of neuro-restorative agents for treatment of neural injury. We focus on cell-based therapies and select from a variety of statins. In addition, we show that cell-based and pharmacological-based therapies enhance brain plasticity and promote recovery of function after stroke and intracerebral hemorrhage (ICH).

Injured brain recapitulates ontogeny. Cerebral tissue around the infarction expresses developmental genes, many of which are present only during embryonic or neonatal stages of development. Brain response to injury undergoes remodeling with induction of angiogenesis, neurogenesis, and synaptogenesis. The attempt at remodeling, although expressed as a partial improvement in patients with stroke and ICH, is clearly insufficient to promote substantial recovery in many patients. The goal of restorative therapies should be to activate and amplify this endogenous restorative brain plasticity process to potentiate functional recovery. The logic of restorative therapy is to treat intact or marginally compromised tissue and not injured or dying tissue. Thus, these treatments can be made available for all neurological injury. Once demonstrated to be effective for treatment of a large middle cerebral artery occlusion (MCAo), these restorative treatments can be applied to many types of injury, including ICH, traumatic brain injury, and neurodegenerative disease such as experimental autoimmune encephalomyelitis and multiple sclerosis.

Keywords: Stroke; intracerebral hemorrhage; cell-based therapy; bone marrow mesenchymal cells; statins; restorative therapy.

Cell-based therapy for stroke and intracerebral hemorrhage (ICH)

The primary action of cell-based therapy in inducing recovery of function after brain injury is to stimulate endogenous restorative mechanisms [12, 14, 26, 33, 37] and not to replace tissue. The cells, whether they be bone marrow mesenchymal [2, 20, 30], neurospheres [13, 35], umbilical cord blood [3, 22], or fetal or embry-onic cells [17, 21], when injected into the adult do not repopulate adult brain tissue; they produce an array of factors including angiogenic and neurotrophic factors that initiate the restorative cascade of recovery [8, 10, 26, 34].

There are various routes of cell administration [2, 15, 16, 36]. Early in the era of cell treatment, the cells were placed directly into the parenchymal tissue, mostly adjacent to areas of damage [15, 30]. It was subsequently shown that these cells could be injected using a vascular route, that they then migrate to the boundary of the lesion and distribute in the microvasculature encompassing the brain lesion [10, 20, 30, 31].

In our studies of stroke, we induce middle cerebral artery occlusion (MCAo) by the placement of a mono-filament into the internal carotid artery to transiently (2 h) [2] or permanently block the MCA [20]. This produces a massive unilateral infarction that encompasses nearly the entire territory of the MCA and results in major and persistent neurological deficits. We have treated this type of lesion with a number of different restorative cell types. We will focus the present data on treatment with bone marrow mesenchymal cells (MSCs).

All animals were subjected to a battery of outcome measures, which include a modified neurological score and adhesive removal tests, among others. Our data show that there is significant and persistent therapeutic benefit when MSCs are administered via a vascular route 1 [2], 7 [2], or 30 days [31] after stroke onset. Some of the treated animals have been permitted to survive for 1 year, at which time significant functional benefit persists [30]. This treatment approach has been extended to models of ICH [28]; 0.1 cc autologous blood is injected into the striatum. This evokes major neurological deficits

Correspondence: Michael Chopp, PhD, Department of Neurology, Henry Ford Hospital, 2799 W. Grand Boulevard, Detroit, MI 48202, USA. e-mail: chopp@neuro.hfh.edu

and has been employed as a standard rodent model of ICH. MSCs were administered 24 h after injection and functional outcome was significantly improved.

A major question is: what underlies this functional improvement? How is the brain being altered so that benefit becomes evident? Here, we will briefly discuss 3 changes in the brain in response to administration of MSCs.

The central hypothesis is that cells evoke restorative responses within the injured brain. Exogenously administered cells act as catalysts to amplify intrinsic restorative processes. To test this, we injected human bone MSCs into rodents subjected to MCAo and measured angiogenic and neurotrophic factors, vascular endothelial growth factor (VEGF). Human and animal forms of VEGF can be readily distinguished [5]. Performing ELISA assays, we found that there was an increase in rodent VEGF in response to the human cells. This suggests that the injected cells stimulate the parenchymal cells to produce VEGF. Immunohistochemical labeling of VEGF demonstrates that the astrocytes express VEGF, and it is possible that the astrocytes are producing a response trophic factors [12]. Parenchymal cells produce a wide array of trophic factors and cytokines in response to MSCs in brain, including brain-derived neurotropic factor (BDNF), fibroblastic growth factor, and endothelial growth factor, among others [24]. *In vitro* studies from our laboratory also demonstrate that production of factors by MSCs, which stimulate the parenchymal cells, are dependent on the microenvironment of the MSCs [8, 26]. For example, the production of stimulatory factors by MSCs is dependent on the calcium levels within the environment [9]. MSC gene is also altered by the environment in which theses cells are placed [8, 26]. Co-culture experiments with normal and ischemic tissue extracts reveal significantly different MSC gene profiles [8, 26]. Thus, there is a dynamic coupling between injected cells and the brain tissue environment, which likely dictates the changes in response to cell therapy.

Establishing that MSCs stimulate production of many trophic factors, we next investigated how the brain uses these factors and how the is brain altered. A major mechanism in brain repair and plasticity is the induction of angiogenesis. MSCs significantly increase angiogenesis in the boundary of ischemic brain [5]. Vascular density in the penumbral regions of ischemic brain is significantly upregulated. Angiogenic vessels are critically important in brain remodeling. Newly-formed vessels produce an array of factors that can contribute to brain plasticity. Among the factors produced by newly-formed vessels are BDNF, which is a potent neurotrophic factor, and matrix metalloproteinases, which are chemotactic for endogenous neural stem cells. Angiopoietin 1 and its receptor, Tie2, are also upregulated in ischemic brain in response to MSC therapy [33]. These factors are responsible for the maturation and stabilization of this newly-formed vasculature. We also note that it is not only angiogenesis that may be increased by the exogenously administered cells; vasculogenesis and arteriogenesis likely occur and promote brain recovery.

Complementing the increase in angiogenesis is the amplification of neurogenesis in the ischemic and injured brain after treatment of stroke [6] and ICH [28] with cell-based therapy. There are 2 primary regions of neurogenesis in the injured brain: the subventricular zone (SVZ) and the subgranular layer of the hippocampus [1]. The SVZ is the primary neurogenic region in response to stroke. In the normal uninjured brain, cells generated within the SVZ migrate along the rostral migratory stream to the olfactory bulb. However, after an injury such as stroke, the cells originating within the SVZ migrate to the region of injury, where they localize in the boundary region and integrate into tissue and stimulate synaptogenesis [39]. The SVZ cells contribute to improved neurological function. Treatment of stroke and ICH with MSCs significantly amplifies the generation of SVZ cells [6, 28]. These cells also selectively migrate to the compromised vasculature in the boundary region of the brain, where they form a vascular niche, a domain, a microenvironment, which couples brain plasticity, synaptogenesis, and neurogenesis [35]. SVZ cells also stimulate angiogenic endothelial cells, which subsequently attract additional neuroblasts from the SVZ and provide them with trophic factors. The SVZs also promote angiogenesis and augment synaptic connections and activity.

White matter changes in brain

Treatment of stroke stimulates the production of progenitor oligodendrocytes and mature oligodendrocytes. These cells produce myelin and are essential for viability of the white matter tracks in the central nervous system (CNS). Thus, we investigated the changes in white matter tracks in the brain after stroke and treatment with MSCs [18, 20, 29]. After stroke, the thickness of the ipsilateral corpus callosum was significantly increased [18]. After treatment of stroke with MSCs, both ipsilateral and contralateral corpus callosum were significantly increased compared with non-treated stroke animals. MSCs also cause white matter growth and near-encapsulation of the ischemic lesion. Axonal fibers permeate scar tissue around the infarct and project around and into the lesional tissue. This is also observed on MRI using fiber tracking techniques [13]. White matter bundles within the injured striatum were significantly altered by MSCs. After stroke, white matter bundles in the striatum are disrupted and the numbers of intact white matter bundles are significantly reduced. MSCs greatly increase the numbers of intact white matter bundles compared with non-treated animals. These substantial changes in white-matter architecture in response to cell treatment can be monitored using MRI tractography techniques. Particularly, methods such as diffusion tensor imaging (DTI) and fractional anisotropy (FA) provide an index of tissue structure [13]. The diffusion constant can be used to survey and characterize the structure of injured cerebral tissue. When the diffusion constant is isotropic, there is cavitation of the cerebral tissue, no structure. We have found that the MRI parameter FA is highly correlated to functional outcome. Higher FA values along the boundary of the ischemic tissue indicate better functional recovery. White matter changes are also prominent in the spinal cord in response to MSC treatment of stroke.

Thus, treatment of stroke and ICH with cell-based therapies stimulates changes in the brain, which interact to promote functional benefit. The injected cells produce many factors that stimulate neuro-restorative factors in parenchymal cells, which alter brain architecture, angiogenesis, neurogenesis, produce white matter changes, and promote functional recovery from stroke and ICH.

Pharmacological based therapies for the treatment of stroke and ICH

Our laboratory has investigated multiple approaches to stimulate functional recovery after neural injury. Included among these are, nitric oxide (NO) donors [10], cyclic guanosine monophosphate (cGMP) upregulated by phosphodiesterase 5 inhibitors [38], statins [19], erythropoietin [32], and carbamylated erythropoietin [25] and high density lipoproteins, among others. These data demonstrate that there are key molecular triggers that promote brain remodeling. In this study, we focus on statins as restorative therapeutic agents.

Statins, hydroxymethylglutaryl coenzyme A reductase inhibitors, are pleiotropic agents that have been most notably used for the reduction of cholesterol, primarily reducing low density lipoprotein, the bad cholesterol [11]. However, these agents have many protective and restorative effects that go well beyond the beneficial effects on cholesterol. Statins also increase NO and cGMP and stimulate signal transduction pathways, which lead to recovery of neurological function following neural injury.

We have employed statins in the treatment of stroke [7], ICH [27], and traumatic brain injury (TBI) [23], demonstrating a robust therapeutic benefit as restorative agents. Statins given 1 day after stroke, ICH, or TBI significantly enhance many of the neuro-restorative factors noted above, including angiogenesis, neurogenesis, and synaptogenesis. The response of stroke, ICH, and TBI to statins also shows a prominent dose-response with low doses (e.g., 1 mg/kg), demonstrating significantly improved functional benefit; high doses (e.g., 8 mg/kg) show no benefit, and possibly a reversal of benefit [27]. These *in vivo* data are also evident in the *in vivo* dose-response of angiogenesis after treatment with statins, with low-dose showing a robust angiogenesis and high-dose a diminution. *In vitro* data show similar profiles [7]. Studies in cell culture of primary neurons show a statin dose-dependent effect on neurite outgrowth and endothelial cell angiogenic tubule formation [4]. Statins are relatively safe drugs with many benefits and can be easily translated into the clinic for neuro-restorative treatments. Based on the extensive preclinical studies in the treatment of multiple models of neural injury with statins, Dr. Don Seyfried of Henry Ford Hospital has initiated a Phase I study for the treatment of ICH patients with statins.

Conclusions and summary

For decades, the focus of much research for the treatment of ICH and stroke has been on neuroprotection. The results of these studies have not been promising and there are essentially no neuroprotective agents on the market for clinical use, save thrombolysis within a 3-hour therapeutic window for stroke. This failure may, to an extent, be attributed to the need to treat very early after the onset of injury. For treatment to be effective, cerebral perfusion must also be adequate to support treatment and the metabolic viability the tissue, and to inhibit the often-inexorable cascade of events that simply destroy brain tissue.

The goals of our research have been to reduce or minimize brain damage and sequelae. In restorative therapy, we treat the intact tissue. Treatment can be initiated many hours, days, or weeks after injury. The goal of this treatment is to stimulate endogenous restorative events present, but at low levels, within the injured brain. Here, we have focused on some of our studies on the use of MSCs as a cell-based therapy and statins as a pharmacological based-therapy to remodel brain and enhance functional recovery after cerebral injury. Our data bring promise that the era of stimulating recovery of neurological function by cell or drug treatment is at hand.

Acknowledgments

Funding of this study was provided by the National Institutes of Health/ National Institute of Neurological Disorders, Center for Stroke Research, Grant P01NS023393, and Treatment for Neural Injury with MSC's, Grant P01NS042345.

References

1. Alvarez-Buylla A, Lim DA (2004) For the long run: maintaining germinal niches in the adult brain. Neuron 41: 683–686
2. Chen J, Li Y, Wang L, Zhang Z, Lu D, Lu M, Chopp M (2001) Therapeutic benefit of intravenous administration of bone marrow stromal cells after cerebral ischemia in rats. Stroke 32: 1005–1011
3. Chen J, Sanberg PR, Li Y, Wang L, Lu M, Willing AE, Sanchez-Ramos J, Chopp M (2001) Intravenous administration of human umbilical cord blood reduces behavioral deficits after stroke in rats. Stroke 32: 2682–2688
4. Chen J, Zhang ZG, Li Y, Wang Y, Wang L, Jiang H, Zhang C, Lu M, Katakowski M, Feldkamp CS, Chopp M (2003) Statins induce angiogenesis, neurogenesis, and synaptogenesis after stroke. Ann Neurol 53: 743–751
5. Chen J, Zhang ZG, Li Y, Wang L, Xu YX, Gautam SC, Lu M, Zhu Z, Chopp M (2003) Intravenous administration of human bone marrow stromal cells induces angiogenesis in the ischemic boundary zone after stroke in rats. Circ Res 92: 692–699
6. Chen J, Li Y, Zhang R, Katakowski M, Gautam SC, Xu Y, Lu M, Zhang Z, Chopp M (2004) Combination therapy of stroke in rats with a nitric oxide donor and human bone marrow stromal cells enhances angiogenesis and neurogenesis. Brain Res 1005: 21–28
7. Chen J, Zacharek A, Li A, Cui X, Roberts C, Lu M, Chopp M (2008) Atorvastatin promotes presenilin-1 expression and Notch1 activity and increases neural progenitor cell proliferation after stroke. Stroke 39: 220–226
8. Chen X, Li Y, Wang L, Katakowski M, Zhang L, Chen J, Xu Y, Gautam SC, Chopp M (2002) Ischemic rat brain extracts induce human marrow stromal cell growth factor production. Neuropathology 22: 275–279
9. Chen XG, Li Y, Wang L, Katakowski M, Zhang LJ, Chen J, Xu YX, Gautam SC, Chopp M (2002) Calcium promotes secretion of growth factors from human bone marrow stromal cells (hMSCs) and tube formation of human brain microvessel endothelial cells. Stroke 33: 401
10. Cui X, Chen J, Zacharek A, Li Y, Roberts C, Kapke A, Savant-Bhonsale S, Chopp M (2007) Nitric oxide donor upregulation of stromal cell-derived factor-1/chemokine (CXC motif) receptor 4 enhances bone marrow stromal cell migration into ischemic brain after stroke. Stem Cells 25: 2777–2785
11. Davignon J, Montigny M, Dufour R (1992) HMG-CoA reductase inhibitors: a look back and a look ahead. Can J Cardiol 8: 843–864
12. Gao Q, Li Y, Chopp M (2005) Bone marrow stromal cells increase astrocyte survival via upregulation of phosphoinositide 3-kinase/threonine protein kinase and mitogen-activated protein kinase kinase/extracellular signal-regulated kinase pathways and stimulate astrocyte trophic factor gene expression after anaerobic insult. Neuroscience 136: 123–134
13. Jiang Q, Zhang ZG, Ding GL, Silver B, Zhang L, Meng H, Lu M, Pourabdillah-Nejed DS, Wang L, Savant-Bhonsale S, Li L, Bagher-Ebadian H, Hu J, Arbab AS, Vanguri P, Ewing JR, Ledbetter KA, Chopp M (2006) MRI detects white matter reorganization after neural progenitor cell treatment of stroke. Neuroimage 32: 1080–1089
14. Li Y, Jiang N, Powers C, Chopp M (1998) Neuronal damage and plasticity identified by microtubule-associated protein 2, growth-associated protein 43, and cyclin D1 immunoreactivity after focal cerebral ischemia in rats. Stroke 29: 1972–1981
15. Li Y, Chopp M, Chen J, Wang L, Gautam SC, Xu YX, Zhang Z (2000) Intrastriatal transplantation of bone marrow nonhematopoietic cells improves functional recovery after stroke in adult mice. J Cereb Blood Flow Metab 20: 1311–1319
16. Li Y, Chen J, Chen XG, Wang L, Gautam SC, Xu YX, Katakowski M, Zhang LJ, Lu M, Janakiraman N, Chopp M (2002) Human marrow stromal cell therapy for stroke in rat: neurotrophins and functional recovery. Neurology 59: 514–523
17. Li Y, Yang XY, Chen J, Wang Y, Zhang C, Chen XG, Katakowski M, Mikkelsen T, Lu M, Chopp M (2002) Transplantation of a new composite of neural cells and marrow stromal cells into rat brain after stroke. Neurosci Res Commun 31: 155–163
18. Li Y, Chen J, Zhang CL, Wang L, Lu D, Katakowski M, Gao Q, Shen LH, Zhang J, Lu M, Chopp M (2005) Gliosis and brain remodeling after treatment of stroke in rats with marrow stromal cells. Glia 49: 407–417
19. Liu XS, Zhang ZG, Zhang L, Morris DC, Kapke A, Lu M, Chopp M (2006) Atorvastatin downregulates tissue plasminogen activator-aggravated genes mediating coagulation and vascular permeability in single cerebral endothelial cells captured by laser microdissection. J Cereb Blood Flow Metab 26: 787–796
20. Liu Z, Li Y, Qu R, Shen L, Gao Q, Zhang X, Lu M, Savant-Bhonsale S, Borneman J, Chopp M (2007) Axonal sprouting into the denervated spinal cord and synaptic and postsynaptic protein expression in the spinal cord after transplantation of bone marrow stromal cell in stroke rats. Brain Res 1149: 172–180
21. Lu D, Li Y, Mahmood A, Wang L, Rafiq T, Chopp M (2002) Neural and marrow-derived stromal cell sphere transplantation in a rat model of traumatic brain injury. J Neurosurg 97: 935–940
22. Lu D, Sanberg PR, Mahmood A, Li Y, Wang L, Sanchez-Ramos J, Chopp M (2002) Intravenous administration of human umbilical cord blood reduces neurological deficit in the rat after traumatic brain injury. Cell Transplant 11: 275–281
23. Lu D, Qu C, Goussev A, Jiang H, Lu C, Schallert T, Mahmood A, Chen J, Li Y, Chopp M (2007) Statins increase neurogenesis in the dentate gyrus, reduce delayed neuronal death in the hippocampal CA3 region, and improve spatial learning in rat after traumatic brain injury. J Neurotraum 24: 1132–1146
24. Mahmood A, Lu D, Chopp M (2004) Intravenous administration of marrow stromal cells (MSCs) increases the expression of growth factors in rat brain after traumatic brain injury. J Neurotraum 21: 33–39
25. Mahmood A, Lu D, Qu C, Goussev A, Zhang ZG, Lu C, Chopp M (2007) Treatment of traumatic brain injury in rats with erythropoietin and carbamylated erythropoietin. J Neurosurg 107: 392–397
26. Qu R, Li Y, Gao Q, Shen L, Zhang J, Liu Z, Chen X, Chopp M (2007) Neurotrophic and growth factor gene expression profiling of

mouse bone marrow stromal cells induced by ischemic brain extracts. Neuropathology 27: 355–363

27. Seyfried D, Han Y, Lu D, Chen J, Bydon A, Chopp M (2004) Improvement in neurological outcome after administration of ator-vastatin following experimental intracerebral hemorrhage in rats. J Neurosurg 101: 104–107

28. Seyfried D, Ding J, Han Y, Li Y, Chen J, Chopp M (2006) Effects of intravenous administration of human bone marrow stromal cells after intracerebral hemorrhage in rats. J Neurosurg 104: 313–318

29. Shen LH, Li Y, Chen J, Zhang J, Vanguri P, Borneman J, Chopp M (2006) Intracarotid transplantation of bone marrow stromal cells increases axon-myelin remodeling after stroke. Neuroscience 137: 393–399

30. Shen LH, Li Y, Chen J, Cui Y, Zhang C, Kapke A, Lu M, Savant-Bhonsale S, Chopp M (2007) One-year follow-up after bone marrow stromal cell treatment in middle-aged female rats with stroke. Stroke 38: 2150–2156

31. Shen LH, Li Y, Chen J, Zacharek A, Gao Q, Kapke A, Lu M, Raginski K, Vanguri P, Smith A, Chopp M (2007) Therapeutic benefit of bone marrow stromal cells administered 1 month after stroke. J Cereb Blood Flow Metab 27: 6–13

32. Wang L, Zhang Z, Wang Y, Zhang R, Chopp M (2004) Treatment of stroke with erythropoietin enhances neurogenesis and angio-genesis and improves neurological function in rats. Stroke 35: 1732–1737

33. Zacharek A, Chen J, Cui X, Li A, Li Y, Roberts C, Feng Y, Gao Q, Chopp M (2007) Angiopoietin1/Tie2 and VEGF/Flk1 induced by MSC treatment amplifies angiogenesis and vascular stabilization after stroke. J Cereb Blood Flow Metab 27: 1684–1691

34. Zhang ZG, Zhang L, Jiang Q, Zhang R, Davies K, Powers C, Bruggen N, Chopp M (2000) VEGF enhances angiogenesis and promotes blood-brain barrier leakage in the ischemic brain. J Clin Invest 106: 829–838

35. Zhang RL, Zhang L, Zhang ZG, Morris D, Jiang Q, Wang L, Zhang LJ, Chopp M (2003) Migration and differentiation of adult rat subventricular zone progenitor cells transplanted into the adult rat striatum. Neuroscience 116: 373–382

36. Zhang ZG, Jiang Q, Jiang F, Ding G, Zhang R, Wang L, Zhang L, Robin AM, Katakowski M, Chopp M (2004) In vivo magnetic resonance imaging tracks adult neural progenitor cell targeting of brain tumor. Neuroimage 23: 281–287

37. Zhang C, Li Y, Chen J, Gao Q, Zacharek A, Kapke A, Chopp M (2006) Bone marrow stromal cells upregulate expression of bone morphogenetic proteins 2 and 4, gap junction protein connexin-43 and synaptophysin after stroke in rats. Neuroscience 141: 687–695

38. Zhang L, Zhang Z, Zhang RL, Cui Y, LaPointe MC, Silver B, Chopp M (2006) Tadalafil, a long-acting type 5 phosphodiesterase isoenzyme inhibitor, improves neurological functional recovery in a rat model of embolic stroke. Brain Res 1118: 192–198

39. Zhang RL, LeTourneau Y, Gregg SR, Wang Y, Toh Y, Robin AM, Zhang ZG, Chopp M (2007) Neuroblast division during migration toward the ischemic striatum: a study of dynamic migratory and proliferative characteristics of neuroblasts from the subventricular zone. J Neurosci 27: 3157–3162

Acta Neurochir Suppl (2008) 105: 85–87
© Springer-Verlag 2008
Printed in Austria

Deficiency of CD18 gene reduces brain edema in experimental intracerebral hemorrhage in mice

E. Titova[5], C. G. Kevil[2], R. P. Ostrowski[1], H. Rojas[1], S. Liu[1], J. H. Zhang[1,3,4], J. Tang[1]

[1] Department of Physiology and Pharmacology, Loma Linda University, Loma Linda, CA, USA
[2] Department of Pathology, Louisiana State University Health Sciences Center, Shreveport, Louisiana, USA
[3] Department of Neurosurgery, Loma Linda University, Loma Linda, CA, USA
[4] Department of Anesthesiology, Loma Linda University, Loma Linda, CA, USA
[5] Department of Anesthesiology, Krasnoyarsk State Medical University, Krasnoyarsk, Russia

Summary

Experimental studies of intracerebral hemorrhage (ICH) point toward leukocytes as a major contributor to ICH-induced brain injury. Leukocyte and endothelial cell adhesion molecules are responsible for injurious neutrophil-endothelial cell interactions in vasculature. Since deficiency of leukocyte-expressed CD18 protects against ischemia-reperfusion injury, we hypothesized that such deficiency may have similar effect in ICH-induced injury. Our aim was to investigate whether CD18 deficiency affords neuroprotection by decreasing ICH-induced brain injury, thereby improving neurological function and reducing mortality.

A total of 20 males wild-type CD18$^{+/+}$ mice and 12 CD18$^{-/-}$ knockout mice were used in our study. ICH was induced by collagenase injection. Mortality, neurological function, and brain edema were measured at 24 h after ICH. Data were analyzed by ANOVA, Chi-square, and Student t-test. Differences of $p < 0.05$ were considered statistically significant.

Our study showed that the increase in brain water content caused by ICH was significantly smaller in CD18 knockout mice compared with wild-type mice ($p < 0.05$, Student t-test). This result correlated with a tendency toward improvement of neurological function and a decrease in mortality. We conclude that CD18 deficiency significantly reduces brain edema after ICH, which corresponds with a trend toward reduction in neurological deficit and mortality.

Keywords: CD18$^{-/-}$; integrins; inflammation; intracerebral hemorrhage; collagenase; edema; mice.

Introduction

Inflammation plays an extremely important role in intracerebral hemorrhage (ICH)-induced brain injury. Both animal models and human studies show inflammatory response occurring in and around blood clot. This response is mainly characterized by infiltration of leuko-

cytes and macrophages, which, along with activation of microglia, peaks at 48–72 h after ICH onset [2, 15].

Leukocyte and endothelial cell adhesion molecules are responsible for neutrophil-endothelial cell interactions in vasculature, and are necessary for leukocyte recruitment. Interactions between β_2 integrins (CD18) and intercellular adhesion molecule-1 (ICAM-1) are responsible for firm adhesion of neutrophils to the endothelium in the acute stage of inflammation [12]. Leukocyte-expressed CD18 is extremely important, since deficiency of CD18 plays a great role in lessening of ischemia-reperfusion injury [5, 6]. However it is still unknown how neutrophil-endothelial cell interactions contribute in ICH-induced brain injury.

We used mice genetically engineered with a targeted mutation of CD18, the common β_2 subunit of CD11/CD18 integrins. We tested our hypothesis that CD18 gene-targeted deficiency decreases ICH-induced brain injury, thereby improving neurological function and reducing mortality.

Materials and methods

Animals

All procedures for these studies were approved by the Animal Care and Use Committee at Loma Linda University and were in compliance with the Guide for the Care and Use of Laboratory Animals. A total of 32, 19- to 22-week-old male mice (24.4 ± 4.8 g) were used in our study: 20 wild-type C57BL/6J, and 12 CD18 knockout mice (C57BL/6J-Itgb2tm2bay).

Mice were housed in a specific pathogen-free facility with controlled temperature and humidity, with 12-h light/dark cycles, and were allowed free access to food and water. All neurological tests were performed during the light cycle.

Correspondence: Jiping Tang, MD, Department of Physiology and Pharmacology, Loma Linda University Medical Center, 11041 Campus Street, Risley Hall Room 133, Loma Linda, CA 92354, USA. e-mail: jtang@llu.edu

Experimental design

Mice were divided into wild-type and CD18$^{-/-}$ knockout groups. All animals were sacrificed one day after ICH induction, when neurological testing was performed. Brain samples were collected for measurements of brain edema and hemorrhage volume. Evaluation of neurological deficit was carried out by investigators blinded to mice type. Mortality was examined 24 h after stroke onset.

ICH induction

We performed the collagenase-induced ICH model as previously described [9]. Briefly, under ketamine (100 mg/kg, i.p.) and xylazine (5 mg/kg, i.p.) anesthesia, a 27-gauge needle was inserted stereotaxically into the right basal ganglia (coordinates: 0.09 mm posterior, 0.4 mm ventral, and 0.12 mm lateral to the bregma). Then the collagenase (0.075 U in 0.5 μL of saline; VII-S, Sigma-Aldrich, St. Louis, MO) was infused into the brain over 2 min at a rate 0.25 μL/min with a micro-infusion pump (Harvard Apparatus, Holliston, MA). The needle was left in place for additional 10 min after injection to prevent the possible leakage of collagenase solution.

Neurological deficit

Neurological evaluation was conducted using a 28-point neurological scoring system developed by Clark *et al.* [1] at 24 h after ICH. The examiner had no knowledge of procedure or mice type. The neurobehavioral study consisted of 7 tests with a score of 0–4 for each test. The 7 tests are: 1) Body symmetry (open bench top); 2) Gait (open bench top); 3) Climbing (gripping surface, 45° angle); 4) Circling behavior (open bench top); 5) Front limb symmetry (mouse suspended by its tail); 6) Compulsory circling (front limbs on bench, rear suspended by tail); and 7) Whisker response (light touch from behind). The score given to each mouse at the completion of the evaluation is the sum of all 7 individual test scores. The minimum neurological score was "0" for healthy mouse and the maximum was "28" for mouse with greatest focal deficit.

Brain water content

Brain water content was measured and calculated as previously described [9]. For calculations the following formula was used: [(WW-DW)/WW] × 100%.

Hemorrhage volume

Hemoglobin assay was conducted as described previously [9]. The ipsilateral hemispheres were homogenized, centrifuged, and Drabkin's reagent (400 μL; Sigma-Aldrich) was added to the resultant supernatants. Absorbance was determined by means of a spectrophotometer at wavelength of 540 nm. The amount of blood in each brain was calculated using a standard curve generated from known blood volumes.

Statistical analysis

Quantitative data are expressed as mean ± SEM. Statistical comparisons were conducted using ANOVA, Chi-square, and Student *t*-test for intergroup comparisons. Differences of $p < 0.05$ were considered statistically significant.

Results

Neurological evaluation

Intracerebral collagenase injection induced significant neurological deficit in the ICH model for both wild-type

and CD18$^{-/-}$ mice (Table 2). Neurological examination revealed tendency toward a decrease in neurological deficit in CD18$^{-/-}$ mice 24 h after ICH onset, but the difference was not significant when compared with wild-type mice ($p > 0.05$, Student *t*-test).

Brain water content

Brain water content increased markedly after collagenase injection in all ICH mice (Table 1), especially in the ipsilateral hemisphere ($p < 0.05$ ipsilateral vs. contralateral, ANOVA). Brain water content was significantly reduced in CD18 null mice when compared with wild-type 24 h after ICH onset (Student *t*-test, $p < 0.05$). No water content changes were observed in cerebellum between all groups ($p > 0.05$, ANOVA).

Mortality

Mortality was reduced in CD 18$^{-/-}$ mice compared with wild-type mice (Table 2); however, this reduction

Table 1. *Percent brain edema in wild-type and CD18$^{-/-}$ knockout mice after intracerebral hemorrhage*

Mice	Right hemisphere	Left hemisphere	Cerebellum
Wild-type	80.339 ± 0.204	78.659 ± 0.243	77.198 ± 0.070
CD18$^{-/-}$	79.623 ± 0.221*	78.189 ± 0.143	77.237 ± 0.063

* $p < 0.05$ vs. wild-type; unpaired *t*-test, mean ± SEM.

Table 2. *Differences in neurological function, mortality, and hemorrhage volume between wild-type and CD18$^{-/-}$ knockout mice after intracerebral hemorrhage*

Mice	Neurological function	Mortality	Hemorrhage volume (mg/hemisphere)
Wild-type	6.33 ± 1.92; n = 20	45% (9/20)	3.69 ± 0.76, n = 5
CD18$^{-/-}$	10.13 ± 2.10, n = 12	33.3% (4/12)	3.77 ± 0.64, n = 3

$p > 0.05$, unpaired *t*-test, mean ± SEM.

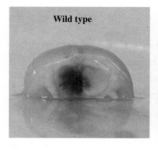 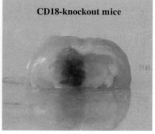

Fig. 1. Representative photographs of brains with hemorrhage in wild-type and CD18$^{-/-}$ knockout mice. Hemorrhage volume did not differ between groups

was not significant ($p > 0.05$, Chi-square and Fisher tests).

Hemorrhage volume

We did not find a statistically significant difference in hemorrhage volume between wild-type and CD18 null mice (Table 2 and Fig. 1), which confirms the consistency of our model ($n = 5$ in wild-type group and $n = 3$ in knockout group).

Discussion

The inflammatory response in areas surrounding lesion brain tissues is extremely important for cell survival or death [8, 10]. Neutrophils are the first peripheral leukocytes to migrate into the brain parenchyma, of which recruitment starts within the first hours after stroke, peaks within 2–3 days, and dissipates after 1 week [10, 15]. Large numbers of neutrophils have been observed migrating out of surrounding blood vessels at the periphery of the hematoma in both collagenase and blood injection models in experimental ICH and in patient autopsy [2, 4].

CD18$^{-/-}$ mutant mice display a phenotype resembling that seen in humans with leukocyte adhesion deficiency (LAD-1). LAD-1 is characterized by the absence of β_2 integrins (CD11/CD18) on leukocytes and the inability of leukocytes, in particular neutrophilic granulocytes, to emigrate from the bloodstream toward sites of inflammation [16]. Neutrophils from CD18$^{-/-}$ mice do not express CD11/CD18 adhesion complexes [14].

The β_2 integrins mediate firm adhesion of polymorphonuclear leukocytes (PMNs) to the endothelial cells, which represents a prerequisite for PMN extravasation and, as was shown in previous studies, β_2 integrins are involved in the control of the lifetime of emigrating PMNs by triggering apoptosis [11]. As previously reported, β_2 integrins regulate adhesion-dependent injury responses on venular endothelium after ischemia reperfusion through adhesion events involving activated endothelial cells and leukocytes [6, 7]. These processes could lead to alteration of blood–brain barrier permeability and brain edema, and may contribute to hematoma expansion [3, 13].

Concordantly, our present results suggest that CD18 deficiency significantly diminished brain edema formation in the collagenase model of ICH. A trend toward reduced mortality and improved neurological status after collagenase-induced ICH was also found in CD18 deficient mice. Further study is required to better understand the mechanism involved in CD18 regulation of ICH.

Acknowledgment

This work was supported by a grant from the National Institutes of Health (NS052492) to Jiping Tang.

References

1. Clark W, Gunion-Rinker L, Lessov N, Hazel K (1998) Citicoline treatment for experimental intracerebral hemorrhage in mice. Stroke 29: 2136–2140
2. Gong C, Hoff JT, Keep RF (2000) Acute inflammatory reaction following experimental intracerebral hemorrhage in rat. Brain Res 871: 57–65
3. Hu B, Liu C, Zivin JA (1999) Reduction of intracerebral hemorrhaging in a rabbit embolic stroke model. Neurology 53: 2140–2145
4. Huang J, Upadhyay UM, Tamargo RJ (2006) Inflammation in stroke and focal cerebral ischemia. Surg Neurol 66: 232–245
5. Jones SP, Trocha SD, Strange MB, Granger DN, Kevil CG, Bullard DC, Lefer DJ (2000) Leukocyte and endothelial cell adhesion molecules in a chronic murine model of myocardial reperfusion injury. Am J Physiol Heart Circ Physiol 279: H2196–H2201
6. Kakkar AK, Lefer DJ (2004) Leukocyte and endothelial adhesion molecule studies in knockout mice. Curr Opin Pharmacol 4: 154–158
7. Suzuki K, Masawa N, Takatama M (2001) The pathogenesis of cerebrovascular lesions in hypertensive rats. Med Electron Microsc 34: 230–239
8. Szymanska A, Biernaskie J, Laidley D, Granter-Button S, Corbett D (2006) Minocycline and intracerebral hemorrhage: influence of injury severity and delay to treatment. Exp Neurol 197: 189–196
9. Tang J, Liu J, Zhou C, Ostanin D, Grisham MB, Neil Granger D, Zhang JH (2005) Role of NADPH oxidase in the brain injury of intracerebral hemorrhage. J Neurochem 94: 1342–1350
10. Wang J, Doré S (2007) Inflammation after intracerebral hemorrhage. J Cereb Blood Flow Metab 27: 894–908
11. Weinmann P, Scharffetter-Kochanek K, Forlow SB, Peters T, Walzog B (2003) A role for apoptosis in the control of neutrophil homeostasis in the circulation: insights from CD18-deficient mice. Blood 101: 739–746
12. Winn R, Vedder N, Ramamoorthy C, Sharar S, Harlan J (1998) Endothelial and leukocyte adhesion molecules in inflammation and disease. Blood Coagul Fibrinolysis 9(Suppl 2): S17–S23
13. Wu G, Xi G, Huang F (2006) Spontaneous intracerebral hemorrhage in humans: hematoma enlargement, clot lysis, and brain edema. Acta Neurochir Suppl 96: 78–80
14. Wu H, Prince JE, Brayton CF, Shah C, Zeve D, Gregory SH, Smith CW, Ballantyne CM (2003) Host resistance of CD18 knockout mice against systemic infection with Listeria monocytogenes. Infect Immun 71: 5986–5993
15. Xi G, Keep RF, Hoff JT (2006) Mechanisms of brain injury after intracerebral haemorrhage. Lancet Neurol 5: 53–63
16. Yakubenia S, Wild MK (2006) Leukocyte adhesion deficiency II. Advances and open questions. FEBS J 273: 4390–4398

Acta Neurochir Suppl (2008) 105: 89–93
© Springer-Verlag 2008
Printed in Austria

Tissue inhibitor of matrix metalloproteinases-3 (TIMP-3) lacks involvement in bacterial collagenase-induced intracerebral hemorrhage in mouse

M. Grossetete[1], G. A. Rosenberg[2]

[1] Department of Neurology, University of New Mexico Health Sciences Center, Albuquerque, New Mexico, USA
[2] Departments of Neurology, Neurosciences, Cell Biology and Physiology, University of New Mexico Health Sciences Center, Albuquerque, New Mexico, USA

Summary

Intracerebral hemorrhage (ICH) leads to delayed cell death in the regions around the hemorrhagic mass. Apoptosis has been identified in the dying cells, but the mechanism involved is unclear. Others and us have shown that matrix metalloproteinases (MMPs) are increased in ICH and could directly contribute to cell death. Tissue inhibitor to metalloproteinases-3 (TIMP-3) facilitates apoptosis in cancer cells and neurons by inhibiting the shedding of tumor necrosis factor-α (TNF-α) death receptors, Fas and p55TNF receptor 1, by MMP-3 and TNF-α converting enzyme (TACE), respectively. Therefore, TIMP-3 may contribute to cell death in ICH. We adapted the bacterial collagenase-induced hemorrhage (CIH) model to the mouse. Adult C57Bl/6 and *Timp-3* knockout mice had CIH. Expression of mRNA for TIMP-3 was determined by real-time PCR. Hemorrhage volume and numbers of apoptotic cells were measured by unbiased stereology. *Timp-3* mRNA was similar in the knockout and wild-type mice prior to injury and induction of CIH failed to cause an increase in Timp-3 mRNA in the wild-type. Furthermore, there were no differences found in the hemorrhage size or in the numbers of apoptotic cells between the *Timp-3* knockout or wild-type. We were unable to prove the hypothesis that TIMP-3 is involved cell death in CIH in the mouse.

Keywords: Matrix metalloproteinases; tissue inhibitor of metalloproteinases-3; intracerebral hemorrhage; collagenase-induced intracerebral hemorrhage; mouse.

Introduction

Edema, growth of the hemorrhage, and delayed cell death contribute to the poor prognosis associated with intracerebral hemorrhage (ICH) as compared to that of patients with comparably sized ischemic strokes [8]. The endogenous production of matrix metalloproteinases (MMPs) and the recruitment of MMP-laden leukocytes has been implicated in the progressive injury [10]. A delayed apoptotic cell death has been observed in experimental models of ICH, but the factors involved in the inflammatory cell death are uncertain. We hypothesized that tissue inhibitor of metalloproteinases-3 (TIMP-3) was involved in apoptosis after ICH. To test the hypothesis, we used the bacterial collagenase-induced hemorrhage (CIH) model that was developed in our laboratory [11]. TIMP-3 is one of four inhibitors of the MMPs; it is unique because it is bound to the extracellular matrix where it acts to regulate a number of cell surface events [1]. We showed that TIMP-3 expression at both the mRNA and protein levels occur early in stroke [13]. Neuronal death is attenuated following mild ischemia in the *Timp-3* knockout mouse [14]. These data suggest that TIMP-3 may be involved in cell death in ICH. Therefore, we adapted the CIH model to the mouse and examined the involvement of TIMP-3 in CIH, utilizing *Timp-3* knockout and wild-type mice. We characterized the time course of *Timp-3* mRNA, MMP activity in the *Timp-3* knockout, and the role of TIMP-3 in hemorrhage volume and cell death following ICH.

Materials and methods

Stereotactic injection of bacterial collagenase or saline

Animal studies were approved by the Institutional Animal Care and Use Committee (IACUC) and conformed to NIH standards for use of animals in research. The methods used have been described in detail previously [3]. *Timp-3* knockout mice were a gift of Dr. Rama Khokha [6]. Corresponding wild-types were produced by breeding *Timp-3* heterozygotic mice for the homozygotic wild-type genotypes, which were then backcrossed at least 10 generations to produce homozygotic wild-type breeders on a C57Bl/6 background. C57Bl/6 were purchased as controls for the wild-type.

Correspondence: Gary A. Rosenberg, MD, Department of Neurology, MSC10 5620, University of New Mexico Health Sciences Center, Albuquerque, New Mexico 87131-0001, USA. e-mail: grosenberg@salud.unm.edu

Male mice weighing 24–30 g were anesthetized with 2.5% Halothane delivered in 70% nitrous oxide/30% oxygen. Bacterial collagenase (0.5 µL of 0.0375 U Type VII-S; Sigma-Aldrich Corp., St. Louis, MO, USA) or sterile normal saline (Sigma-Aldrich) was injected over two minutes; the needle was left in place another 2 min.

Quantitative TaqMan real-time PCR

Comparison of the time course of *Timp-3* mRNA in mice following 12, 24, 48, and 72 h of CIH or saline injection was performed for *Timp-3* normalized to *Rpl-32*. The mRNA levels were quantitated using the TaqMan real-time PCR assay (Applied Biosystems, Foster City, CA, USA). *Timp-3* and *Rpl-32* mRNA levels in the reaction mixtures were calculated from a standard curve generated by amplification of known concentrations of TIMP-3 and rpl-32 plasmid DNA using the GeneAmp 5700 Sequence Detection System (Applied Biosystems). Plasmids for TIMP-3 and rpl-32 were created using pGEM-T Easy Vector Systems II (Promega, Madison, WI, USA).

Stereological analysis of apoptotic cell counts and hemorrhage volume

Stereological evaluation of TdT-mediated dUTP-biotin nick end-labeling (TUNEL) positive cells was performed, using the optical fractionator method of stereology for CIH in wild-type and *Timp-3* knockout mice. Immunohistochemical analysis of TUNEL positive cells was performed on slide mounted sections (20 µm) using NeuroTACS II (Trevigen Inc., Gaithersburg, MD, USA).

Gelatin-substrate zymography

Brain tissue samples were separated on 10% sodium dodecylsulfate-polyacrylamide gel electrophoresis (SDS-PAGE) gels containing 1%

gelatin (Sigma-Aldrich). After electrophoresis, the gels were washed in 2.5% Triton X-100 (Sigma-Aldrich) to remove the SDS (Fisher Scientific). Following incubation, gels were stained with Coomassie R-250 dye (Sigma-Aldrich) and proteolytic bands were visualized as regions of clear lysis following differentiation in 10% acetic acid. Gels were dried between two sheets of cellophane and scanned with an AGFA Duoscan scanner (AGFA Corp., Ridgefield Park, NJ, USA) followed by densitometric analysis using AlphaEase software (Alpha Innotech Corp., San Leandro, CA, USA).

Immunohistochemical analysis of ICH

At 24 h, anaesthetized mice were perfused transcardially with 2% para-formaldehyde solution containing lysine, and sodium periodate (PLP) (Sigma-Aldrich). The brains were then post-fixed overnight in PLP at 4 °C, cryoprotected in a solution of 30% sucrose (Sigma-Aldrich) at 4 °C, and frozen sections were cut on a cryostat at 16 µm. For immunolabeling, rabbit anti-human TIMP-3 (1:1500, Chemicon), biotin conjugated goat anti-rabbit (1:500, Jackson ImmunoResearch Laboratories, West Grove, PA, USA) and the chromogen diaminobenzidine were utilized with osmium tetroxide enhancement.

Results

Timp-3 mRNA in knockout and wild-type mice after CIH

There were no differences in mRNA levels for *Timp-3*, *Mmp-2, and Mmp-9* between the C57Bl/6 controls and the wild-type (Fig. 1A). We then induced hemorrhagic lesions with bacterial collagenase and measured mRNA;

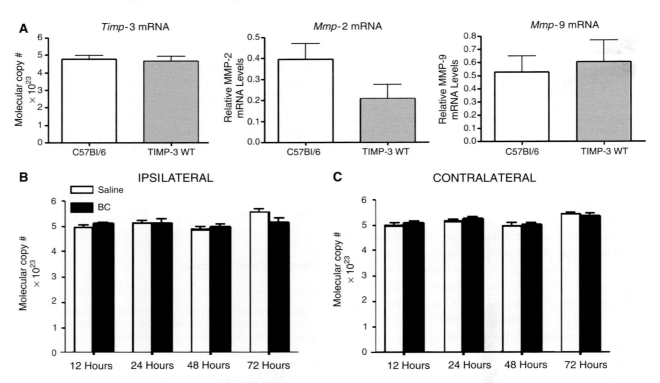

Fig. 1. A) *Timp-3*, *Mmp-2* and *Mmp-9* mRNA levels are similar in C57Bl/6 control and *Timp-3* wild-type mice. B) Time course analysis for *Timp-3* mRNA following CIH shows similarity of the saline-injected and bacterial collagenase-injected mice in the injected hemisphere, and in the contralateral side (C)

we found similar levels of mRNA in knockout and wild-type after CIH, suggesting that *Timp-3* mRNA expression was not altered in CIH in mice. The contribu-

tion of TIMP-3 following the hemorrhagic insult was evaluated by comparing *Timp-3* mRNA levels following either saline or BC intracerebral injection over the time

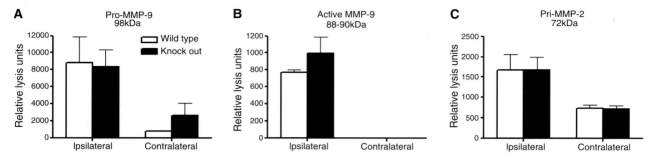

Fig. 2. A) The data from the gelatin zymograms at 72 h after CIH shows similar amounts of latent MMP-9 (98 kDa) in the *Timp-3* knockout and wild-type. B) No differences were seen in the active form of MMP-9 (88 kDa) between knockout and wild-type. C) Latent MMP-2 production was similar and activated forms were not seen

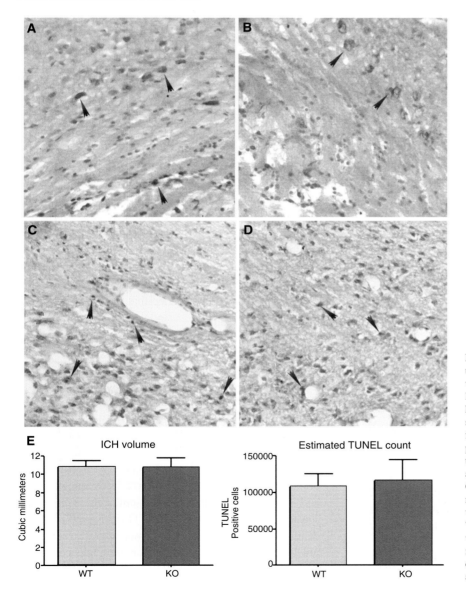

Fig. 3. TIMP-3 following 24 h CIH and unbiased stereological analysis of ICH volume and TUNEL-positive cells following 72 h in wild-type and *Timp-3* knockouts. (A–D) Coronal sections representative of mid-lesion at bregma stained for TIMP-3. Arrowheads indicate TIMP-3 positive cells (40×). (A, C) Ipsilateral to hemorrhage at lateral corpus callosum and border of ICH, respectively. (B, D) Contralateral to hemorrhage of same representative regions. (E) *Timp-3* wild-type versus *Timp-3* knockout mice following 72 h of BC-induced ICH. Hemorrhage volume is not affected in *Timp-3* null mice. The number of TUNEL positive cells is unaffected between the wild-type and knockout

course of 12 to 72 h. The mRNA levels were evaluated in both the ipsilateral injected and contralateral non-injected striata. No increase in mRNA production was observed over the time course measured (Fig. 1B and C).

Gelatinase expression in Timp-3 knockout and wild-mice after CIH

We were unable to detect any differences in the MMP-2 or -9 levels or in their activity between knockout and wild-type; production and activation were similar in the *Timp-3* deficient mice compared to wild-type (Fig. 2). These data suggest that cell death in ICH is not modulated in the same manner as in ischemic stroke where *Timp-3* deficient mice had reduced cell death.

Effect of TIMP-3 on hemorrhage volume and cell death in CIH

Because TIMP-3 may have an effect on cell death independent of an effect on the gelatinases, we investigated the effect of TIMP-3 protein on hemorrhage volume and cell death by comparing *Timp-3* knockout to wild-type mice 72 h after ICH. We found similar hemorrhage volumes and numbers of TUNEL positive cells between the knockout and wild type (Fig. 3E). Additionally, immunohistochemical analysis of TIMP-3 in 24 h CIH C57Bl/6 mice showed similar intensity and staining patterns (Fig. 3A–D).

Discussion

Cell death after ICH occurs by necrosis from ischemia around the lesion or by apoptosis initiated by the inflammatory response [2]. TIMP-3 has been shown to induce apoptosis in cerebral ischemia by blocking the shedding of death receptors from the cell surface [14]. We tested the hypothesis that TIMP-3 contributes to cell death in ICH. We found that the TIMP-3 protein and *Timp-3* mRNA levels were not altered after CIH in the wild-type and that production and activation of MMP-2 and MMP-9 were similarly unaffected in the knockout. Using the *Timp-3* knockout mouse, which was protected from apoptosis after an ischemic injury, we found no differences between the knockout and the wild-type after CIH. More importantly, we were unable to demonstrate a contribution of TIMP-3 to either an increase in brain hemorrhage volume or TUNEL-positive cells.

TIMP-3 is bound to the extracellular matrix where it exerts a number of effects, including enhancing apoptosis in cancer cells [12]. MMP-3 and tumor necrosis factor-α converting enzyme (TACE) act as sheddases, releasing the death receptors, Fas and p55TNF receptor 1, from the cell surface, which protects the cells. TIMP-3 inhibits the sheddases and facilitates apoptosis. We were unable to show that a similar mechanism is occurring in the mouse after CIH. This suggests that a different mechanism is involved in CIH in the mouse. Ischemia leads to expression of a complex set of molecules secondary to the hypoxic stimulus. There is increasing evidence that the main lesion in ICH is inflammation due to the presence of blood products and infiltrating leukocytes [5]. We found recently that inflammation around the site of the bleed led to the release of large amounts of MMP-9 from neutrophils and induction of MMP-3 in microglia/macrophages. One interpretation of the lack of an effect of TIMP-3 in the CIH in mouse is that there is an absence of a strong hypoxic stimulus.

Evidence for apoptotic cell death appears in experimental hemorrhage models including micro-balloon inflation, autologous blood injection, and bacterial collagenase injection [4, 9, 15]. Apoptotic cells were found to be distributed both within the matrix of the hematoma and in the perihematomal region in animal models, and apoptosis has been observed in perihematomal human tissue following ICH. TUNEL-positive cells are found to be mainly neurons and astrocytes within and around the hemorrhage in the BC-induced hemorrhage model [7]. Autologous blood injection resulted in greater than 95% neuronal TUNEL-positive cells around the clot [2]. Cell culture studies showed that BC was not toxic to neurons and suggested that the blood itself was toxic [7].

The presence of TIMP-3 in the adult brain under normal conditions is very low, and following cerebral ischemia it becomes elevated in the cortical neurons that undergo death in the 90 min focal ischemia model in the rat [1]. However, unlike the induction seen for *Timp-3* mRNA following 90-min of middle cerebral artery occlusion in rat, our data show that *Timp-3* mRNA levels are unaltered following saline injection or BC injection from 12 to 72 h. Additionally, hemorrhage volume and cell death were unaltered between wild-type and *Timp-3* null mice 72 h after collagenase injection. These data indicate that unlike TIMP-3 mediated cell death in ischemic neurons, hemorrhagic stroke does not induce TIMP-3 formation nor modulate cell death in this model.

Acknowledgements

Supported by grants from the National Institutes of Health RO1 NS045847 to GAR and F31 NS051144-01A1 to MG from the NIH Minority Biomedical Research Support Program (GM060201) at the University of New Mexico.

References

1. Cunningham LA, Wetzel M, Rosenberg GA (2005) Multiple roles for MMPs and TIMPs in cerebral ischemia. Glia 50: 329–339
2. Gong C, Boulis N, Qian J, Turner DE, Hoff JT, Keep RF (2001) Intracerebral hemorrhage-induced neuronal death. Neurosurgery 48: 875–882
3. Grossetete M, Rosenberg GA (2008) Matrix metalloproteinase inhibition facilitates cell death in intracerebral hemorrhage in mouse. J Cereb Blood Flow Metab 28: 752–763
4. Hickenbottom SL, Grotta JC, Strong R, Denner LA, Aronowski J (1999) Nuclear factor-kappaB and cell death after experimental intracerebral hemorrhage in rats. Stroke 30: 2472–2477
5. Jiang Y, Wu J, Hua Y, Keep RF, Xiang J, Hoff JT, Xi G (2002) Thrombin-receptor activation and thrombin-induced brain tolerance. J Cereb Blood Flow Metab 22: 404–410
6. Leco KJ, Waterhouse P, Sanchez OH, Gowing KL, Poole AR, Wakeham A, Mak TW, Khokha R (2001) Spontaneous air space enlargement in the lungs of mice lacking tissue inhibitor of metalloproteinases-3 (TIMP-3). J Clin Invest 108: 817–829
7. Matsushita K, Meng W, Wang X, Asahi M, Asahi K, Moskowitz MA, Lo EH (2000) Evidence for apoptosis after intercerebral hemorrhage in rat striatum. J Cereb Blood Flow Metab 20: 396–404
8. Mendelow AD, Gregson BA, Fernandes HM, Murray GD, Teasdale GM, Hope DT, Karimi A, Shaw MD, Barer DH (2005) Early surgery versus initial conservative treatment in patients with spontaneous supratentorial intracerebral haematomas in the international surgical trial in intracerebral haemorrhage (STICH): a randomised trial. Lancet 365: 387–397
9. Qureshi AI, Suri MF, Ostrow PT, Kim SH, Ali Z, Shatla AA, Guterman LR, Hopkins LN (2003) Apoptosis as a form of cell death in intracerebral hemorrhage. Neurosurgery 52: 1041–1047
10. Rosenberg GA, Dencoff JE, McGuire PG, Liotta LA, Stetler-Stevenson WG (1994) Injury-induced 92-kDa gelatinase and urokinase expression in rat brain. Lab Invest 71: 417–422
11. Rosenberg GA, Mun-Bryce S, Wesley M, Kornfeld M (1990) Collagenase-induced intracerebral hemorrhage in rats. Stroke 21: 801–807
12. Smith MR, Kung H, Durum SK, Colburn NH, Sun Y (1997) TIMP-3 induces cell death by stabilizing TNF-alpha receptors on the surface of human colon carcinoma cells. Cytokine 9: 770–780
13. Wallace JA, Alexander S, Estrada EY, Hines C, Cunningham LA, Rosenberg GA (2002) Tissue inhibitor of metalloproteinase-3 is associated with neuronal death in reperfusion injury. J Cereb Blood Flow Metab 22: 1303–1310
14. Wetzel M, Li L, Harms KM, Roitbak T, Ventura PB, Rosenberg GA, Khokha R, Cunningham LA (2008) Tissue inhibitor of metalloproteinases-3 facilitates Fas-mediated neuronal cell death following mild ischemia. Cell Death Differ 15: 143–151
15. Xue M, Del Bigio MR (2000) Intracerebral injection of autologous whole blood in rats: time course of inflammation and cell death. Neurosci Lett 283: 230–232

Acta Neurochir Suppl (2008) 105: 95–97
© Springer-Verlag 2008
Printed in Austria

Radial glia marker expression following experimental intracerebral hemorrhage

T. Nakamura[1,2], **Y. Kuroda**[3], **N. Okabe**[1], **S. Shibuya**[4], **N. Kawai**[2], **T. Tamiya**[2], **G. Xi**[5], **R. F. Keep**[5], **T. Itano**[1], **S. Nagao**[2]

[1] Department of Neurobiology, Kagawa University Faculty of Medicine, Miki, Kagawa, Japan
[2] Department of Neurological Surgery, Kagawa University Faculty of Medicine, Miki, Kagawa, Japan
[3] Department of Emergency and Critical Care Medicine, Kagawa University Faculty of Medicine, Miki, Kagawa, Japan
[4] Department of Orthopedic Surgery, Kagawa University Faculty of Medicine, Miki, Kagawa, Japan
[5] Department of Neurosurgery, University of Michigan Medical School, Ann Arbor, Michigan, USA

Summary

In this study, we examine 3CB2 expression, a marker of radial glia, after intracerebral hemorrhage (ICH). Adult male Sprague-Dawley rats received an intracaudate injection of 100 μL autologous whole blood. Animals were sacrificed, and 3CB2 expression was quantified on Western blot. Single and double labeled immunohistochemistry was used to identify which cells express 3CB2. Neurobehavioral examinations (forelimb placing test) were performed as an evaluation of function. By Western blot, 3CB2 was strongly expressed at day 3 and expression persisted for at least 1 month. By immunohistochemistry, 3CB2 immunoreactivity was present in large numbers of astrocytes surrounding the hematoma at day 3 after ICH. At 1 month later, 3CB2 immunoreactivity was co-localized with a neuronal marker (TUC-4). Neurobehavioral function in the 1 month after ICH group was significantly improved compared with that of 3 days after ICH. The ICH-induced 3CB2 expression in astrocytes may reflect an early response of these cells to injury, while the delayed expression in neurons might be a part of the adaptative response to injury, perhaps leading to recovery of neurobehavioral function.

Keywords: 3CB2; radial glia; intracerebral hemorrhage; behavior; rat.

Introduction

Radial glia prolifereate actively during neurogenesis, inducing migration of neurons [4]. One recent study reported that radial glia not only serve as a guide for neurons, but also have properities of neural progenitor cells [7]. Radial glia can be detected by immunoassay using 3CB2 [8]. The effect of intracerebral hemorrhage (ICH) on 3CB2 expression has not been examined. ICH induces perihematomal edema and causes neurological deficits. The mechanisms of brain injury after ICH are not fully understood but are different from ischemic stroke. We examine ICH-induced 3CB2 upregulation in the rat and whether the temporal profile of 3CB2 expression may correlate with marked recovery of function that occurs with time in that species [2].

Materials and methods

Animal preparation and intracerebral infusion

Animal protocols were approved by the Animal Committee of the Kagawa University. Male Sprague-Dawley rats (CLEA, Tokyo, Japan), each weighing 300–400 g, were used for all experiments. Rats were allowed free access to food and water. The animals were anesthetized with pentobarbital (40 mg/kg, i.p.) and the right femoral artery was catheterized to sample blood for intracerebral infusion. The rats were positioned in a stereotaxic frame (Narishige Instruments, Tokyo, Japan) and a cranial burr-hole (1 mm) was drilled near the right coronal suture 3.5 mm lateral to the midline. A 27-gauge needle was inserted stereotaxically into the right basal ganglia (coordinates: 0.2 mm anterior, 5.5 mm ventral, and 3.5 mm lateral to the bregma). Autologous whole blood (100 μL) was infused at a rate of 10 μL/min with the use of a microinfusion pump (Terumo, Tokyo, Japan).

Experimental group

We evaluated the time course of 3CB2 expression after ICH. Rats received an intracaudate injection of 100 μL autologous whole blood. Some rats were sacrificed at day 3 and at 1 month after ICH, and brains were processed for Western blotting ($n = 3$, per time point) to quantify 3CB2 expression. The others were sacrificed at day 3 and at 1 month after ICH for single and double labeled immunochemistry to identify which cells express 3CB2 ($n = 3$, per time point). The following were examined: 3CB2, glial fibrillary acidic protein (GFAP, an astrocyte marker), and TUC-4 (a neuronal precursor marker). In

Correspondence: Takehiro Nakamura, Departments of Neurobiology and Neurological Surgery, Kagawa University Faculty of Medicine, 1750-1 Ikenobe, Miki, Kita, Kagawa 761-0173, Japan. e-mail: tanakamu@kms.ac.jp

the sham group, rats were sacrificed at day 3 and at 1 month after needle insertion (no injection) for immunohistochemistry ($n = 3$, per time point).

Western blot analysis

Animals were anesthetized before undergoing intracardiac perfusion with saline. The brains were then removed and a 3-mm thick coronal brain slice was cut approximately 4 mm from the frontal pole. The slice was separated into ipsilateral and contralateral basal ganglia. Briefly, 50 μg proteins for each were separated by sodium dodecyl sulfate polyacrylamide gel electrophoresis and transferred to a Hybond-C pure nitrocellulose membrane (Amersham Biosciences, Piscataway, NJ, USA). The membranes were blocked in Carnation nonfat milk. Membranes were probed with a 1:1000 dilution of the primary antibody (mouse anti-3CB2; Developmental Studies Hybridoma Bank, University of Iowa, Iowa City, IA, USA) and a 1:1500 dilution of the second antibody (peroxidase-conjugated goat anti-mouse antibody; BioRad Laboratories, Hercules, CA, USA). The antigen-antibody complexes were visualized with a chemiluminescence system (Amersham Biosciences) and exposed to film. The relative densities of bands (55 kDa) were analyzed with NIH Image software (National Institutes of Health, Bethesda, MD, USA).

Histological examination

Rats were anesthetized and underwent intracardiac perfusion with 4% paraformaldehyde in 0.1 mol/L (pH 7.4) phosphate-buffered saline. The brains were removed and kept in 4% paraformaldehyde for 6 h, then immersed in 25% sucrose for 3 to 4 days at 4 °C. Brains were then placed in OCT embedding compound (Sakura Finetek USA Inc., Torrance, CA, USA) and sectioned on a cryostat (18 μm thick). Using the avidin-biotin complex technique, sections were incubated in 1:10 goat or horse serum for 30 min, rinsed, and incubated overnight with the primary antibody. The primary antibodies were mouse anti-3CB2 monoclonal antibody, goat anti-GFAP polyclonal antibody (Santa Cruz Biotechnology, Santa Cruz, CA, USA), and rabbit anti-TUC-4 polyclonal antibody (Chemicon International Inc., Temecula, CA, USA). Normal mouse or rabbit IgG was used as negative control. Sections were incubated with 1:1000 dilution of biotinylated horse anti-mouse IgG, rabbit anti-goat IgG, or goat anti-rabbit IgG (Vector Laboratories, Burlingame, CA, USA) for 90 min and then incubated with avidin-biotinylated horseradish peroxidase (Vector Laboratories) for 90 min.

For immunofluorescent double labeling, each primary antibody was incubated overnight at 4 °C. Rhodamine conjugated goat anti-rabbit (1:100) and fluorescein isothiocyanate (FITC) labeled horse anti-mouse (1:100) second antibodies were incubated with sections for 2 h at room temperature. The double labeling was analyzed by a fluorescence microscope (Carl Zeiss Inc., Germany) with the use of a rhodamine filter and a FITC filter.

Neurobehavioral tests (forelimb placing test)

Forelimb placing was scored using the vibrissae-elicited forelimb placing test [2]. Animals were held by their bodies to allow their forelimbs to hang free. Independent testing of each forelimb was induced by brushing the respective vibrissae on the corner of a table top once per trial for 10 trials. A score of 1 was given each time the rat placed its forelimb onto the edge of the table in response to vibrissae stimulation. Percent successful placing responses were determined for impaired forelimb and non-impaired forelimb.

Statistical analysis

All data in this study are presented as mean ± SD. Data were analyzed using ANOVA or Student *t*-test. Significance levels were measured at $p < 0.05$.

Results

3CB2 expression after ICH

By Western blot analysis, 3CB2 expression in the ipsilateral basal ganglia was significantly increased at 3 days after ICH ($p < 0.01$; Fig. 1), and expression persisted for at least 1 month ($p < 0.05$; Fig. 1). 3CB2 immunoreactivity was present in large numbers of astrocytes (GFAP-positive) surrounding the lesion at 3 days after ICH (Table 1). However, not all 3CB2-positive glia-like cells were GFAP-positive. At 1 month, 3CB2 immunoreactivity was co-lo-

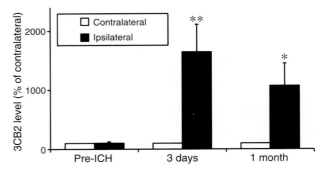

Fig. 1. Western blot analysis of 3CB2 expression in contralateral and ipsilateral basal ganglia at day 3 and 1 month after ICH ($n = 3$ in each group). Values are mean ± SD. *$p < 0.05$ and **$p < 0.01$ compared with contralateral basal ganglia

Table 1. *Immunoreactivity in different cell types after intracerebral hemorrhage*

Time point	3CB2 immunoreactivity	Cell types	Other immunoreactivity
3 days	++	E, A	GFAP
1 month	+	E, N, A	TAC-4, GFAP

+, Moderate; ++, strong; *E* endothelial cell; *A* glia-like cell; *N* neuron-like cell; *GFAP* glial fibrillary acidic protein.

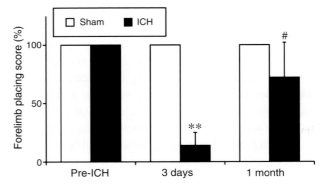

Fig. 2. Forelimb placing score was measured pre-ICH and at 3 days after ICH (by infusion of 100 μL autologous whole blood) or in sham controls (needle insertion without infusion). Values are expressed as mean ± SD; $n = 5$; **$p < 0.01$ compared with sham group, and #$p < 0.05$ compared with score at day 3

calized with TUC-4 (Table 1). In the sham group, a few astrocytic 3CB2-positive cells were observed only around the needle track at 3 days after ICH (data not shown).

Neurobehavioral test

There was an improvement in ICH-induced forelimb placing score, with a significant improvement at 1 month after ICH compared with that at 3 days after ICH ($p < 0.05$; Fig. 2).

Discussion

We investigated the early and chronic phase of 3CB2 expression after ICH by Western blotting and immunohistochemical staining. Increased expression of 3CB2 immunoreactivity was observed at 3 days and it lasted for at least 1 month following ICH. Early expression of 3CB2 occurred in astrocytes, but there was delayed expression in neurons.

3CB2 expression in early and chronic phase

3CB2 upregulation has been detected in a number of pathological conditions including traumatic brain injury [6], spinal cord injury [9], and in the kindling model [10]. As in ICH, this upregulation is prolonged in these different injury models, lasting at least 1 month [6, 9, 10].

Early after ICH (3 days), 3CB2 was expressed in astrocytes around the injury site. These astrocytes were mostly, but not solely, GFAP-positive. We previously demonstrated that some nestin-positive glia after ICH were also GFAP-positive [5].

Increased GFAP expression after brain damage is a hallmark of reactive astrocytes, and this cytoskeletal protein contributes to a barrier effect of the glial scar for axon extension [3].

At 1 month following ICH, 3CB2 was expressed in some neuron-like cells localized to the injury site. The fact that these cells have neuron-like properties was confirmed by immunofluorescent double-labeling of 3CB2 and TUC-4. Our previous study showed that nestin immunoreactivity was co-localized with neuron-specific enolase [5]. The appearance of 3CB2-positive cells was similar to that found in nestin-positive cells. Englund *et al.* [1] have indicated that nestin or GFAP-positive cells migrate extensively within white matter tracts after progenitor cell transplantation. These results suggest that some precursor cell marker expression after ICH may reflect active proliferation of neural precursor cells,

migration of those cells through white matter, and possibility have some capacity for self-repair in rodent brain after ICH.

Neurobehavioral function after ICH

ICH can cause neurobehavioral impariment clinically and also experimentally [2]. In this study, we showed that neurobehavioral function at 1 month after ICH was significantly improved compared with that of 1 day after ICH. This result suggests improvement of neurological function following ICH. The improvement of function after ICH may reflect the remodeling changes in the damaged brain.

Conclusions

The ICH-induced 3CB2 expression in astrocytes may reflect an early response of these cells to injury, while the delayed expression in neurons might be a part of the adaptative response to injury leading to recovery of neurobehavioral function.

Acknowledgments

This study was supported by a Grant-in-Aid for Scientific Research from the Japanese Society for the Promotion of Science.

References

1. Englund U, Björklund A, Wictorin K (2002) Migration patterns and phenotypic differentiation of long-term expanded human neural progenitor cells after transplantation into the adult rat brain. Brain Res Dev Brain Res 134: 123–141
2. Hua Y, Schallert T, Keep RF, Wu J, Hoff JT, Xi G (2002) Behavioral tests after intracerebral hemorrhage in the rat. Stroke 33: 2478–2484
3. McGraw J, Hiebert GW, Steeves JD (2001) Modulating astrogliosis after neurotrauma. J Neurosci Res 63: 109–115
4. Mission JP, Takahashi T, Caviness VS Jr (1991) Ontogeny of radial and other astroglial cells in murine cerebral cortex. Glia 4: 138–148
5. Nakamura T, Xi G, Hua Y, Hoff JT, Keep RF (2003) Nestin expression after experimental intracerebral hemorrhage. Brain Res 981: 108–117
6. Nakamura T, Miyamoto O, Auer RN, Nagao S, Itano T (2004) Delayed precursor cell markers expression in hippocampus following cold-induced cortical injury in mice. J Neurotrauma 21: 1747–1755
7. Parnavelas JG, Nadarajah B (2001) Radial glial cells. Are they really glia? Neuron 31: 881–884
8. Prada FA, Dorado ME, Quesada A, Prada C, Schwarz U, de la Rosa EJ (1995) Early expression of a novel radial glia antigen in the chick embryo. Glia 15: 389–400
9. Shibuya S, Miyamoto O, Itano T, Mori S, Norimatsu H (2003) Temporal progressive antigen expression in radial glia after contusive spinal cord injury in adult rats. Glia 42: 172–183
10. Tanaka S, Miyamoto O, Janjua NA, Miyazaki T, Takahashi F, Konishi R, Itano T (2005) Stage and region dependent expression of a radial glial marker in commissural fibers in kindled mice. Epilepsy Res 67: 61–72

Acta Neurochir Suppl (2008) 105: 99–100
© Springer-Verlag 2008
Printed in Austria

Long-term effects of melatonin after intracerebral hemorrhage in rats

R. E. Hartman[1], H. A. Rojas[2], T. Lekic[2], R. Ayer[2], S. Lee[2], V. Jadhav[2], E. Titova[2], J. Tang[2], J. H. Zhang[3]

[1] Department of Psychology, Loma Linda University, Loma Linda, CA, USA
[2] Department of Physiology and Pharmacology, Loma Linda University, Loma Linda, CA, USA
[3] Department of Neurosurgery, Loma Linda University, Loma Linda, CA, USA

Summary

Free radical scavengers have been shown to improve short-term outcome after intracerebral hemorrhage (ICH). The purpose of this study was to evaluate whether melatonin (a potent free radical scavenger and an indirect antioxidant) can improve short- and/or long-term neurological function after ICH, which was induced by collagenase injection into the striatum of adult rats. Melatonin (15 mg/kg) was administered by intraperitoneal injection at 1, 24, 48, and 72 h. Neurological and behavioral testing was performed at several time points from 1 day to 8 weeks post-ICH. Neurological and behavioral deficits were observed in ICH rats at all time points, but the melatonin treatment regimen did not improve performance or level of brain injury.

Keywords: Hemorrhage; collagenase; learning; memory; motor; melatonin.

Introduction

Intracerebral hemorrhage (ICH) represents at least 10–15% of all strokes in the Western population [13] and is often fatal. The collagenase-induced ICH rat model was originally described by Rosenberg *et al.* [14] and has been extensively used to evaluate the injury mechanisms and potential treatment regimens after ICH. However, the long-term effects after ICH in this model are not well understood. There are several published studies that have tested the behavioral effects of various therapeutic strategies following collagenase-induced ICH within the basal ganglia [1, 3, 5, 9, 10, 12], with most using motor tasks as the sole behavioral outcome measure to assess the efficacy of treatment strategies. However, cognitive deficits following ICH in humans are among the most prominent and troubling [7, 11, 15], with increasing evidence suggesting that the basal ganglia play a role in cognitive skills such as learning and memory. Our study examined whether melatonin reduces infarct size and/or neurological and cognitive deficits after collagenase-induced ICH in rats.

Materials and methods

Intracerebral hemorrhage

Adult male Sprague-Dawley rats were divided into sham-operated controls and ICH groups and anesthetized. Injecting collagenase (VII-S; Sigma-Aldrich, St. Louis, MO) into the basal ganglia with a microinfusion pump (Harvard Apparatus, Holliston, MA) induced ICH, as previously described [16]. The needle was left in place for an additional 10 min after injection to prevent collagenase leakage. Sham surgery was performed with needle insertion alone.

Melatonin treatment

After surgery, ICH rats were divided into 2 groups (ICH + vehicle; ICH + 15 mg/kg melatonin). Intraperitoneal injections were administered at 1, 24, 48, and 72 h post-ICH. Sham rats were given vehicle injections.

Behavioral testing

A number of behavioral tests were administered through 8 weeks post-ICH, including a battery of neurological tests [6], accelerating Rotarod, open field, and water maze. This battery of tests allowed for repeated testing of a number of behavioral domains, including neurological reflexes, sensorimotor coordination and balance, motor learning, general activity levels, cued learning, spatial learning, short- and long-term memory, swim speed, and turn bias.

Histology

Brains were removed at 10 weeks post-ICH, sliced into 10 μm thick sections, stained with cresyl violet Nissl stain, and infarct size was evaluated (Table 1).

Correspondence: Richard E. Hartman, PhD, Department of Psychology, Loma Linda University, 11130 Anderson St. 119, Loma Linda, CA 92354, USA. e-mail: behavioralneuroscience@gmail.com

Table 1. *Infarct size (percent of contralateral hemisphere)*

Treatment group	Infarct size
Sham + Vehicle	0
ICH + Vehicle	10 ± 3
ICH + 15 mg/kg melatonin	12 ± 4

Results

Neurobehavioral testing

Although behavioral deficits, including cued and spatial learning, spatial memory, and sensorimotor coordination were observed in ICH rats throughout the 8-week test period, the melatonin treatment regimen produced no significant change in behavior.

Histology

Treatment with melatonin did not produce any significant changes in the area of injury produced by collagenase-induced ICH.

Discussion

The collagenase-induced ICH model produces lesions in the dorsolateral and middle regions of the striatum [8], which are important areas for the control of skilled motor function [17]. This model often produces a functional impairment of fine motor control of the distal forelimb and paw as revealed by the staircase test [3]. Neurological deficits in this model are most severe from 24–72 h after ICH induction and are typically attenuated by 1 month [4, 5, 14]. However, long-term neurological deficits have been shown when evaluating rotational bias in response to amphetamine and contralateral stepping [2]. In the current study, this model of ICH produced detectable cognitive and motor deficits in rats over an 8 week time period. Along with histological analysis of infarct volume, this characterization provides a suitable baseline for the analysis of therapeutic intervention strategies. However, melatonin, at the dose and frequency tested, did not improve infarct size or neurological function of rats after ICH induction. It is possible the melatonin regimen was ineffective at reducing the oxidative damage produced by ICH, or that processes other than oxidative stress were responsible for the behavioral deficits and brain damage. It remains to be determined whether other antioxidant agents can prevent the long-term behavioral deficits that were characterized in this model.

Acknowledgement

This study is partially supported by a grant from the National Institutes of Health (NIHNS53407) to JHZ.

References

1. Altumbabic M, Peeling J, Del Bigio MR (1998) Intracerebral hemorrhage in the rat: effects of hematoma aspiration. Stroke 29: 1917–1923
2. Chesney JA, Kondoh T, Conrad JA, Low WC (1995) Collagenase-induced intrastriatal hemorrhage in rats results in long-term locomotor deficits. Stroke 26: 312–317
3. Clarke J, Ploughman M, Corbett D (2007) A qualitative and quantitative analysis of skilled forelimb reaching impairment following intracerebral hemorrhage in rats. Brain Res 1145: 204–212
4. Del Bigio MR, Yan HJ, Buist R, Peeling J (1996) Experimental intracerebral hemorrhage in rats. Magnetic resonance imaging and histopathological correlates. Stroke 27: 2312–2320
5. Del Bigio MR, Yan HJ, Campbell TM, Peeling J (1999) Effect of fucoidan treatment on collagenase-induced intracerebral hemorrhage in rats. Neurol Res 21: 415–419
6. Garcia JH, Wagner S, Liu KF, Hu XJ (1995) Neurological deficit and extent of neuronal necrosis attributable to middle cerebral artery occlusion in rats. Statistical validation. Stroke 26: 627–635
7. King JT Jr, DiLuna ML, Cicchetti DV, Tsevat J, Roberts MS (2006) Cognitive functioning in patients with cerebral aneurysms measured with the mini mental state examination and the telephone interview for cognitive status. Neurosurgery 59: 803–811
8. Kirik D, Rosenblad C, Björklund A (1998) Characterization of behavioral and neurodegenerative changes following partial lesions of the nigrostriatal dopamine system induced by intrastriatal 6-hydroxydopamine in the rat. Exp Neurol 152: 259–277
9. MacLellan CL, Davies LM, Fingas MS, Colbourne F (2006) The influence of hypothermia on outcome after intracerebral hemorrhage in rats. Stroke 37: 1266–1270
10. Masuda T, Hida H, Kanda Y, Aihara N, Ohta K, Yamada K, Nishino H (2007) Oral administration of metal chelator ameliorates motor dysfunction after a small hemorrhage near the internal capsule in rat. J Neurosci Res 85: 213–222
11. Nys GM, van Zandvoort MJ, de Kort PL, Jansen BP, de Haan EH, Kappelle LJ (2007) Cognitive disorders in acute stroke: prevalence and clinical determinants. Cerebrovasc Dis 23: 408–416
12. Peeling J, Del Bigio MR, Corbett D, Green AR, Jackson DM (2001) Efficacy of disodium 4-[(tert-butylimino)methyl]benzene-1,3-disulfonate N-oxide (NXY-059), a free radical trapping agent, in a rat model of hemorrhagic stroke. Neuropharmacology 40: 433–439
13. Qureshi AI, Tuhrim S, Broderick JP, Batjer HH, Hondo H, Hanley DF (2001) Spontaneous intracerebral hemorrhage. N Engl J Med 344: 1450–1460
14. Rosenberg GA, Mun-Bryce S, Wesley M, Kornfeld M (1990) Collagenase-induced intracerebral hemorrhage in rats. Stroke 21: 801–807
15. Thajeb P, Thajeb T, Dai D (2007) Cross-cultural studies using a modified mini mental test for healthy subjects and patients with various forms of vascular dementia. J Clin Neurosci 14: 236–241
16. Titova E, Ostrowski RP, Sowers LC, Zhang JH, Tang J (2007) Effects of apocynin and ethanol on intracerebral haemorrhage-induced brain injury in rats. Clin Exp Pharmacol Physiol 34: 845–850
17. Whishaw IQ, O'Connor WT, Dunnett SB (1986) The contributions of motor cortex, nigrostriatal dopamine and caudate-putamen to skilled forelimb use in the rat. Brain 109: 805–843

Acta Neurochir Suppl (2008) 105: 101–104
© Springer-Verlag 2008
Printed in Austria

Management of delayed edema formation after fibrinolytic therapy for intracerebral hematomas: preliminary experimental data

V. Rohde[1], N. Uzma[1], R. Thiex[2], U. Samadani[1]

[1] Department of Neurosurgery, Georg-August-University, Goettingen, Germany
[2] Department of Neurosurgery, Technical University, Aachen, Germany

Summary

Objective. Fibrinolytic therapy for spontaneous intracerebral hemorrhage using recombinant tissue plasminogen activator (rtPA) is considered a viable alternative to microsurgical hematoma removal. However, experimental data suggest that rtPA is neurotoxic and evokes a late perihematomal edema. We present preliminary data focusing on the avoidance of late edema formation after lysis of an intracerebral hematoma in a porcine model.

Methods. Twenty pigs underwent placement of a frontal intracerebral hematoma with a minimum volume of 1 mL. Half of the pigs were subjected to rtPA clot lysis and MK-801 injection for blockage of the NMDA receptor-mediated rtPA-enhanced excitotoxic pathway. The remaining 10 pigs received desmoteplase (DSPA) for clot lysis, which is known to be a less neurotoxic fibrinolytic agent than rtPA. MRI on the day of surgery and on postoperative days 4 and 10 was used to assess hematoma and edema volumes.

Results. Late edema formation could be prevented in both the MK-801/rtPA and DSPA pigs.

Conclusion. The benefits of fibrinolytic therapy for intracerebral hematomas appear to be counterbalanced by late edema formation. MK-801 infusion as an adjunct to rtPA lysis, or the use of DSPA instead of rtPA, prevents late edema and therefore has the potential to further improve results after clot lysis.

Keywords: Intracerebral hemorrhage; fibrinolysis; tissue plasminogen activator; desmoteplase; excitotoxicity.

Introduction

With mortality rates between 27 and 70%, spontaneous supratentorial intracerebral hemorrhage (ICH) carries the worst prognosis of the 3 types of stroke. Several randomized prospective trials have shown that craniotomy and microsurgical clot removal fail to improve the poor prognosis [4, 12, 13, 27]. It had been assumed that surgical trauma contributed to the dismal results, which led to the development of minimally-invasive techniques, especially for frame-based and frameless stereotaxy, hematoma puncture, and subsequent fibrinolytic therapy with recombinant tissue plasminogen activator (rtPA) [9, 17, 19, 21]. However, recent data suggest that rtPA might be neurotoxic in the presence of an intracerebral hematoma. In our own experiments, fibrinolytic therapy in experimental ICH resulted in delayed perifocal edema [18]. Delayed edema is hypothesized to be caused by promotion of excitotoxic pathways initiated by perihematomal ischemia, or a reduction in the activity of protease nexin-1 (PN-1) and plasminogen-activator inhibitor-1 (PAI-1), which inhibit both rtPA and edema-evoking thrombin. The purpose of our investigation was to elucidate the pathways that might be responsible for the delayed edema and to propose potential therapeutic alternatives.

Materials and methods

Animal preparation

The protocol for pig intracranial hemorrhage has been described in detail [18]. Briefly, 20 male pigs weighing 30–35 kg were sedated with a 1:6 mixture of atropine (0.3–0.5 mg/kg) and azaperone (7–10 mg/kg). The animals were further anesthetized with pentobarbital (15–20 mg/kg) administered via a line in an ear vein. After endotracheal intubation, the pigs were mechanically ventilated and vital parameters kept at physiological levels. The hematoma was induced under intracranial pressure control by injecting autologous venous blood into a preformed right frontal cavity created by balloon dilatation.

After hematoma induction, magnetic resonance imaging (MRI) scans were performed on a 1.5T system on all animals. T2-weighted fluid attenuated inversion recovery (FLAIR) turbo spin-echo images were used to quantitate edema and T2*-weighted gradient echo images were acquired for hematoma measurement. Pigs with a hematoma size of less

Correspondence: Veit Rohde, MD, Department of Neurosurgery, Medical Faculty – Georg-August-University Goettingen, Robert-Koch-Strasse 40, 37085 Goettingen, Germany. e-mail: veit.rohde@med.uni-goettingen.de

than $1 cm^3$ on MRI were excluded. The scans were repeated on days 4 and 10. Our previous studies have shown that changes in FLAIR intensity correlate with areas of perihematomal edema and inflammatory infiltration [20].

Experimental groups

Ten animals underwent fibrinolytic therapy of the hematoma with rtPA (Actilyse, Thomae GmbH, Biberach, Germany) administered via the Rickham reservoir directly following initial MR imaging. The amount of rtPA given in milligrams was equal to the maximum diameter of the hematoma measured in centimeters on $T2^*$-weighted gradient echo sequences [19]. In the remaining 10 pigs, desmoteplase (DSPA) (Paion, Aachen, Germany), in a dosage equivalent to the lytic properties of rtPA, was used as the fibrinolytic agent.

In the 10 rtPA pigs, the NMDA receptor-antagonist MK-801 (M107, Sigma-Aldrich, Germany), which inhibits the excitotoxic pathway, was administered intravenously at a dosage of 0.3 mg/kg body weight immediately after hematoma induction (before the first MRI) and then again at 24 h and 72 h postoperatively.

Statistical analysis

All values are presented as mean ± standard deviation. For comparison of hematoma and edema volume changes during the study period, the 1-tailed paired *t*-test was used. Differences were considered significant at probability values of less than 0.05.

Results

MK-801/rtPA pigs

The mean hematoma size in the 10 animals measured $1.29 \pm 0.26 cm^3$ and decreased to $0.57 \pm 0.34 cm^3$ on day 4 ($p < 0.001$) and to $0.37 \pm 0.25 cm^3$ on day 10 ($p < 0.001$), respectively. The mean edema volume on FLAIR images measured $0.73 \pm 0.54 cm^3$ directly after surgery and increased to $1.29 \pm 0.76 cm^3$ on day 4 ($p < 0.08$) and $1.29 \pm 1.76 cm^3$ on day 10 ($p < 0.35$).

DSPA pigs

The mean hematoma size in the 10 animals was $1.21 \pm 0.34 cm^3$. DSPA lysis reduced the hematoma volume to $0.55 \pm 0.31 cm^3$ on day 4 ($p < 0.001$) and to $0.30 \pm 0.15 cm^3$ on day 10 ($p < 0.001$). The mean edema volume on the day of surgery was $0.63 \pm 0.28 cm^3$ and increased to $1.44 \pm 0.52 cm^3$ on day 4 ($p < 0.001$), but dropped again to $0.94 \pm 1.4 cm^3$ on day 10 ($p < 0.24$).

Comparison of MK-801/rtPA and DSPA pigs

The initial hematoma volume in both groups of pigs was comparable. Furthermore, the fibrinolytic effect of rtPA and DSPA was equivalent, with almost similar reductions in the initial hematoma volume on postoperative days 4 and 10. The edema volume in both the MK-801 and DSPA groups increased until day 4. Then, the edema volume remained stable in the MK-801 group but dropped in the DSPA group, as seen on day 10.

Discussion

The optimal therapy for spontaneous intracerebral hemorrhage has yet to be determined. The few prospective randomized trials comparing microsurgical clot removal with conventional medical therapy failed to support surgery. Even when surgery is performed, mortality rates are as high as 40–67% [4, 12]. Frame-based stereotactic or neuronavigationally-guided hematoma puncture and subsequent clot lysis with tPA has been proposed as a therapeutic alternative. In several prospective clinical series, promising results have been published, with mortality rates between 10 and 25% [9, 17, 19]. These good results have been attributed to the less-invasive nature of the procedure, diminishing operative trauma to the brain overlying the hematoma.

Studies on fibrinolytic therapy in experimental intracerebral hematoma are rare. Wagner and coworkers demonstrated that fibrinolysis with rtPA and subsequent aspiration of lysed clot reduces the amount of the perifocal edema in a pig model on postoperative day 1 [24]. Using a similar porcine model, our studies confirm the positive effect of clot lysis on diminishing early edema, and demonstrate increased hemorrhage site edema on day 10. This delayed edema was significantly larger than that seen in an untreated control group [18].

rtPA neurotoxicity

Two hypothetical pathways may account for the increase in delayed edema. 1) Experimental studies of focal cerebral ischemia using tPA knockout and wild-type mice showed that tPA induces neuronal death by enhancing the excitotoxic pathway [25]. Similar findings were reported in mice experiments using unilateral intrahippocampal injection of kainic acid [22, 23]. The NMDA receptor plays a dominant role in this excitotoxic pathway. tPA amplifies the NMDA-induced increase in intracellular calcium concentration and potentially provokes cell death by cleavage of a fragment from the NR1 subunit of the NMDA receptor [11, 15]. 2) Blood degradation products, especially thrombin, are well known factors contributing to the development of perihematomal edema [3, 6, 7, 14, 26]. Thrombin is inhibited by PN-1 and PAI-1. Figueroa and coworkers showed that addition of rtPA attenuates the inhibition of thrombin by competing for PN-1 and PAI-1 [2]. It seems possible that the relative increase in thrombin concentration causes delayed perihematomal edema.

Anti-neurotoxic options

Prior to our current study there was little evidence that rtPA mediated up regulation of excitotoxic pathways or that attenuation of the PN-1/PAI-1-induced inhibition of thrombin contributed to the development of delayed edema in successfully lysed experimental hematomas. Our recent experiments clearly indicate that at least the first pathway is involved in late edema formation. MK-801 is a non-competitive blocker of the NMDA receptor and, therefore, of the excitotoxic pathway, as proven by reduction of the infarct size in experiments on focal ischemia. Similarly, NMDA receptor blockade attenuates the neurotoxic effect of external tPA with inhibition of calcium overload [1, 5]. In our previous series [18], the mean edema volume on day 10 was $3.33 \, cm^3 \pm 3.2 \, cm^3$ in rtPA pigs, but only $1.29 \pm 1.76 \, cm^3$ in rtPA and MK-801 treated pigs, despite comparable initial hematoma volumes and fibrinolytic effects. This significant reduction in edema volume by MK-801 suggests that activation of the excitotoxic pathway by exogenous tPA plays a substantial role in delayed edema formation.

DSPA is an alternative lytic agent derived from the saliva of the blood-feeding vampire bat. In 2 models of neurodegeneration, DSPA was found not to promote kainite- or NMDA-mediated neurotoxicity [8, 10, 16]. Our study demonstrates once again that DSPA as a fibrinolytic agent is not neurotoxic, even if given in an extravasated fashion. Delayed edema volume in the DSPA pigs, at $0.94 \, cm^3$, was lower than that on day 4, while in rtPA pigs the highest edema volume was observed on day 10.

We have preliminary evidence that PN-1/PAI-1-induced inhibition of thrombin additionally contributes to the development of delayed edema in successfully lysed experimental hematomas; PAI-1 injection after induction of the hematoma and rtPA clot lysis reduces delayed edema formation while only mildly reducing the lytic potential of rtPA (Samadani and Rohde, unpublished data).

Conclusion

Our work demonstrates that MK-801 may be a useful adjunct to diminish delayed edema after rtPA clot lysis. Additionally, DSPA fibrinolysis, when used in lieu of rtPA, may have a similar effect. These agents have the potential to further improve outcomes after stereotactic

hematoma puncture and fibrinolytic therapy by blockage or avoidance of the neurotoxic properties of the injected rtPA. These data are preliminary and further investigations are necessary, as the effects of MK-801 and DSPA have not been compared with a direct, but with a previous control group. PAI-1 injection after clot lysis with rtPA offers a third modality for controlling delayed edema formation.

References

1. Buchan AM, Slivka A, Xue D (1992) The effect of the NMDA receptor antagonist MK-801 on cerebral blood flow and infarct volume in experimental focal stroke. Brain Res 574: 171–177
2. Figueroa BE, Keep RF, Betz AL, Hoff JT (1998) Plasminogen activators potentiate thrombin-induced brain injury. Stroke 29: 1202–1208
3. Huang FP, Xi G, Keep RF, Hua Y, Nemoianu A, Hoff JT (2002) Brain edema after experimental intracerebral hemorrhage: role of hemoglobin degradation products. J Neurosurg 96: 287–293
4. Juvela S, Heiskanen O, Poranen A, Valtonen S, Kuurne T, Kaste M, Troupp H (1989) The treatment of spontaneous intracerebral hemorrhage. A prospective randomized trial of surgical and conservative treatment. J Neurosurg 70: 755–758
5. Kilic E, Bähr M, Hermann DM (2001) Effects of recombinant tissue plasminogen activator after intraluminal thread occlusion in mice: role of hemodynamic alterations. Stroke 32: 2641–2647
6. Lee KR, Colon GP, Betz AL, Keep RF, Kim S, Hoff JT (1996) Edema from intracerebral hemorrhage: the role of thrombin. J Neurosurg 84: 91–96
7. Lee KR, Kawai N, Kim S, Sagher O, Hoff JT (1997) Mechanisms of edema formation after intracerebral hemorrhage: effects of thrombin on cerebral blood flow, blood–brain barrier permeability, and cell survival in a rat model. J Neurosurg 86: 272–278
8. Liberatore GT, Samson A, Bladin C, Schleuning WD, Medcalf RL (2003) Vampire bat salivary plasminogen activator (desmoteplase): a unique fibrinolytic enzyme that does not promote neurodegeneration. Stroke 34: 537–543
9. Lippitz BE, Mayfrank L, Spetzger U, Warnke JP, Bertalanffy H, Gilsbach JM (1994) Lysis of basal ganglia haematoma with recombinant tissue plasminogen activator (rtPA) after stereotactic aspiration: initial results. Acta Neurochir (Wien) 127: 157–160
10. López-Atalaya JP, Roussel BD, Ali C, Maubert E, Petersen KU, Berezowski V, Cecchelli R, Orset C, Vivien D (2007) Recombinant Desmodus rotundus salivary plasminogen activator crosses the blood–brain barrier through a low-density lipoprotein receptor-related protein-dependent mechanism without exerting neurotoxic effects. Stroke 38: 1036–1043
11. Matys T, Strickland S (2003) Tissue plasminogen activator and NMDA receptor cleavage. Nature Med 9: 371–373
12. Mendelow AD, Gregson BA, Fernandes HM, Murray GD, Teasdale GM, Hope DT, Karimi A, Shaw MD, Barer DH; STICH investigators (2005) Early surgery versus initial conservative treatment in patients with spontaneous supratentorial intracerebral haematomas in the International Surgical Trial in Intracerebral Haemorrhage (STICH): a randomised trial. Lancet 365: 387–397
13. Morgenstern LB, Frankowski RF, Shedden P, Pasteur W, Grotta JC (1998) Surgical treatment for intracerebral hemorrhage (STICH): a single-center, randomized clinical trial. Neurology 51: 1359–1363
14. Nakamura T, Keep RF, Hua Y, Schallert T, Hoff JT, Xi G (2004) Deferoxamine-induced attenuation of brain edema and neurological

deficits in a rat model of intracerebral hemorrhage. J Neurosurg 100: 672–678

15. Nicole O, Docagne F, Ali C, Margaill I, Carmeliet P, MacKenzie ET, Vivien D, Buisson A (2001) The proteolytic activity of tissue-plasminogen activator enhances NMDA receptor-mediated signaling. Nature Med 7: 59–64

16. Reddrop C, Moldrich RX, Beart PM, Farso M, Liberatore GT, Howells DW, Petersen KU, Schleuning WD, Medcalf RL (2005) Vampire bat salivary plasminogen activator (desmoteplase) inhibits tissue-type plasminogen activator-induced potentiation of excitotoxic injury. Stroke 36: 1241–1246

17. Rohde V, Rohde I, Reinges MH, Mayfrank L, Gilsbach JM (2000) Frameless stereotactically guided catheter placement and fibrinolytic therapy for spontaneous intracerebral hematomas: technical aspects and initial clinical results. Minim Invasive Neurosurg 43: 9–17

18. Rohde V, Rohde I, Thiex R, Ince A, Jung A, Dückers G, Gröschel K, Röttger C, Küker W, Müller HD, Gilsbach JM (2002) Fibrinolysis therapy achieved with tissue plasminogen activator and aspiration of the liquefied clot after experimental intracerebral hemorrhage: rapid reduction in hematoma volume but intensification of delayed edema formation. J Neurosurg 97: 954–962

19. Schaller C, Rohde V, Meyer B, Hassler W (1995) Stereotactic puncture and lysis of spontaneous intracerebral hemorrhage using recombinant tissue-plasminogen activator. Neurosurgery 36: 328–335

20. Thiex R, Küker W, Müller HD, Rohde I, Schröder JM, Gilsbach JM, Rohde V (2003) The long-term effect of recombinant tissue-plas-

minogen-activator (rt-PA) on edema formation in a large-animal model of intracerebral hemorrhage. Neurol Res 25: 254–262

21. Thiex R, Rohde V, Rohde I, Mayfrank L, Zeki Z, Thron A, Gilsbach JM, Uhl E (2004) Frame-based and frameless stereotactic hematoma puncture and subsequent fibrinolytic therapy for the treatment of spontaneous intracerebral hemorrhage. J Neurol 251: 1443–1450

22. Tsirka SE, Gualandris A, Amaral DG, Strickland S (1995) Excitotoxin-induced neuronal degeneration and seizure mediated by tissue plasminogen activator. Nature 377: 340–344

23. Tsirka SE, Rogove AD, Strickland S (1996) Neuronal cell death and tPA. Nature 384: 123–124

24. Wagner KR, Xi G, Hua Y, Zuccarello M, de Courten-Myers GM, Broderick JP, Brott TG (1999) Ultra-early clot aspiration after lysis with tissue plasminogen activator in a porcine model of intracerebral hemorrhage: edema reduction and blood–brain barrier protection. J Neurosurg 90: 491–498

25. Wang YF, Tsirka SE, Strickland S, Stieg PE, Soriano SG, Lipton SA (1998) Tissue plasminogen activator (tPA) increases neuronal damage after focal cerebral ischemia in wild-type and tPA-deficient mice. Nat Med 4: 228–231

26. Xi G, Keep RF, Hoff JT (2006) Mechanisms of brain injury after intracerebral haemorrhage. Lancet Neurol 5: 53–63

27. Zuccarello M, Brott T, Derex L, Kothari R, Sauerbeck L, Tew J, Van Loveren H, Yeh HS, Tomsick T, Pancioli A, Khoury J, Broderick J (1999) Early surgical treatment for supratentorial intracerebral hemorrhage: a randomized feasibility study. Stroke 30: 1833–1839

Acta Neurochir Suppl (2008) 105: 105–112
© Springer-Verlag 2008
Printed in Austria

Erythropoietin attenuates intracerebral hemorrhage by diminishing matrix metalloproteinases and maintaining blood–brain barrier integrity in mice

Y. Li[1], M. E. Ogle[1], G. C. Wallace IV[1], Z.-Y. Lu[1], S. P. Yu[1,2], L. Wei[1]

[1] Department of Pathology and Laboratory Medicine, Medical University of South Carolina, Charleston, SC, USA
[2] Department of Pharmaceutical and Biomedical Sciences, Medical University of South Carolina, Charleston, SC, USA

Summary

The protective mechanism of recombinant human erythropoietin (rhEPO) on blood–brain barrier (BBB) after brain injury is associated with the attenuation of neuro-inflammation. We hypothesize that rhEPO treatment after intracerebral hemorrhage (ICH) modulates matrix metalloproteinase (MMP) activity, maintains BBB integrity, and reduces BBB breakdown-associated inflammation.

Adult male 129S2/sv mice were subjected to autologous whole blood-induced ICH. rhEPO or saline was administered intraperitoneally immediately after surgery and for 3 more days until day of sacrifice. BBB permeability was measured by Evans blue leakage, and edema was assessed by brain water content. Immunofluorescence and Western blotting were performed to detect expression of tight junction marker occludin, type IV collagen, MMPs, tissue inhibitor of metalloproteinase (TIMP), and glial fibrillary acidic protein. rhEPO prevented Evans blue leakage, reduced brain edema, and preserved expression of occludin and collagen IV. rhEPO treatment decreased MMP-2 expression, increased TIMP-2 expression, and reduced the number of reactive astrocytes in the brain compared to saline control.

We conclude that rhEPO reduces MMP activity, BBB disruption, and the glial cell inflammatory reaction 3 days after ICH. Our study provides additional evidence for the mechanism of rhEPO's neurovascular protective effects and a potential clinical application in the treatment of ICH.

Keywords: Intracerebral hemorrhage; recombinant human erythropoietin; blood–brain barrier; matrix metalloproteinase; tissue inhibitor of metalloproteinase; anti-inflammatory; neurovascular protection.

Introduction

Intracerebral hemorrhage (ICH), a high mortality and morbidity subtype of stroke, makes up approximately 10% to 15% of all strokes, of which the pathological mechanisms are not yet fully clarified. Only a few randomized clinical trials have been executed after the first American Heart Association guidelines for the man-agement of spontaneous ICH were published in 1999. Tremendous effort has been dedicated to understanding the basic science mechanisms of ICH, although they are still largely unknown. Information thus far concludes that the massive damage induced by ICH results from the effects of hematoma, which causes local obstruction of the microcirculation, resulting in ischemia and compression of the distant structures [10]. The inflammation surrounding the blood clot also contributes to delayed neuronal death [17]. It has also been demonstrated that ICH is followed by disruption of the blood–brain barrier (BBB), which is accompanied by edema surrounding the lesion area [21]. Disruption of the BBB initiates the neuro-inflammatory response and tissue injury after ICH [3].

The BBB is composed of endothelial cells, astrocyte end-feet, and pericytes, restricting the passage of toxins and maintaining homeostasis of the neuro-parenchymal microenvironment [6]. Endothelial cell tight junctions comprise the first border line against external structures from entering the brain. The basal lamina, which wraps the endothelial cells and pericytes and is contiguous with the plasma membranes of astrocytic end-feet and endothelial cells, provides a charge barrier and may impede influx of larger molecules. Matrix metalloproteinases (MMPs) contribute to BBB disruption during central nervous system (CNS) pathological circumstances by digesting the components of the basal lamina, such as heparin sulfate, laminin, fibronectin, and type IV collagen [14]. In the acute phase of ischemia, MMP expression is up-regulated [3], which degrades the BBB and leads to brain edema and secondary injury to the brain [4]. Increased BBB permeability consequently

Correspondence: Ling Wei, M.D., Department of Anesthesiology, Emory University, Atlanta, GA 30322, USA. e-mail: weil@musc.edu results in the infiltration of leukocytes and macrophages into the brain and an accelerated inflammatory response, a proposed component of the cell death mechanism after ICH. Inhibition of MMPs exerted neuroprotection following mouse ICH [18].

The novel neuroprotectant, recombinant human erythropoietin (rhEPO) [5, 8, 19], has exhibited potential effects in BBB protection in different neurovascular diseases [9, 11, 15]. Anti-inflammation has recently been reported [7, 16, 20] as one of the possible neuroprotective mechanisms of rhEPO. We hypothesize that rhEPO suppresses MMP activation after ICH and maintains the integrity of the BBB, thus attenuating neuro-inflammatory responses, which may be another neuroprotective mechanism.

Materials and methods

Induction of ICH by autologous whole blood and drug administration

All animal experiments and surgical procedures were approved by the University Animal Research Committee and met National Institutes of Health standards. Male 129S2/Sv mice (20–25 g; Harlan, Indianapolis, IN, USA) were subjected to intraperitoneal injection of 4% chloral hydrate anesthesia, and were positioned in a mouse stereotaxic frame (myNeurolab.com, St. Louis, MO). A 1-mm cranial burr hole was drilled stereotaxically near the bregma and above the right basal ganglia (AP: -0.2 mm; ML: $+2.0$ mm). A 26-gauge needle was inserted into the hole at a depth of 3.5 mm (DV: $+3.5$ mm). Autologous whole blood (20 µl) drawn from the tail vein was infused at a rate of 5 µl/min using a microinfusion pump (Stoelting Co., Wood Dale, IL, USA). After waiting an extra 2 min following the infusion, the needle was slowly withdrawn, the burr hole was filled with bone wax, and the skin incision was closed with suture. During surgery and recovery periods, body temperature was monitored and maintained at $37.0 \pm 0.5\,^{\circ}\text{C}$ using a temperature control unit and heating pads.

rhEPO (5000 U/kg; Amgen Inc., Thousand Oaks, CA, USA) or saline was injected intraperitoneally immediately after surgery and continued once per day after insult for 3 days. Animals were sacrificed by decapitation 3 days after ICH. The brain was immediately removed and mounted in optimal cutting temperature compound (Sakura Finetek USA, Inc. Torrance, CA) at $-80\,^{\circ}\text{C}$ for further processing.

Macroscopic evaluation of alterations in BBB permeability and brain edema

In order to visualize the BBB leakage, sterilized 2% Evans blue (Sigma-Aldrich, St. Louis, MO) solution was administered intravenously at a dosage of 0.1 mL per animal 6 hours before sacrifice. Brains were removed and coronal sections were used to examine the Evans blue extravasation by photographing under the TRITC (red) excitation wavelength at 1.25× fluorescent microscopy (BX5; Olympus, Japan). Adobe Photoshop CS 8.0 software (Adobe Systems Inc., San Jose, CA, USA) was used to make an image mosaic. The leakage volume was morphometrically measured based on the Evans blue leakage area using our previous protocol [9]. The leakage ratio and volume were measured by an image analyzer (SigmaScan Pro 5; Systat Software Inc., San Jose, CA, USA).

To evaluate the effects of brain edema following ICH, tissue sections from rhEPO and saline groups were assayed for water content at 72 h after injury by using wet weight/dry weight ratios [9].

Western blot assay

For each group, 3 animals were used to collect ipsilateral tissue samples from the lesion border. Each sample was run in 3 independent assays. Western blotting procedure is the standard procedure in our laboratory [8] and was repeated 3 times with new samples collected from different animals. In total, 9 different animals were used in each group. The following antibodies were used: mouse anti-occludin (1:500; Invitrogen, Carlsbad, CA, USA), rabbit anti-MMP-2 (1:1000, AB19167; Chemicon International, Temecula, CA, USA), rabbit anti-tissue inhibitor of metalloproteinase (TIMP)-2 (1:1000, AB801; Chemicon International), and rabbit anti-glial fibrillary acidic protein (GFAP) (1:1000; Biomeda Corp., Burlingame, CA). Mouse anti-β-actin (Sigma-Aldrich) was used as the protein loading control. The protein band was quantified and analyzed using Image J software (National Institutes of Health, Bethesda, MD, USA). The intensity of each band was first measured and then subtracted by the background. The expression ratio of each target protein was then normalized against β-actin.

Immunofluorescence staining

Coronal fresh frozen sections were sliced 10-µm thick using a cryostat vibratome (Ultapro 5000, St. Louis, MO). After the slides were completely air dried, slices were fixed in 10% buffered formalin phosphate for 10 min, followed by 0.2% Triton-100 for 5 min and washed with phosphate-buffered saline 3 times between each step. Slides were blocked in 1% gelatin from cold water fish before incubation with primary antibodies overnight at $4\,^{\circ}\text{C}$. The primary antibodies were as follows: mouse anti-occludin (1:500; Invitrogen), goat anti-collagen IV (1:1000; Santa Cruz Biotechnology, Santa Cruz, CA, USA), rabbit anti-MMP-2 (1:1000, AB19167; Chemicon), rabbit anti-TIMP-2 (1:1000, AB801; Chemicon), and mouse anti-GFAP (1:800; Biomeda Corp.). After rinsing with phosphate-buffered saline, brain sections were then treated with secondary antibodies Alexa Fluor 488 anti-mouse, anti-rabbit, or anti-goat IgG (Molecular Probes, Eugene, OR), Cy3-conjugated anti-mouse or anti-rabbit IgG (Jackson ImmunoResearch Laboratories, West Grove, PA, USA) for 1.5 h at room temperature. Hoechst 33342 (Molecular Probes) was used to stain all nuclei. Brain sections were mounted and cover-slipped, imaged and photographed under a fluorescent microscope (BX51; Olympus) and laser scanning confocal microscope (Carl Zeiss Microimaging Inc., Thornwood, NY, USA).

Statistical analysis

Student's two-tailed t-test was used to compare the 2 experimental groups. Changes were identified as significant if $p < 0.05$. Mean values were reported together with the standard error of mean (Mean $\pm$ SE).

Results

rhEPO reduced Evans blue leakage and brain edema induced by ICH

The area of Evans blue leakage on a single section was much less in the rhEPO group (Fig. 1B) than saline group (Fig. 1A) as revealed by the mosaic images taken under a fluorescent microscope. There was a significant reduction (36.6%) in the rhEPO group compared to the saline group in the indirect ratio of Evans blue leakage (Fig. 1C).

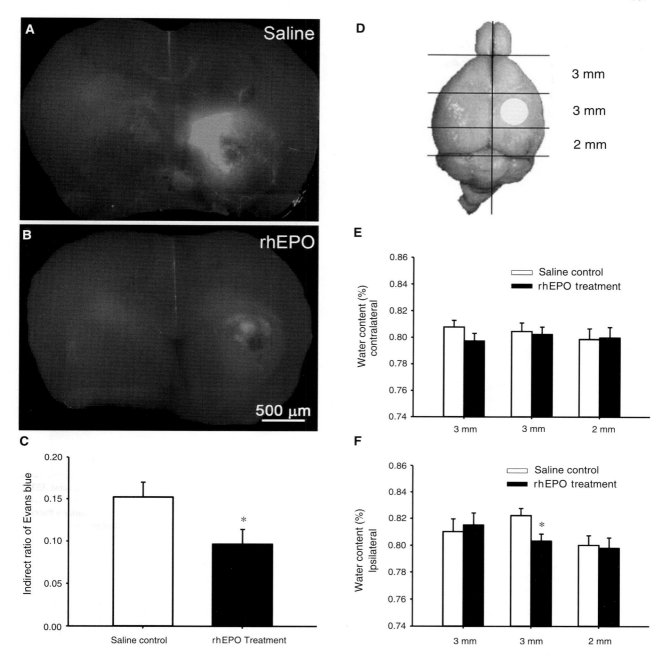

Fig. 1. rhEPO reduced Evans blue leakage and brain edema 3 days after ICH. (A, B) Images of Evans blue leakage. There was a greatly reduced area of Evans blue dye (*red*) in rhEPO treatment group (B) compared to saline group (A). (C) Ratio of Evans blue leakage. There was significant reduction in the indirect ratio of Evans blue leakage in rhEPO group compared to saline group ($N = 5$). $^*p < 0.05$. (D) Sectioning scheme used to compare edema in different regions of brain. White circle represents lesion area. (E, F) Water content for contralateral and ipsilateral hemispheres was calculated separately ($N = 6$). On the contralateral side, there was no significant difference between rhEPO and saline group in corresponding sections (E). On the ipsilateral side, there was significant reduction of water content in the second 3-mm section of the rhEPO group compared to saline (F). $^*p < 0.05$

Water content was used to represent brain edema (Fig. 1D). There was no significant difference between the rhEPO and saline group in any of the sections on the contralateral side (Fig. 1E). A higher percentage of water content was seen on the ipsilateral side than the contra-lateral side in general. On the ipsilateral side, there was a significant reduction of water content in the second 3-mm section but not in the first 3-mm or the 2-mm sections in the rhEPO group as compared to saline control (Fig. 1F).

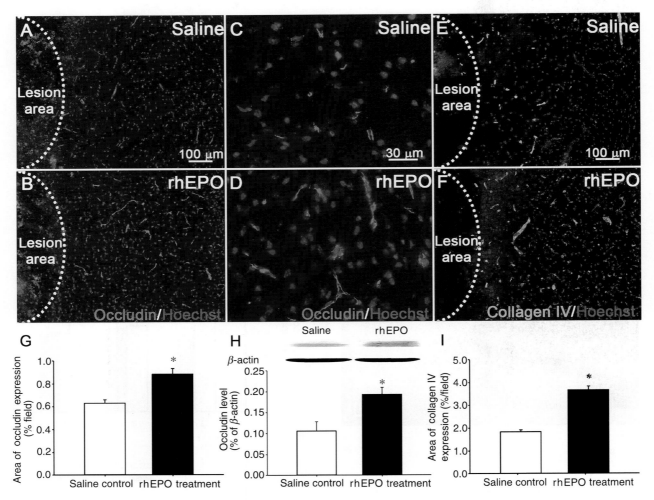

Fig. 2. rhEPO maintained distribution of occludin and collagen IV expression 3 days after ICH. (A–D) Expression of occludin (*red*) against Hoechst (*blue*) was detected in saline group (A and C) and rhEPO group (B and D) at both lower (A and B) and higher magnification (C and D) ($N = 9$). (E, F) Expression of collagen IV (*green*) against Hoechst (*blue*) was detected in saline group (E) and rhEPO group (F) ($N = 9$). *Dash-lines* mark the boundary of ICH-induced lesion area in A, B, E, and F. (G) The area of occludin expression showed significantly more expression in the rhEPO group compared to saline group. *$p < 0.01$. Panel H: Western blot and densitometry analysis of occludin expression 3 days after ICH in rhEPO and saline groups ($N = 9$). Compared with saline group, expression of occludin in rhEPO group was significantly greater. *$p < 0.05$. (I) Collagen IV expression was significantly greater in rhEPO group than in saline group. *$p < 0.01$

rhEPO maintained structural integrity after ICH

The integrity of the BBB endothelial cell tight junction was visualized by immunofluorescence staining of occludin in both lower and higher magnification images on the border of ICH injury in saline (Fig. 2A and C) and rhEPO groups (Fig. 2B and D). The expression level was also quantified by Western blot. Morphologically, occludin expression was less abundant and shorter and in length and width in the saline group as compared to the rhEPO group, where expression was much more robust and stronger. The area of occludin expression was significantly greater (40%) in the rhEPO group than

Fig. 3. rhEPO down-regulated MMPs, up-regulated TIMPs, and attenuated activated astrocytes 3 days after ICH. (A, B) MMP-2 (*red*), GFAP (*green*), and Hoechst (*blue*) triple-staining revealed less MMP-2 and GFAP expression in rhEPO groups (B) compared to saline (A). (C, D) TIMP-2 (*red*), GFAP (*green*) and Hoechst (*blue*) triple-staining showed less GFAP but more TIMP-2 in rhEPO treatment group (D) than saline group (C). Panel E: Western blots for MMP-2 and TIMP-2 3 days after ICH ($N = 9$). (F, G) Densitometry analysis of MMP-2 (F) and TIMP-2 (G) expression 3 days after ICH. Compared to saline group, there was significantly lower expression of MMP-2 but greater expression of TIMP-2 in rhEPO group. *$p < 0.05$. (H) Western blots for GFAP expression ($N = 9$). Significantly lower expression of GFAP was shown in rhEPO group as compared to saline group. *$p < 0.01$

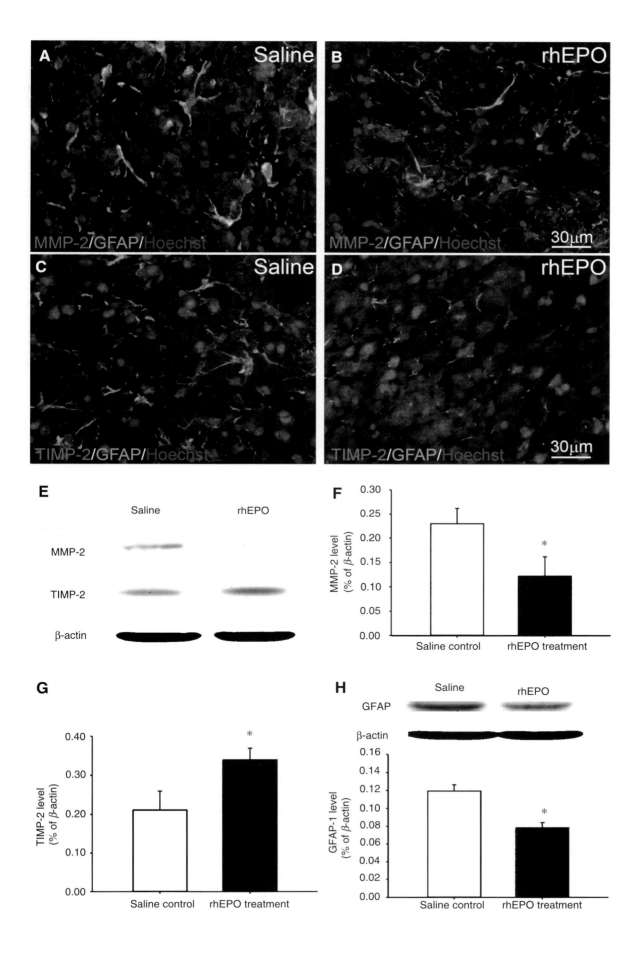

in the saline group (Fig. 2G). Occludin expression was also significantly greater in the rhEPO group when compared to saline control as detected by Western blot (Fig. 2H).

The structural integrity of BBB endothelial cells was also shown by immunofluorescence staining of collagen IV in the saline (Fig. 2E) and rhEPO groups (Fig. 2F). Three days after ICH, there was a much more abundant and stronger and expression of collagen IV on cerebral endothelial cells in the rhEPO group as compared to saline control. Its expression area was significantly greater in the rhEPO group (Fig. 2I).

rhEPO reduced MMP expression, increased TIMP expression, and reduced inflammatory reactions after ICH

Immunofluorescence staining at the border of ICH showed less MMP-2 but more TIMP-2 expression in the rhEPO treatment group (Fig. 3B and D) compared to saline control (Fig. 3A and C). Western blotting showed significantly lower expression of MMP-2 but greater expression of TIMP-2 in the rhEPO group as compared to saline group (Fig. 3E–3G). Immunofluorescence staining of GFAP at the border showed less abundant and weaker GFAP expression in the rhEPO group (Fig. 3B and D) than in saline group (Fig. 3A and C). Swollen astrocytes were barely detected in the rhEPO group. Western blotting revealed significantly lower expression of GFAP in the rhEPO group compared to saline group (Fig. 3H).

Discussion

Our study demonstrates that rhEPO significantly maintains BBB integrity in the acute phase after ICH. It also reveals the effects of rhEPO on suppression of MMP activity and the attenuation of neuro-inflammation with rhEPO treatment 3 days after ICH in an autologous whole blood-induced mouse model. Our study also indicates that exogenous administration of rhEPO attenuates neuro-inflammation by diminishing MMP activities and maintaining BBB after ICH.

It is well known that the degree of cell death and behavioral deficits after cerebral injury are highly dependent on the severity of BBB disruption, which makes the maintenance and protection of BBB one of the therapeutic strategies in many neurological diseases [6]. It has been shown that rhEPO protects against BBB disruption after seizure and global and focal ischemia [2, 9, 15]. We

first demonstrated the protective effect of rhEPO on BBB in a mouse ICH model. Damage to BBB was visualized and quantified by Evans blue leakage. The 2% Evans blue dye, which was administered intravenously, was detected under TRICT excitation wavelength. rhEPO treatment induced a significantly smaller leakage area, indicating decreased permeability of BBB 3 days after ICH with rhEPO treatment. To further support this data, relative water content was used to evaluate brain edema, which is an important clinical endpoint in ICH studies. Ipsilateral brain sections with ICH-induced damage had significantly less water content in the rhEPO treatment animals compared to saline control. These results demonstrate that rhEPO reduces BBB permeability and the consequential brain edema 3 days following ICH.

To maintain the barrier function of BBB, intracellular junction proteins play extraordinarily important roles. Among these proteins, tight junctions are exclusively recruited as the first defensive line with particular enzymes to prevent the entrance of certain substances [14]. Occludin, a well-accepted tight junction marker, was used to illustrate the integrity of the BBB. In cultured brain microvascular endothelial cells, decreased occludin expression was shown 24 h after being exposed in glutamate, a BBB disrupting agent [1]. Three days after focal ischemia, less abundant occludin was also detected [9]. In our current study, occludin expression was severely disrupted both inside and on the border of the lesion area 3 days after ICH. More abundant and better organized occludin-positive microvessels were detected in the rhEPO treatment group compared to the saline group. The area of occludin expression was significantly higher in the rhEPO group. These results were confirmed by Western blot. Taken together, rhEPO treatment preserved BBB, partly through maintaining the structure of endothelial cell tight junctions.

As the other key barrier that prevents larger molecules influx, the integrity of the basal lamina was detected as well. Anatomically, basal lamina forms a layer that wraps the endothelial cells and pericytes. Compared to the saline group, rhEPO treatment prevented type IV collagen degradation 3 days after ICH, as more abundant, longer, and thicker collagen IV expression was seen in the rhEPO treatment group. There was an almost doubled expression area of collagen IV in rhEPO group compared to saline group, which indicated the preservation of type IV collagen/basal lamina from degradation, therefore maintaining BBB integrity.

Our data demonstrated rhEPO's protective effects on the BBB in ICH from various angles. To further investigate the mechanisms, we focused our hypothesis on MMPs, as they have been implicated in degradation of the basal lamina degrader, which leads to BBB disruption [14]. Recently it has been reported that MMPs also degrade tight junction proteins, which leads to BBB disruption as well. Inhibition of MMPs reversed the disruption of tight junction proteins in focal ischemic rat [22]. MMPs are a subfamily of metalloproteinases, which have many members. They are recognized as matrix-degrading enzymes in BBB disruption, extracellular matrix remodeling, and inflammation [3]. MMP activity is regulated by TIMP [4]. In the CNS, most cell types are able to express MMPs and TIMPs after a variety of stimuli or injuries, including neurons, glia, and endothelial cells. An increasing amount of work has been done to characterize MMP/TIMP expression in ischemic stroke, but not in ICH. Bacterial collagenase-induced ICH is closely related to MMPs [13]. Up-regulation of MMP-2 and MMP-9, as well as acute brain injury after ICH, was ameliorated after a broad-spectrum MP inhibitor [18]. In our current study, expression of MMP-2 after ICH was significantly down-regulated by rhEPO treatment, while TIMP-2 expression was up-regulated 3 days after ICH in rhEPO animals. Our data indicate that rhEPO attenuates MMP expression and, thus, preserves both the endothelial cell tight junctions and the basal lamina, which may be involved in protection against BBB damage in the acute phase after ICH.

rhEPO has been well-demonstrated as an anti-inflammatory agent that exhibits potential for treatment of brain injury [16, 23]. Neuroprotection with rhEPO treatment after ICH was indicated by a decrease in TUNEL-positive cells compared to control groups 3 days after insult and better functional recovery at longer time points, which were achieved by reducing perihematomal inflammation [7]. The neuro-inflammatory response has cellular and molecular components. In terms of molecular inflammation, adhesion molecules, chemokines, and cytokines are the most common subtypes. MMPs are also thought to take part in brain inflammation. At the cellular level, inflammation is related to the elicitation and activation of certain types of cells into the injury area. Neutrophils, lymphocytes, and monocytes occur in the circulation, whereas astrocytes and microglia are seen in the injured brain [12]. In our present study, the less GFAP accumulation on the border of the ICH lesion area and a less-swollen morphology in the rhEPO treatment group indicated a lower inflammatory response to injuries. Since the level of inflammatory response in and

around the injured areas limited the severity of apoptosis, the attenuation of inflammation by rhEPO treatment 3 days after ICH provides further evidence of its anti-inflammation and anti-apoptosis functions.

Overall, our current study demonstrated that rhEPO attenuated neuro-inflammation after ICH by diminishing the activation of MMPs and preserving BBB integrity.

Acknowledgment

This work was supported by National Institutes of Health grants NS 37372, NS 045155, and NS 045810, and by NIH C06 RR015455 from the Extramural Research Facilities Program of the National Center for Research Resources.

References

1. András IE, Deli MA, Veszelka S, Hayashi K, Hennig B, Toborek M (2007) The NMDA and AMPA/KA receptors are involved in glutamate-induced alterations of occludin expression and phosphorylation in brain endothelial cells. J Cereb Blood Flow Metab 27: 1431–1443

2. Bahcekapili N, Uzüm G, Gökkusu C, Kuru A, Ziylan YZ (2007) The relationship between erythropoietin pretreatment with blood–brain barrier and lipid peroxidation after ischemia/reperfusion in rats. Life Sci 80: 1245–1251

3. Cunningham LA, Wetzel M, Rosenberg GA (2005) Multiple roles for MMPs and TIMPs in cerebral ischemia. Glia 50: 329–339

4. Gasche Y, Soccal PM, Kanemitsu M, Copin JC (2006) Matrix metalloproteinases and diseases of the central nervous system with a special emphasis on ischemic brain. Front Biosci 11: 1289–1301

5. Genc S, Koroglu TF, Genc K (2004) Erythropoietin as a novel neuroprotectant. Restor Neurol Neurosci 22: 105–119

6. Hawkins BT, Davis TP (2005) The blood–brain barrier/neurovascular unit in health and disease. Pharmacol Rev 57: 173–185

7. Lee ST, Chu K, Sinn DI, Jung KH, Kim EH, Kim SJ, Kim JM, Ko SY, Kim M, Roh JK (2006) Erythropoietin reduces perihematomal inflammation and cell death with eNOS and STAT3 activations in experimental intracerebral hemorrhage. J Neurochem 96: 1728–1739

8. Li Y, Lu Z, Keogh CL, Yu SP, Wei L (2007) Erythropoietin-induced neurovascular protection, angiogenesis, and cerebral blood flow restoration after focal ischemia in mice. J Cereb Blood Flow Metab 27: 1043–1054

9. Li Y, Lu ZY, Ogle M, Wei L (2007) Erythropoietin prevents blood–brain barrier damage induced by focal cerebral ischemia in mice. Neurochem Res 32: 2132–2141

10. Ma B, Zhang J (2006) Nimodipine treatment to assess a modified mouse model of intracerebral hemorrhage. Brain Res 1078: 182–188

11. Martinez-Estrada OM, Rodriguez-Millán E, González-De Vicente E, Reina M, Vilaró S, Fabre M (2003) Erythropoietin protects the in vitro blood–brain barrier against VEGF-induced permeability. Eur J Neurosci 18: 2538–2544

12. Nilupul Perera M, Ma HK, Arakawa S, Howells DW, Markus R, Rowe CC, Donnan GA (2006) Inflammation following stroke. J Clin Neurosci 13: 1–8

13. Power C, Henry S, Del Bigio MR, Larsen PH, Corbett D, Imai Y, Yong VW, Peeling J (2003) Intracerebral hemorrhage induces

macrophage activation and matrix metalloproteinases. Ann Neurol 53: 731–742

14. Rosenberg GA (2002) Matrix metalloproteinases in neuroinflammation. Glia 39: 279–291
15. Uzüm G, Sarper Diler A, Bahcekapili N, Ziya Ziylan Y (2006) Erythropoietin prevents the increase in blood–brain barrier permeability during pentylentetrazol induced seizures. Life Sci 78: 2571–2576
16. Villa P, Bigini P, Mennini T, Agnello D, Laragione T, Cagnotto A, Viviani B, Marinovich M, Cerami A, Coleman TR, Brines M, Ghezzi P (2003) Erythropoietin selectively attenuates cytokine production and inflammation in cerebral ischemia by targeting neuronal apoptosis. J Exp Med 198: 971–975
17. Wang J, Doré S (2007) Inflammation after intracerebral hemorrhage. J Cereb Blood Flow Metab 27: 894–908
18. Wang J, Tsirka SE (2005) Neuroprotection by inhibition of matrix metalloproteinases in a mouse model of intracerebral haemorrhage. Brain 128: 1622–1633
19. Wei L, Han BH, Li Y, Keogh CL, Holtzman DM, Yu SP (2006) Cell death mechanism and protective effect of erythropoietin after focal ischemia in the whisker-barrel cortex of neonatal rats. J Pharmacol Exp Ther 317: 109–116

20. Xue YQ, Zhao LR, Guo WP, Duan WM (2007) Intrastriatal administration of erythropoietin protects dopaminergic neurons and improves neurobehavioral outcome in a rat model of Parkinson's disease. Neuroscience 146: 1245–1258
21. Yang GY, Betz AL, Chenevert TL, Brunberg JA, Hoff JT (1994) Experimental intracerebral hemorrhage: relationship between brain edema, blood flow, and blood–brain barrier permeability in rats. J Neurosurg 81: 93–102
22. Yang Y, Estrada EY, Thompson JF, Liu W, Rosenberg GA (2007) Matrix metalloproteinase-mediated disruption of tight junction proteins in cerebral vessels is reversed by synthetic matrix metalloproteinase inhibitor in focal ischemia in rat. J Cereb Blood Flow Metab 27: 697–709
23. Yatsiv I, Grigoriadis N, Simeonidou C, Stahel PF, Schmidt OI, Alexandrovitch AG, Tsenter J, Shohami E (2005) Erythropoietin is neuroprotective, improves functional recovery, and reduces neuronal apoptosis and inflammation in a rodent model of experimental closed head injury. FASEB J 19: 1701–1703

Acta Neurochir Suppl (2008) 105: 113–117
© Springer-Verlag 2008
Printed in Austria

Hyperbaric oxygen for experimental intracerebral hemorrhage

Z. Qin[1,3], **G. Xi**[1], **R. F. Keep**[1], **R. Silbergleit**[2], **Y. He**[1], **Y. Hua**[1]

[1] Department of Neurosurgery, University of Michigan Medical School, Ann Arbor, MI, USA
[2] Department of Emergency Medicine, University of Michigan Medical School, Ann Arbor, MI, USA
[3] Department of Neurosurgery, Huashan Hospital, Fudan University, Shanghai, China

Summary

Acute brain edema formation contributes to brain injury after intracerebral hemorrhage (ICH). It has been reported that hyperbaric oxygen (HBO) is neuroprotective in cerebral ischemia, subarachnoid hemorrhage, and brain trauma. In this study, we investigated the effects of HBO on brain edema following ICH in rats.

Male Sprague-Dawley rats received intracerebral infusion of autologous whole blood, thrombin, or ferrous iron. HBO (100% O_2, 3.0 ATA for 1 h) was initiated 1 h after intracerebral injection. Control rats were exposed to air at room pressure. Brains were sampled at 24 or 72 h for water content, ion measurement, and Western blot analysis. We found that 1 session of HBO reduced perihematomal brain edema ($p < 0.05$) 24 h after ICH. HBO also reduced heat shock protein-32 (HSP-32) levels ($p < 0.05$) in ipsilateral basal ganglia 24 h after ICH. However, HBO failed to attenuate thrombin-induced brain edema and exaggerated ferrous iron-induced brain edema ($p < 0.05$). Three sessions of HBO also failed to reduce brain edema 72 h after ICH.

In summary, HBO reduced early perihematomal brain edema and HSP-32 levels in brain. HBO-related brain protection does not occur through reduction in thrombin toxicity because HBO failed to attenuate thrombin-induced brain edema. Our results also indicate that HBO treatment after hematoma lysis for ICH may be harmful, since HBO amplifies iron-induced brain edema.

Keywords: Hyperbaric oxygen; cerebral hemorrhage; thrombin; iron; heme oxygenase.

Introduction

Spontaneous intracerebral hemorrhage (ICH), originating from a variety of sources, causes instantaneous mass effect, disruption of surrounding brain, and often an early neurological death [13, 28]. There is currently no proven therapy for ICH. Brain injury after ICH appears to involve several phases [26], including an early phase involving the clotting cascade and thrombin production [5, 23] and a later phase involving erythrocyte lysis and toxicity from iron [4, 22].

Heme oxygenase-1 (HO-1) is a stress protein and a key enzyme for degradation of heme in hemoglobin [27]. HO-1 is upregulated after ICH [20]. An inhibitor of HO, tin-mesoporphyrin reduces perihematomal edema in pigs [19]. In a previous study, we showed that hemoglobin-induced brain edema is also attenuated by another HO inhibitor, tin-protoporphyrin, in a rat model of ICH [4].

Hyperbaric oxygen (HBO) treatment is neuroprotective in cerebral ischemia and brain trauma [2, 14, 17, 29]. Early use of HBO reduces blood–brain barrier (BBB) disruption, brain edema, and infarct volume after experimental cerebral ischemia [6, 9]. In another study, we also showed that HBO treatment attenuated hemorrhagic transformation after transient cerebral ischemia [12].

In the present study, we investigated the effect of HBO therapy on brain injury after ICH.

Materials and methods

Animal preparation and intracerebral injection

The animal protocol was approved by the University of Michigan Committee on the Use and Care of Animals. Male Sprague-Dawley rats (Charles River Laboratories, Portage, MI) weighing 300–350 g were used in this study. Rats were allowed free access to food and water before and after the experiment. Animals were anesthetized by intraperitoneal injection of pentobarbital (45 mg/kg). The right femoral artery was catheterized to monitor arterial blood pressure, to obtain blood for intracerebral injection, and for analysis of blood pH, PaO_2, $PaCO_2$, hematocrit, and glucose levels. Rectal temperature was maintained at 37.0–37.5 °C using a feedback-controlled heating pad. Animals were then positioned in a stereotactic frame (David Kopf Instruments,

Correspondence: Ya Hua, MD, Department of Neurosurgery, University of Michigan Medical School, 109 Zina Pitcher Place, R5018 Biomedical Science Research Building, Ann Arbor, MI 48109-2200, USA. e-mail: yahua@umich.edu

Tujunga, CA), and a cranial burr hole (1 mm) was drilled in the right coronal suture 3.5 mm lateral to the midline. Autologous whole blood, thrombin, or ferrous iron was infused into the right basal ganglia using a microinfusion pump (Harvard Apparatus, South Natick, MA) through a 26-gauge needle (coordinates: 0.2 mm anterior, 5.5 mm ventral, and 3.5 mm lateral to the bregma). The needle was removed, the burr hole was filled with bone wax, and the skin incision was closed with suture.

Experimental groups

There were 3 parts to our study. In the first part, rats received an intracaudate injection of autologous whole blood (100 μL) and underwent HBO treatment for 1 h each day beginning 1 h after intracerebral injection. Rats were killed 24 or 72 h later to obtain brain water content, ion measurements, and Western blot analysis. In the second part of the study, rats received intracaudate injection of thrombin (5 units in 50 μL saline) and the rats were treated with HBO 1 h later. Rats were killed at 24 h for brain edema measurements. In the third part, rats received intracaudate injection of ferrous iron (1 mM, 50 μL) and had HBO treatment 1 h later. Brains were sampled for brain water content measurement at 24 h.

HBO administration

Animals in HBO treatment groups were placed in a small rodent HBO chamber (Marine Dynamics Corp., Long Beach, CA). HBO-treated animals were pressurized over 15 min to a plateau pressure of 3 ATA with 100% oxygen supplied continuously and maintained for 60 min. Decompression was then carried out over 25–30 min. Control animals were also placed into the HBO chamber but received normobaric room air.

Brain water content measurement

Animals were re-anesthetized (pentobarbital 60 mg/kg, i.p.) and decapitated after ICH to measure brain water and ion content, as described previously [22]. The brains were removed and a coronal tissue slice (~3 mm thick) was cut 4 mm from the frontal pole using a blade. The brain tissue slice was divided into 2 hemispheres along the midline, and each hemisphere was dissected into cortex and basal ganglia. The cerebellum served as control. Five tissue samples from each brain were obtained: the ipsilateral and contralateral cortex, the ipsilateral and contralateral basal ganglia, and the cerebellum. Brain samples were immediately weighed on an electronic analytical balance (model AE 100; Mettler Instrument, Highstown, NJ) to obtain wet weight (WW). The dry weight (DW) of samples was determined after the tissues were heated for 24 h at 100 °C in a gravity oven (Blue M Electric Co., Watertown, WI). Tissue water content (%) was then calculated as: $100 \times (WW - DW)/WW$. The dehydrated samples were then digested in 1 mL of 1 mol/L nitric acid for 1 week. Sodium content was measured using an automatic flame photometer (model IL 943; Instrumentation Laboratory, Lexington, MA). Sodium ion content was expressed in micro-equivalents per gram of dehydrated brain tissue (μEq/gm DW).

Western blot analysis

Animals were re-anesthetized and underwent transcardiac perfusion with 0.1 M phosphate-buffered saline (PBS) until colorless perfusion fluid was obtained from the right atrium. A coronal brain section was then cut as described for brain water and ion content. The ipsilateral and contralateral basal ganglia were sampled, immersed in 0.5 mL of Western blot sample buffer, and sonicated. Protein concentration

was determined by Bio-Rad protein assay kit (Bio-Rad Laboratories, Hercules, CA). Western blot analysis was performed as described previously [24]. Fifty μg of protein for each sample were separated using sodium dodecyl sulfate polyacrylamide gel electrophoresis after being denatured by boiling at 95 °C for 5 min, and then transferred to pure nitrocellulose membrane. The membranes were blocked in Carnation nonfat milk and probed with polyclonal rabbit anti-heat shock protein-32 (HSP-32) at 1:2000 dilution (Stress Gen Biotechnologies, San Diego, CA) overnight, then immunoprobed by a second antibody (peroxidase-conjugated goat anti-rabbit antibody; Bio-Rad Laboratories). The antigen-antibody complexes were demonstrated with a chemiluminescence system (Amersham Pharmacia, Piscataway, NJ) and exposed to photosensitive film (X-OMAT; Kodak, Rochester, NY). Relative densities of the band were analyzed using NIH Image software, version 1.62 (National Institutes of Health, Bethesda, MD).

Statistical analysis

Data are expressed as mean ± standard deviation (SD). Statistical significance was analyzed using 2-tailed Student *t*-test or ANOVA with Scheffe's multiple comparison tests. Probability value of $p < 0.05$ was considered statistically significant.

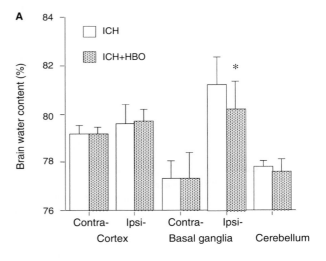

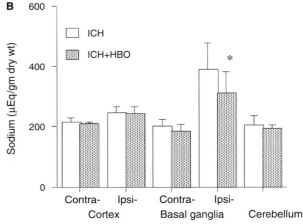

Fig. 1. Bar graph showing (A) water content and (B) sodium ion levels in different areas of rat brain 24 h after ICH. Values are mean ± SD, $n = 10$, *$p < 0.05$ vs. ICH

Results

One session of HBO treatment started at 1 h after ICH reduced brain water content in the ipsilateral basal ganglia 24 h later (80.2 ± 1.1 vs. 81.2 ± 1.1% in the control, $p < 0.05$; Fig. 1A). The reduction of water content was accompanied by a reduction in sodium ion accumulation (310 ± 68 vs. 388 ± 86 µEq/gm DW in control, $p < 0.05$; Fig. 1B). However, 3 consecutive sessions of HBO treatment failed to reduce brain water content at 72 h after ICH (82.1 ± 0.9 vs. 82.4 ± 0.8% vs. control, $p > 0.05$).

Thrombin infusion (5 units) resulted in marked brain edema. HBO treatment did not reduce thrombin-induced brain edema at 24 h (84.7 ± 1.5 vs. 84.7 ± 1.1% in control, $p > 0.05$; Fig. 2A) and sodium ion accumula-

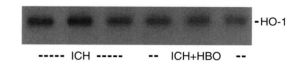

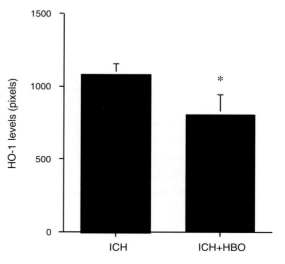

Fig. 3. HO-1 protein levels in ipsilateral basal ganglia measured by Western blot 24 h after ICH treated with or without HBO. Values are mean ± SD, $n = 3$, $^*p < 0.05$ vs. ICH

tion (701 ± 136 vs. 721 ± 141 µEq/gm DW, $p > 0.05$). Interestingly, HBO therapy significantly exaggerated ferrous iron-induced brain edema at 24 h (84.9 ± 0.8 vs. 82.2 ± 1.9% in control, $p < 0.05$; Fig. 2B) and sodium ion accumulation (706 ± 136 vs. 451 ± 143 µEq/gm DW, $p < 0.05$).

Western blot analysis showed that 1 session of HBO therapy reduced HO-1 levels in the ipsilateral basal ganglia (807 ± 137 vs. 1082 ± 72 pixels in control, $p < 0.05$; Fig. 3).

Discussion

In this study, we found that a single session of HBO attenuates perihematomal brain edema at 24 h after ICH. HBO treatment also reduced HO-1 protein levels in the ipsilateral basal ganglia after ICH. However, 3 sessions of repeated administration of HBO every 24 h did not reduce perihematomal brain edema at 72 h. In addition, HBO failed to attenuate thrombin-induced brain edema and exaggerated brain edema induced by ferrous iron.

It is still controversial whether secondary ischemia contributes to brain injury after ICH [28]. Cerebral blood flow (CBF) has been measured by single-photon emission computerized tomography in patients with ICH [7]. A zone of low CBF was found around the clot soon

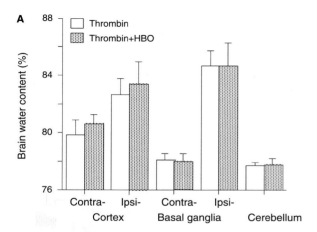

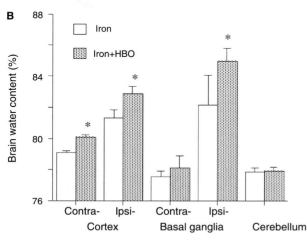

Fig. 2. (A) Brain water content 24 h after intracerebral infusion of thrombin (5 units in 50 µL saline) into right basal ganglia. HBO-treated rats received single HBO therapy. Values are mean ± SD, $n = 4$–5. (B) Brain water content 24 h after intracerebral injection of ferrous iron (1 mM in 50 µL saline). Rats were treated with HBO or normobaric room air 1 h after ferrous iron injection. Values are mean ± SD, $n = 5$, $^*p < 0.05$ vs. iron alone

after the ictus. This zone resolved within 48 h. Tanaka *et al.* [18] also reported CBF reduction after ICH. In a positron emission tomography study, however, Zazulia *et al.* [30] could not find secondary ischemic injury following ICH. Using diffusion-weighted magnetic resonance imaging and proton magnetic resonance spectroscopic imaging, widespread ischemia was not found around an intracerebral clot [1]. Experimental studies in animals have shown that CBF adjacent to a hematoma decreases [8], but the reduction is temporary and modest [11]. It is well known that HBO dramatically increases the oxygen content of blood, thereby increasing oxygen delivery to the brain [16, 31]. It is unclear, however, whether a modest reduction in CBF causes brain injury following ICH, and whether an increased oxygen level around hematoma can reduce acute brain damage.

HBO might also affect the level of proteins that are regulated by oxygen levels. The transcription factor, hypoxia inducible factor-1α, senses changes in oxygen levels and plays a critical role in the regulation of a number of proteins, including HO-1 [15]. HO-1, also known as heat shock protein-32 (HSP-32), is a key enzyme of heme degradation and is upregulated significantly after ICH. In the current study, we found that HBO reduces brain HO-1 protein levels around hematoma. Inhibition of HO is associated with reduction in perihematomal brain edema in rats [4] and pigs [19], but it is unclear whether reduced brain edema in the HBO-treated group results from lower levels of HO-1.

Our previous studies demonstrated that thrombin and iron are 2 major factors contributing to brain edema following ICH [3]. Thrombin causes BBB disruption and contributes to acute brain edema formation. Our current results show that HBO therapy fails to reduce thrombin-induced brain edema at 24 h. Iron also plays an important role in edema formation after ICH [10, 21]. In this study we found that HBO therapy exaggerates iron-induced brain edema. Ferrous iron can be converted into ferric iron, and HBO may accelerate this process, which exacerbates free radical production in the brain. We also found that 3 sessions of HBO failed to attenuate brain edema, possibly due to HBO-enhanced iron toxicity, since red blood cells start to lyse at 2–3 days after ICH [22, 25].

In summary, HBO reduced early perihematomal brain edema. HBO-induced brain protection does not occur through reduction in thrombin or iron toxicity. Our results also indicate that HBO treatment after hematoma lysis may be harmful.

Acknowledgments

This study was supported by grants NS-017760, NS-039866, and NS-047245 from the National Institutes of Health (NIH) and 0755717Z from American Heart Association (AHA). The content is solely the responsibility of the authors and does not necessarily represent the official views of the NIH or AHA.

References

1. Carhuapoma JR, Wang PY, Beauchamp NJ, Keyl PM, Hanley DF, Barker PB (2000) Diffusion-weighted MRI and proton MR spectroscopic imaging in the study of secondary neuronal injury after intracerebral hemorrhage. Stroke 31: 726–732
2. Henninger N, Kuppers-Tiedt L, Sicard KM, Gunther A, Schneider D, Schwab S (2006) Neuroprotective effect of hyperbaric oxygen therapy monitored by MR-imaging after embolic stroke in rats. Exp Neurol 201: 316–323
3. Hua Y, Keep RF, Hoff JT, Xi G (2007) Brain injury after intracerebral hemorrhage: the role of thrombin and iron. Stroke 38 (2 Suppl): 759–762
4. Huang FP, Xi G, Keep RF, Hua Y, Nemoianu A, Hoff JT (2002) Brain edema after experimental intracerebral hemorrhage: role of hemoglobin degradation products. J Neurosurg 96: 287–293
5. Lee KR, Colon GP, Betz AL, Keep RF, Kim S, Hoff JT (1996) Edema from intracerebral hemorrhage: the role of thrombin. J Neurosurg 84: 91–96
6. Lou M, Eschenfelder CC, Herdegen T, Brecht S, Deuschl G (2004) Therapeutic window for use of hyperbaric oxygenation in focal transient ischemia in rats. Stroke 35: 578–583
7. Mayer SA, Lignelli A, Fink ME, Kessler DB, Thomas CE, Swarup R, Van Heertum RL (1998) Perilesional blood flow and edema formation in acute intracerebral hemorrhage: a SPECT study. Stroke 29: 1791–1798
8. Mendelow AD, Bullock R, Teasdale GM, Graham DI, McCulloch J (1984) Intracranial haemorrhage induced at arterial pressure in the rat. Part 2: Short term changes in local cerebral blood flow measured by autoradiography. Neurol Res 6: 189–193
9. Mink RB, Dutka AJ (1995) Hyperbaric oxygen after global cerebral ischemia in rabbits reduces brain vascular permeability and blood flow. Stroke 26: 2307–2312
10. Nakamura T, Keep RF, Hua Y, Schallert T, Hoff JT, Xi G (2004) Deferoxamine-induced attenuation of brain edema and neurological deficits in a rat model of intracerebral hemorrhage. J Neurosurg 100: 672–678
11. Nath FP, Kelly PT, Jenkins A, Mendelow AD, Graham DI, Teasdale GM (1987) Effects of experimental intracerebral hemorrhage on blood flow, capillary permeability, and histochemistry. J Neurosurg 66: 555–562
12. Qin Z, Karabiyikoglu M, Hua Y, Silbergleit R, He Y, Keep RF, Xi G (2007) Hyperbaric oxygen-induced attenuation of hemorrhagic transformation after experimental focal transient cerebral ischemia. Stroke 38: 1362–1367
13. Qureshi AI, Ling GS, Khan J, Suri MF, Miskolczi L, Guterman LR, Hopkins LN (2001) Quantitative analysis of injured, necrotic, and apoptotic cells in a new experimental model of intracerebral hemorrhage. Crit Care Med 29: 152–157
14. Rockswold SB, Rockswold GL, Defillo A (2007) Hyperbaric oxygen in traumatic brain injury. Neurol Res 29: 162–172
15. Sharp FR, Bernaudin M (2004) HIF1 and oxygen sensing in the brain. Nat Rev Neurosci 5: 437–448
16. Sheffield PJ (1998) Measuring tissue oxygen tension: a review. Undersea Hyperb Med 25: 179–188

17. Singhal AB (2007) A review of oxygen therapy in ischemic stroke. Neurol Res 29: 173–183

18. Tanaka A, Yoshinaga S, Nakayama Y, Kimura M, Tomonaga M (1996) Cerebral blood flow and clinical outcome in patients with thalamic hemorrhages: a comparison with putaminal hemorrhages. J Neurol Sci 144: 191–197

19. Wagner KR, Hua Y, de Courten-Myers GM, Broderick JP, Nishimura RN, Lu SY, Dwyer BE (2000) Tin-mesoporphyrin, a potent heme oxygenase inhibitor, for treatment of intracerebral hemorrhage: in vivo and in vitro studies. Cell Mol Biol (Noisy-le-grand) 46: 597–608

20. Wu J, Hua Y, Keep RF, Schallert T, Hoff JT, Xi G (2002) Oxidative brain injury from extravasated erythrocytes after intracerebral hemorrhage. Brain Res 953: 45–52

21. Wu J, Hua Y, Keep RF, Nakamura T, Hoff JT, Xi G (2003) Iron and iron-handling proteins in the brain after intracerebral hemorrhage. Stroke. 34: 2964–2969

22. Xi G, Keep RF, Hoff JT (1998) Erythrocytes and delayed brain edema formation following intracerebral hemorrhage in rats. J Neurosurg 89: 991–996

23. Xi G, Wagner KR, Keep RF, Hua Y, de Courten-Myers GM, Broderick JP, Brott TG, Hoff JT (1998) The role of blood clot formation on early edema development following experimental intracerebral hemorrhage. Stroke 29: 2580–2586

24. Xi G, Keep RF, Hua Y, Xiang J, Hoff JT (1999) Attenuation of thrombin-induced brain edema by cerebral thrombin preconditioning. Stroke 30: 1247–1255

25. Xi G, Hua Y, Bhasin RR, Ennis SR, Keep RF, Hoff JT (2001) Mechanisms of edema formation after intracerebral hemorrhage: effects of extravasated red blood cells on blood flow and blood–brain barrier integrity. Stroke 32: 2932–2938

26. Xi G, Keep RF, Hoff JT (2002) Pathophysiology of brain edema formation. Neurosurg Clin N Am 13: 371–383

27. Xi G, Fewel ME, Hua Y, Thompson BG Jr, Hoff JT, Keep RF (2004) Intracerebral hemorrhage: pathophysiology and therapy. Neurocrit Care 1: 5–18

28. Xi G, Keep RF, Hoff JT (2006) Mechanisms of brain injury after intracerebral haemorrhage. Lancet Neurol 5: 53–63

29. Yin D, Zhang JH (2005) Delayed and multiple hyperbaric oxygen treatments expand therapeutic window in rat focal cerebral ischemic model. Neurocrit Care 2: 206–211

30. Zazulia AR, Diringer MN, Videen TO, Adams RE, Yundt K, Aiyagari V, Grubb RL Jr, Powers WJ (2001) Hypoperfusion without ischemia surrounding acute intracerebral hemorrhage. J Cereb Blood Flow Metab 21: 804–810

31. Zhang JH, Lo, T, Mychaskiw G, Colohan A (2005) Mechanisms of hyperbaric oxygen and neuroprotection in stroke. Pathophysiology 12: 63–77

Acta Neurochir Suppl (2008) 105: 119–121
© Springer-Verlag 2008
Printed in Austria

Effect of amantadine sulphate on intracerebral hemorrhage-induced brain injury in rats

E. Titova[5], R. P. Ostrowski[1], J. H. Zhang[1,2,3], J. Tang[1,4]

[1] Department of Physiology and Pharmacology, Loma Linda University, Loma Linda, CA, USA
[2] Department of Neurosurgery, Loma Linda University, Loma Linda, CA, USA
[3] Department of Anesthesiology, Loma Linda University, Loma Linda, CA, USA
[4] Department of Physiology, Chongqing Medical University, Chongqing, China
[5] Department of Anesthesiology, Krasnoyarsk State Medical University, Krasnoyarsk, Russia

Summary

Recent studies have shown that amantadine, an uncompetitive N-methyl-d-aspartate receptor antagonist and dopamine agonist, is effective for the treatment of various cerebral disorders and causes relatively mild side effects. In this study, we investigated whether administration of amantadine will provide a neuroprotective effect in the intracerebral hemorrhage (ICH) rat model.

A total of 15 male Sprague Dawley rats (300–380 g) were divided into sham, ICH-untreated, and ICH-treated with amantadine sulphate groups. ICH was induced by collagenase injection. Total dose 6 mg/kg of amantadine sulphate was divided into 3 injections and administered intraperitoneally at 1, 8, and 16 h after ICH. Brain injury was evaluated by investigating neurological function and brain edema at 24 h after ICH.

Our data demonstrates that ICH caused significant neurological deficit associated with marked brain edema. Amantadine did not reduce brain injury after ICH; neurological function and brain edema in the treated group were not different from those of the untreated group.

We conclude that amantadine sulphate does not offer neuroprotection in acute stage of experimental ICH-induced brain injury.

Keywords: Amantadine sulphate; rats; intracerebral hemorrhage; brain edema.

Introduction

Intracerebral hemorrhage (ICH) is a most devastating type of stroke with high mortality, morbidity, and severe disability. The latest clinical trials failed to confirm effectiveness of early surgical intervention as a cure for ICH. The search for the most effective pharmacological therapy is still ongoing.

Numerous pharmacological agents have been tested in ICH. Among others, aminoadamantanes are considered beneficial due to their neuroprotective effects and good therapeutic tolerance in both acute and chronic types of brain diseases. Aminoadamantanes such as 1-aminoadamantane (amantadine) and 1-amino-3,5-dimethyladamantane (memantine) are low-affinity uncompetitive NMDA receptor antagonists and also affect the synthesis, accumulation, release, and re-uptake of catecholamines within the central nervous system (CNS) [2]. As shown recently, Memantine is effective not only for Alzheimer's disease treatment but also in stroke therapy [5, 6, 16]. Despite having a chemical structure very similar to memantine, amantadine has other effects, such as actions at the sigma-1 receptor site, modulation of nicotinic receptors, and enhancement of noradrenergic transmission [9, 10]. This has led to the assumption that, besides the NMDA receptor antagonist effect, which is similar with memantine, additional targets of amantadine in CNS may account for its relatively complex pharmacological effects.

Amantadine, which was originally used for the treatment of influenza A, was later applied in Parkinson's disease. The latest publications suggest that amantadine is effective in the vegetative state and minimal consciousness state [14], and is also beneficial in traumatic brain injury in adults and children [7, 15].

In this study, we tested whether amantadine sulphate, the water soluble acid salt, improves short-term neurological outcomes in an experimental hemorrhage stroke model.

Correspondence: Jiping Tang, MD, Department of Physiology and Pharmacology, Loma Linda University Medical Center, 11041 Campus Street, Risley Hall Room 133, Loma Linda, CA 92354, USA. e-mail: jtang@llu.edu

Materials and methods

Experimental groups

A total of 15 male Sprague Dawley rats (300–380 g) were divided into a sham group ($n = 5$), an ICH-untreated group ($n = 6$), and an ICH group treated with 6 mg/kg of amantadine sulphate ($n = 4$).

Animal preparation

All procedures in this study were approved by the Animal Care and Use Committee at Loma Linda University and complied with the Guide for the Care and Use of Laboratory Animals.

Animals were housed under 12:12 h light/dark cycle with access to water and food *ad libitum*. Anesthesia was induced with 4% isoflurane in the induction chamber and maintained with 2–3% isoflurane in a 30/70% oxygen/air mixture given via mask to spontaneously breathing animals. Rectal temperature was maintained at $37 \pm 0.5\,°C$ with a warming blanket. The right femoral artery was cannulated with a PE-50 polyethylene cannula to monitor mean arterial blood pressure and to measure blood gas and blood glucose levels (1610 pH/Blood Gas Analyzer; Instrumentation Laboratories, Lexington, MA). Measurements of physiological parameters (arterial blood gas and blood glucose level) were taken before ICH induction, during collagenase injection, and after surgery.

For the experimental treatment, we used the infusion form of amantadine sulphate (0.4 mg/mL) produced by Merz Pharmaceuticals GmbH (Germany) for the management of akinetic crisis in patients with Parkinson's disease. The usual recommended dose for human treatment ranges from 200 to 600 mg/day, and is potent enough to increase level of consciousness. Therefore, aiming to mimic a clinical situation, we used a similar proportion, which for rats was calculated to be 6 mg/kg/day. We used the pharmacological form of the drug at a low concentration, considering that the elimination half-life of amantadine is 9.7–14.5 h. To avoid overhydration, we divided total amantadine dose into 3 injections given at 1, 8, and 16 h after ICH. The ICH with vehicle treatment group (untreated) was injected with the same volume of normal saline.

All animals were sacrificed at 24 h after surgery through deep anesthesia with isoflurane inhalation and subsequent decapitation. Brains were collected immediately to measure brain water content.

Surgical procedure

We adapted a collagenase-induced ICH model in rats, previously described by Rosenberg *et al.* [11, 12]. Briefly, anesthetized rats were positioned in a stereotaxic head frame (Kopf Instruments, Tujunga, CA) and a cranial burr-hole (1 mm) was drilled near the right coronal suture 2.9 mm lateral to the midline. A 27-gauge needle was inserted stereotaxically into the right basal ganglia (coordinates: 0.2 mm anterior, 5.6 mm ventral, and 2.9 mm lateral to the bregma). Bacterial collagenase (0.2 U in 1 μL of saline; VII-S, Sigma-Aldrich, St. Louis, MO) in a Hamilton syringe was infused into the brain over 5 min at a rate 0.2 μL/min with a micro-infusion pump (Harvard Apparatus, Holliston, MA). The needle was left in place for additional 10 min after injection to prevent possible leakage of collagenase solution. After removal of the needle, the skull hole was closed with bone wax. The skin incision was closed with suture and the rats were allowed to recover. Sham surgery was performed with only needle insertion.

Neurological deficits and mortality

Twenty-four hours after surgery, each rat was graded neurologically for focal deficits using the 18-point neurological scoring system by Garcia *et al.* [3] (minimum score = 3; maximum score (healthy rat) = 18).

Rating was performed blindly on individual animals and averaged in groups.

Brain water content

Brain water content was measured as described previously [12]. Briefly, rats were decapitated under deep anesthesia. The brains were removed immediately and divided into 3 parts: ipsilateral hemisphere, contralateral hemisphere, and cerebellum. The cerebellum was used as an internal control for brain water content. Tissue samples were weighed on an electronic analytical balance (APX-60; Denver Instrument, Denver, CO) to the nearest 0.1 mg to obtain the wet weight (WW). The tissue was then dried at 100 °C for 24 h to determine the dry weight (DW). Brain water content (%) was calculated as $[(WW - DW)/WW] \times 100$.

Results

All operated animals survived 24 h after surgery. Neurological deficit was detected in all animals with ICH. There was no statistical difference in neurological scores between treated and untreated groups (Fig. 1A).

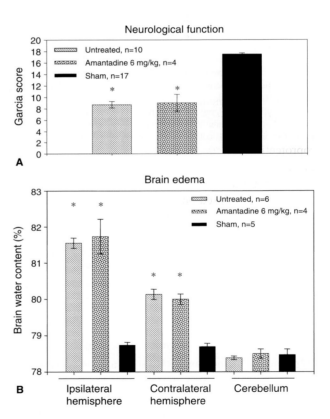

Fig. 1. Amantadine sulphate treatment in ICH. Panel (A) Neurological function was markedly impaired in all ICH-injured animals (*$p < 0.01$ vs. sham; ANOVA). However, there was no difference between treated and untreated groups at 24 h after ICH. Panel (B) Brain edema was significantly higher in all ICH-injured rats when compared with sham-operated animals (*$p < 0.001$ vs. sham, ANOVA). Amantadine sulphate treatment did not result in reduction of brain edema ($p > 0.05$ untreated vs. amantadine; ANOVA)

Brain edema was markedly increased in all animals with ICH, as compared with sham-operated group ($p < 0.05$, ANOVA). We failed to find a statistically significant difference between treated and untreated groups (Fig. 1B).

Discussion

While amantadine is a common and widely-used drug, little is known regarding its biochemical mechanisms and additional therapeutic options. Numerous clinical reports and multicenter studies have shown positive effects of amantadine treatment in unconsciousness patients, patients with acquired brain injury, as well as in pain management [4, 7, 13]. Considering uncompetitive NMDA antagonism, theoretically amantadine may prevent excitotoxic neuronal death after stroke [1]. Moreover, amantadine treatment may have additional advantages such as improving cognitive alertness and awareness in patients because of enhanced dopaminergic pathways [8] and increased catecholamine levels.

The design of our study mimics a clinical situation where acute stage ICH is treated with the infusion form of amantadine sulphate, offered specifically to intensive care departments. The recommended dose ranges from 200 to 600 mg/day was reported as being safe for patients [7]. Although we did not find short-term neuroprotective effects of sulphate amantadine treatment on neurological function and brain edema in an ICH experimental animal model, this result is not entirely disappointing. Based on studies mentioned above, it is clear that a future study with long-term treatment is needed to understand effects of amantadine on brain repair mechanisms and functional performance after ICH.

Acknowledgment

This work was supported by grant NS052492 from the National Institutes of Health to Jiping Tang.

References

1. Chen HS, Lipton SA (2006) The chemical biology of clinically tolerated NMDA receptor antagonists. J Neurochem 97: 1611–1626
2. Danysz W, Parsons CG, Kornhuber J, Schmidt WJ, Quack G (1997) Aminoadamantanes as NMDA receptor antagonists and antiparkinsonian agents – preclinical studies. Neurosci Biobehav Rev 21: 455–468
3. Garcia JH, Wagner S, Liu KF, Hu XJ (1995) Neurological deficit and extent of neuronal necrosis attributable to middle cerebral artery occlusion in rats. Statistical validation. Stroke 26: 627–635
4. Kleinböhl D, Görtelmeyer R, Bender HJ, Hölzl R (2006) Amantadine sulfate reduces experimental sensitization and pain in chronic back pain patients. Anesth Analg 102: 840–847
5. Lee ST, Chu K, Jung KH, Kim J, Kim EH, Kim SJ, Sinn DI, Ko SY, Kim M, Roh JK (2006) Memantine reduces hematoma expansion in experimental intracerebral hemorrhage, resulting in functional improvement. J Cereb Blood Flow Metab 26: 536–544
6. McShane R, Areosa Sastre A, Minakaran N (2006) Memantine for dementia. Cochrane Database Syst Rev CD003154
7. Meythaler JM, Brunner RC, Johnson A, Novack TA (2002) Amantadine to improve neurorecovery in traumatic brain injury-associated diffuse axonal injury: a pilot double-blind randomized trial. J Head Trauma Rehabil 17: 300–313
8. Napolitano E, Elovic EP, Qureshi AI (2005) Pharmacological stimulant treatment of neurocognitive and functional deficits after traumatic and non-traumatic brain injury. Med Sci Monit 11: RA212–RA220
9. Peeters M, Maloteaux JM, Hermans E (2003) Distinct effects of amantadine and memantine on dopaminergic transmission in the rat striatum. Neurosci Lett 343: 205–209
10. Peeters M, Romieu P, Maurice T, Su TP, Maloteaux JM, Hermans E (2004) Involvement of the sigma 1 receptor in the modulation of dopaminergic transmission by amantadine. Eur J Neurosci 19: 2212–2220
11. Rosenberg GA, Mun-Bryce S, Wesley M, Kornfeld M (1990) Collagenase-induced intracerebral hemorrhage in rats. Stroke 21: 801–807
12. Titova E, Ostrowski RP, Sowers LC, Zhang JH, Tang J (2007) Effects of apocynin and ethanol on intracerebral haemorrhage-induced brain injury in rats. Clin Exp Pharmacol Physiol 34: 845–850
13. Whyte J, DiPasquale MC, Vaccaro M (1999) Assessment of command-following in minimally conscious brain injured patients. Arch Phys Med Rehabil 80: 653–660
14. Whyte J, Katz D, Long D, DiPasquale MC, Polansky M, Kalmar K, Giacino J, Childs N, Mercer W, Novak P, Maurer P, Eifert B (2005) Predictors of outcome in prolonged posttraumatic disorders of consciousness and assessment of medication effects: a multicenter study. Arch Phys Med Rehabil 86: 453–462
15. Williams SE (2007) Amantadine treatment following traumatic brain injury in children. Brain Inj 21: 885–889
16. Winblad B, Poritis N (1999) Memantine in severe dementia: results of the 9M-Best Study (Benefit and efficacy in severely demented patients during treatment with memantine). Int J Geriatr Psychiatry 14: 135–146

Experimental intracerebral hemorrhage – model development and characterization

Acta Neurochir Suppl (2008) 105: 125–126
© Springer-Verlag 2008
Printed in Austria

Long-term behavioral characterization of a rat model of intracerebral hemorrhage

R. E. Hartman[1], H. Rojas[2], J. Tang[2], J. Zhang[2]

[1] Department of Psychology, Loma Linda University, Loma Linda, CA, USA
[2] Department of Physiology and Pharmacology, Loma Linda University, Loma Linda, CA, USA

Summary

We tested the behavioral effects of intracerebral hemorrhage (ICH) in adult male rats. ICH was induced by collagenase injection into the basal ganglia and the rats were subjected to a longitudinal behavioral test battery. Both learning and memory deficits were detected shortly after injury. Two months after injury, there were still significant short- and long-term memory deficits. Rotarod testing also revealed long-term sensorimotor coordination deficits. No differences in activity levels were detected at any time. Thus, spontaneous ICH produced detectable cognitive and motor deficits that evolved over the course of 2 months. Along with histological analysis of infarct volume, this characterization provides a suitable baseline for the analysis of therapeutic interventions.

Keywords: Hemorrhage; collagenase; learning; memory; motor.

Introduction

Because cognitive deficits after intracerebral hemorrhage (ICH) in humans are among the most prominent and troubling [7, 8, 11], and because of increasing evidence that the striatum plays a role in learning/memory [1, 2, 9, 10], it is important to characterize both motor and cognitive deficits in animal models of ICH.

Materials and methods

Adult male Sprague-Dawley rats were divided into sham-operated controls and ICH groups.

Intracerebral hemorrhage

Injecting collagenase into the basal ganglia induced ICH, as previously described [12]. Sham surgery was performed with needle insertion alone.

Correspondence: Richard E. Hartman, PhD, Department of Psychology, Loma Linda University, 11130 Anderson St. 119, Loma Linda, CA 92354, USA. e-mail: behavioralneuroscience@gmail.com

Behavioral testing

After 2 weeks and 2 months, the rats were subjected to a battery of behavioral tests, including:

- *Sensorimotor coordination/balance.* The rats were tested using an accelerating Rotarod treadmill.
- *General activity levels/movement patterns.* Activity was assessed similar to previously published protocols [3, 4, 6].
- *Learning/memory.* The water maze tests the learning and memory abilities of rodents [3–6] and requires finding a hidden (submerged) platform in a pool of water using visual cues from around the room. The *cued* (visible platform) task is used to assess sensorimotor and/or motivational deficits that could affect performance during the spatial water maze task. The *spatial* (submerged platform) task required the animal to find the platform based on its relationship to spatial cues in the room. The animals were given 10 trials on each task. The dependent variable was swim distance required to find the escape platform. A probe trial, in which the platform is removed from the water maze, was performed 24 h after the end of the spatial training session, and time spent searching the area that previously contained the platform was measured.

Results

Water maze – early

ICH rats performed significantly worse on both the cued ($p < 0.04$) and spatial ($p < 0.0002$) learning tasks, although there were no differences in probe trial (memory) performance.

Water maze – late

ICH rats performed normally on the cued learning task, and slightly, but not significantly, worse on the spatial learning task. Probe trials revealed memory deficits, however ($p < 0.005$).

Sensorimotor coordination/balance

There were no differences in latency to fall off the Rotarod at the early time point. Therefore, the task was made more difficult (i.e., faster acceleration) for the late time point. The ICH rats performed significantly worse than controls on the accelerating task at the late time point ($p < 0.05$).

General activity levels/movement patterns

There were no differences in general activity levels or movement patterns at either time point.

Discussion

The collagenase injection model of ICH in adult male rat striatum was associated with long-lasting cognitive (spatial memory) and motor (sensorimotor coordination) deficits. This type of repeated behavioral characterization can therefore provide a baseline for the analysis of therapeutic treatments and closely approximates the human condition, in which practice effects are often used as therapeutic strategies.

It is interesting to note that this model produced no observable differences in spontaneous open field activity levels, and that this lack of differences was also reflected in the general observation of home-cage and handling activity. However, testing activity levels in an open field is not a stressful, motivation-driven task like the water maze or Rotarod.

In summary, the collagenase injection model of ICH produced short- and long-term deficits across a broad variety of behavioral domains. Along with histological analysis of infarct size, these tests provide several targets for future tests of short- and long-term efficacy of therapeutic strategies following stroke.

Acknowledgement

This study is partially supported by a grant from the National Institutes of Health (NIHNS53407) to JHZ.

References

1. Benke T, Delazer M, Bartha L, Auer A (2003) Basal ganglia lesions and the theory of fronto-subcortical loops: neuropsychological findings in two patients with left caudate lesions. Neurocase 9: 70–85
2. El Massioui N, Chéruel F, Faure A, Conde F (2007) Learning and memory dissociation in rats with lesions to the subthalamic nucleus or to the dorsal striatum. Neuroscience 147: 906–918
3. Hartman RE, Izumi Y, Bales KR, Paul SM, Wozniak DF, Holtzman DM (2005) Treatment with an amyloid-beta antibody ameliorates plaque load, learning deficits, and hippocampal long-term potentiation in a mouse model of Alzheimer's disease. J Neurosci 25: 6213–6220
4. Hartman RE, Lee JM, Zipfel GJ, Wozniak DF (2005) Characterizing learning deficits and hippocampal neuron loss following transient global cerebral ischemia in rats. Brain Res 1043: 48–56
5. Hartman RE, Shah A, Fagan AM, Schwetye KE, Parsadanian M, Schulman RN, Finn MB, Holtzman DM (2006) Pomegranate juice decreases amyloid load and improves behavior in a mouse model of Alzheimer's disease. Neurobiol Dis 24: 506–515
6. Hartman RE, Wozniak DF, Nardi A, Olney JW, Sartorius L, Holtzman DM (2001) Behavioral phenotyping of GFAP-apoE3 and -apoE4 transgenic mice: apoE4 mice show profound working memory impairments in the absence of Alzheimer's-like neuropathology. Exp Neurol 170: 326–344
7. King JT Jr, DiLuna ML, Cicchetti DV, Tsevat J, Roberts MS (2006) Cognitive functioning in patients with cerebral aneurysms measured with the mini mental state examination and the telephone interview for cognitive status. Neurosurgery 59: 803–811
8. Nys GM, van Zandvoort MJ, de Kort PL, Jansen BP, de Haan EH, Kappelle LJ (2007) Cognitive disorders in acute stroke: prevalence and clinical determinants. Cerebrovasc Dis 23: 408–416
9. Ragozzino ME (2007) The contribution of the medial prefrontal cortex, orbitofrontal cortex, and dorsomedial striatum to behavioral flexibility. Ann N Y Acad Sci 1121: 355–375
10. Sridharan D, Prashanth PS, Chakravarthy VS (2006) The role of the basal ganglia in exploration in a neural model based on reinforcement learning. Int J Neural Syst 16: 111–124
11. Thajeb P, Thajeb T, Dai D (2007) Cross-cultural studies using a modified mini mental test for healthy subjects and patients with various forms of vascular dementia. J Clin Neurosci 14: 236–241
12. Titova E, Ostrowski RP, Sowers LC, Zhang JH, Tang J (2007) Effects of apocynin and ethanol on intracerebral haemorrhage-induced brain injury in rats. Clin Exp Pharmacol Physiol 34: 845–850

Acta Neurochir Suppl (2008) 105: 127–130
© Springer-Verlag 2008
Printed in Austria

Neurological deficits and brain edema after intracerebral hemorrhage in Mongolian gerbils

T. Kuroiwa[1,2], **M. Okauchi**[2], **Y. Hua**[2], **T. Schallert**[2], **R. F. Keep**[2], **G. Xi**[2]

[1] Clinical Laboratory, Namegata District General Hospital, Namegata, Ibaraki, Japan
[2] Crosby Neurosurgical Laboratories, Department of Neurosurgery, University of Michigan Medical School, Ann Arbor, MI, USA

Summary

We examined the time course of neurological deficits in gerbils after an intracerebral hemorrhage (ICH) induced by autologous blood infusion and examined its correlation with the severity of perihematomal edema.

Mongolian gerbils ($n = 15$) were subjected to stereotaxic autologous blood infusion (30 or 60 μL) into the left caudate nucleus. Corner-turn and forelimb-placing tests were performed before, and 1 and 3 days after ICH. Perihematomal water content was measured by tissue gravimetry. Gerbils developed neurological deficits and perihematomal edema at day 1 after ICH. Both neurological deficits and perihematomal edema were significantly greater in animals with 60 μL blood infusion compared to the 30 μL infusion group, and both neurological deficits and edema were also greater at 3 days compared to 1 day after ICH. The severity of neurological deficits paralleled the degree of perihematomal edema. We conclude that the Mongolian gerbil is a suitable model for studies on the behavioral effects of ICH.

Keywords: Mongolian gerbil; intracerebral hemorrhage; autologous blood infusion; perihematomal edema; gravimetry; forelimb-placing test; corner-turn test.

Introduction

Mongolian gerbils are rodents suitable for assessment of neurological deficits and they have been used for many years in neuroscience research [3–5]. We examined neurological deficits in gerbils after intracerebral hemorrhage (ICH) induced by autologous blood infusion into the caudate nucleus. Corner-turn and forelimb-placing tests were applied for the assessment of neurological deficits. We observed close association between post-ICH neurological deficits and perihematomal edema. Both brain edema and neurological deficits were exacer-

Correspondence: Toshihiko Kuroiwa, Clinical Laboratory, Namegata District General Hospital, Inouefujii 98-8 Namegata, Ibaraki 311-3516, Japan. e-mail: tkuroiwa-nsu@umin.ac.jp

bated over 3 days after onset of ICH and varied with hematoma size.

Materials and methods

Adult male Mongolian gerbils ($n = 15$) were used in this study. Under isoflurane anesthesia, gerbils were subjected to either stereotaxic autologous blood infusion (30 or 60 μL) into the left caudate nucleus or a sham-operation (control group) [7]. Corner-turn and forelimb-placing tests were performed before and 1 and 3 days after ICH [5, 6] (Fig. 1). Water content in the perihematomal tissue was measured by tissue gravimetry [1]. All data were expressed as mean ± SEM. *P*-values of less than 0.05 were considered significant.

Results

All gerbils survived autologous blood injection. Animals were sacrificed at day 1 or 3 under isoflurane anesthesia, and the brain removed. The cut surface of the brain showed the hematoma with perihematomal edema. Water content of the perihematomal tissue was significantly increased in both the 30 and 60 μL blood groups at day 1 (water content: 79.6 ± 0.52, 80.7 ± 0.36, and 77.6 ± 0.31% in 30 μL blood, 60 μL blood, and control groups, respectively; Fig. 2A). Perihematomal edema was exacerbated at day 3 after onset of ICH (water content: 81.5 ± 0.62% and 77.4 ± 0.06% in 30 μL blood and control groups, respectively; Fig. 2B).

After ICH, gerbils developed significant neurological deficits at day 1. The rate of left corner turns was 0.23 ± 0.15, 0.03 ± 0.03, and 0.43 ± 0.07 in the 30 μL blood, 60 μL blood, and control groups, respectively (Fig. 2C). Forelimb-placing scores were 0.67 ± 0.17, 0.27 ± 0.15, and 0.93 ± 0.07 in the 30 μL blood, 60 μL blood, and control groups, respectively (Fig. 2E).

T. Kuroiwa *et al.*

Corner turn   Forelimb placing

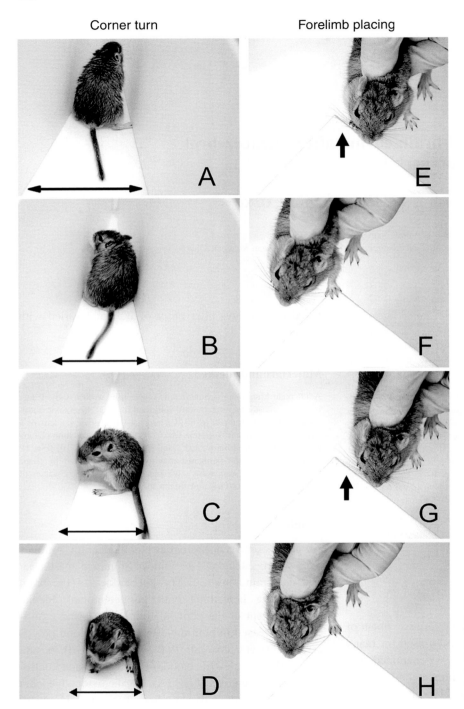

Fig. 1. Corner-turn (A–D) and forelimb-placing (E–H) tests. With the narrowing of the corner (see *arrows*), vibrissae on both sides touch the wall. The animal makes left turn, which is contralateral to the sensory-disturbed side. Forelimb-placing is failed on the right side (see *arrows*), which developed sensorimotor disturbance

Neurological deficits were exacerbated at day 3. Thus, the rate of left corner turns was 0.13 ± 0.15 and 0.47 ± 0.06 in the 30 μL blood and control groups, respectively (Fig. 2D). Forelimb-placing scores were 0.43 ± 0.07 and 0.97 ± 0.03 in 30 μL blood and control groups, respectively (Fig. 2F). Thus, the severity of edema and neurological deficits paralleled injected blood volume, and both increased over 3 days after onset of ICH.

Discussion

We examined neurological deficits and perihematomal edema in a gerbil model of ICH induced by autologous blood infusion into the caudate nucleus. An autologous blood infusion model has been developed using rats and mice [6, 7]. We found Mongolian gerbils are also useful for this model because the animal has a highly sponta-

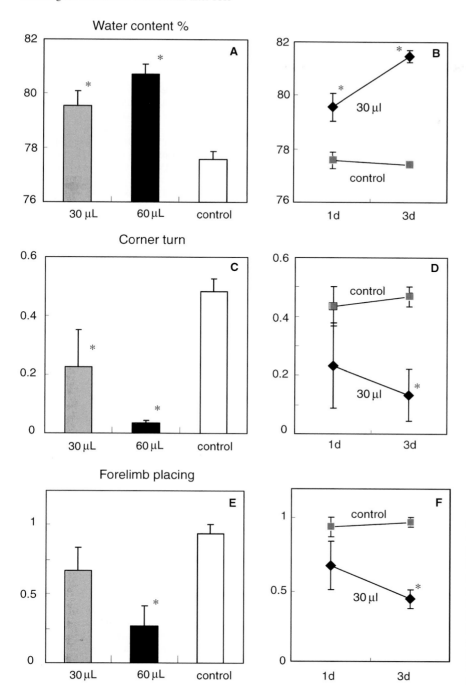

Fig. 2. (A) Water content of perihematomal tissue at 1 day after onset of ICH in 30 μL hematoma (*black*), 60 μL hematoma (*gray*), or sham-operated (*white*) groups. (B) Edema exaggerated at 3 days after onset of ICH. (C) Corner-turn test showed more severe deficit in gerbils with larger hematoma at 1 day after onset of ICH. (D) Neurological deficits were exacerbated at day 3 after onset of ICH. (E, F) Similar change and time course were found in forelimb-placing test. Values are mean ± SEM. *$P < 0.05$ vs. other groups

neous locomotive activity and assessment of neurological deficits is easier than with the other rodents. Two tests that can detect post-ICH neurological deficits in rats [2], forelimb-placing and corner-turn tests, were also useful in this gerbil ICH model. The deficits were exacerbated at day 3 compared to day 1.

Brain edema was assessed using tissue gravimetry with a kerosene/monobrombenzene gradient column [1]. For

this procedure, the sample size was approximately 10 mg, which is suitable for assessment of brain edema development in the rodent brain. We detected significant perihematomal edema at day 1 after onset of ICH. The edema was exacerbated at day 3, which probably corresponds to the delayed brain edema formation observed in rat [7].

These results suggest a close correlation between the severity of behavioral deficits and the degree of brain edema formation. They also suggest that the Mongolian gerbil is a suitable model for ICH studies, particularly those focused on ICH-induced behavioral deficits.

References

1. Fujiwara K, Nitsch C, Suzuki R, Klatzo I (1981) Factors in the reproducibility of the gravimetric method for evaluation of edematous changes in the brain. Neurol Res 3: 345–361
2. Hua Y, Schallert T, Keep RF, Wu J, Hoff JT, Xi G (2002) Behavioral tests after intracerebral hemorrhage in the rat. Stroke 33: 2478–2484
3. Ishibashi S, Kuroiwa T, Endo S, Okeda R, Mizusawa H (2003) Neurological dysfunctions versus regional infarction volume after focal ischemia in Mongolian gerbils. Stroke 34: 1501–1506
4. Lavyne M, Moskowitz M, Zervas N, Wurtman R (1975) Rotational behavior in gerbils following unilateral common carotid artery ligation. J Neural Transm 36: 83–89
5. Lumia AR, Westervelt MO, Rieder CA (1975) Effects of olfactory bulb ablation and androgen on marking and agonistic behavior in male Mongolian gerbils (Meriones unguiculatus). J Comp Physiol Psych 89: 1091–1099
6. Nakamura T, Xi G, Hua Y, Schallert T, Hoff JT, Keep RF (2004) Intracerebral hemorrhage in mice: model characterization and application for genetically modified mice. J Cereb Blood Flow Metab 24: 487–494
7. Xi G, Keep RF, Hoff JT (1998) Erythrocytes and delayed brain edema formation following intracerebral hemorrhage in rats. J Neurosurg 89: 991–996

Acta Neurochir Suppl (2008) 105: 131–134
© Springer-Verlag 2008
Printed in Austria

Rat model of intracerebellar hemorrhage

T. Lekic[1], J. Tang[1], J. H. Zhang[1,2,3]

[1] Department of Physiology and Pharmacology, Loma Linda University, Loma Linda, CA, USA
[2] Department of Neurosurgery, Loma Linda University, Loma Linda, CA, USA
[3] Department of Anesthesiology, Loma Linda University, Loma Linda, CA, USA

Summary

Approximately 15% of all strokes are due to intracerebral hemorrhage (ICH) and of these, 5–10% occur in the cerebellum. The resultant mortality is around 20–30%. However, there is no well-established animal model to address this important clinical problem.

We induced intracerebellar hemorrhage in rats using stereotaxic collagenase injection through a burr-hole into right cerebellum. Dosage-dependent effect of collagenase (0.2, 0.4, and 0.6 U) was tested in male and female rats. Brain edema formation was assessed by brain water content and hemorrhagic volume measured by hemoglobin assay. Wire suspension, inclined plane, beam walking, and neurological deficit score assessed neurological outcome. Marked hematoma was observed in right cerebellum, accompanied by brain edema in a dose-related fashion. When comparing sexes, hemorrhagic volume and neurological deficit scores were significantly increased in females compared to male counterpart. Females had mortality of 16%, while there was no mortality in male rats. Neurological deficits assessed by both beam walking and inclined plane were significantly increased at 0.4 and 0.6 U in females, but only at 0.6 for males. This new cerebellar hemorrhage rat model demonstrated dosage- and sex-dependent changes in hemorrhagic volume, brain edema, and neurological deficits, and could be used to test treatment strategies for ICH.

Keywords: Cerebellum; collagenase; stroke; intracerebellar hemorrhage.

Introduction

Of the 15% of strokes due to intracerebral hemorrhage (ICH) [7], 5–10% of these will occur in the cerebellum [9], with consequent mortality around 20–30% [6]. However, there has yet to be described an adequate animal model to address the important issues of neuroprotection and edema reduction for this important clinical problem.

Materials and methods

All procedures used in our studies were in compliance with the *Guide for the Care and Use of Laboratory Animals* and approved by the Animal Care and Use Committee at Loma Linda University. Aseptic technique was used for all surgeries, and rats were allowed free access to food and water.

Experimental design

A total of 40 Sprague-Dawley rats (290–395 g; Harlan, Indianapolis, IN), 20 male and 20 female, were used in our study. Female rats were one week post-partum. For brain edema and neurological function measurements, rats were divided into sham, 0.2, 0.4, and 0.6 U collagenase, at 4 rats per group. A separate cohort was used for hemorrhagic volume measurements. All animals were euthanized after neurological testing (as described below) at 24 h post-hemorrhage induction, and then samples were collected for hemoglobin assay and brain edema measurements.

Cerebellar hemorrhage induction

Rats were anesthetized with isoflurane and placed prone in a stereotaxic frame (Kopf Instruments, Tujunga, CA). Then, using a collagenase injection ICH model similar to that described previously in rats [8], we used the following modified stereotactic coordinates to localize the right cerebellar hemisphere: 11.64 mm posterior, 3.5 mm ventral, and 2.4 mm lateral to the bregma. A posterior cranial burr-hole (1 mm) was drilled over the right cerebellar hemisphere, into which a 27-gauge needle was inserted at a rate of 1 mm/min. A microinfusion pump (Harvard Apparatus, Holliston, MA) infused the bacterial collagenase (0.2 U in 1 μL saline; VII-S, Sigma-Aldrich, St. Louis, MO) through a Hamilton syringe at a rate of 0.2 μL/min. Needle remained in place for an additional 10 min after injection to prevent "back-leakage". To maintain a core temperature within 37.0 ± 0.5 °C, an electronic thermostat-controlled warming blanket was used throughout the operation. After needle removal, the burr-hole was sealed with bone wax, incision sutured closed, and animals allowed to recover. Sham surgeries consisted of needle insertion alone.

Hemorrhagic volume

At 24 h after induction of cerebellar hemorrhage, a hemoglobin assay was performed as described previously [10]. Briefly, rats were killed by

Correspondence: John H. Zhang, MD, PhD, Department of Physiology and Pharmacology, Loma Linda University School of Medicine, Loma Linda, CA 92354, USA. e-mail: Johnzhang3910@yahoo.com

an overdose of isoflurane and perfused transcardially with 300 mL of "ice-cold" (4 °C) phosphate-buffered saline (PBS). The cerebellum was extracted and dissected free of the brainstem and cerebral hemispheres. This tissue was homogenized (Tissuemiser homogenizer; Fisher Scientific, Pittsburgh, PA) for 60 sec in a test tube with distilled water (total volume, 3 mL). After the centrifugation phase (15,800 *g* for 30 min; Eppendorf Microcentrifuge model 5417R, Hamburg, Germany), Drabkin's reagent (400 μL; Sigma-Aldrich) was added into the 100 μL aliquots of supernatant (4 samples per brain) and allowed to react for 15 min. The solution's absorbance was read using a spectrophotometer (540 nm; Spectronic Genesis 5, Thermo Electron Corp., Waltham, MA), and the amount of blood in each brain was calculated using a curve generated previously using known blood volumes from the same brain region.

Brain water content

Brain edema was measured by methods described previously [10]. Briefly, under deep anesthesia, rats were decapitated, and brains were immediately removed and divided into 4 parts: right and left cerebral hemispheres, brainstem, and cerebellum. The cerebral hemispheres were used as internal controls. These tissue samples were weighed on an electronic analytical balance (APX-60, Denver Instrument, Denver, CO) to the nearest 0.01 mg to obtain the wet weight (WW), and then the tissue was dried at 100 °C for 24 h to determine dry weight (DW). Finally, the brain water content (%) was calculated as (WW–DW)/WW × 100.

Neurological deficit score

Neurological evaluation was conducted using a 6-point neurological scoring system 24 h after collagenase injection. Scoring is based on a vertebrobasilar stroke assessment scale developed by others [11] and used to assess rats in another posterior circulation stroke model [5]. It quantifies limb extensions and dyscoordination (0 = no deficiency, 3 = severely deficient). The examiner had no knowledge of hemorrhagic severity that each rat received.

Wire suspension forelimb testing

This method assessed forelimb strength and balancing ability, as described in greater detail elsewhere [2]. Testing involved a wire 3 mm (diameter) × 40 cm (length) × 100 cm (height), over a 2-inch thick soft cushioned pad and recorded latency before falling (60-sec cut-off), with 2 trials per session and a 10-min inter-trial period.

Inclined plane paradigm

Used previously by others [4] as an indirect measure of overall muscular strength and integrated motor-proprioceptive abilities, testing consisted of a 20 cm (width) × 70 cm (length) × 10 cm (height) box, with a hinge attached to a heavy wooden base so that one end of the box could be lifted to establish an "inclined plane." Angle was recorded by analog protractor attached to the side of the device. Rats were placed right side up and left side up, toward the side of board to be raised. Plane was raised from 10 to 90° at 5° intervals until the animal began to slip backwards. The highest angle achieved was recorded for the 2 trials performed (1 h inter-trial period). The average angle across 2 body positions and both trials was recorded as the final value.

Beam walking ability

This apparatus consisted of a horizontal rod 50 cm (length) × 5 cm (diameter) covered with masking tape to provide firm grip. More detail has

been provided by others [2]. The beam was marked with a ruler into five partitions of 10 cm each, and placed 90 cm above a landing area covered with a 3-inch thick soft cushion. At the beginning of the test, the animal was placed on the middle of the rod, its body axis perpendicular to the beam's longitudinal axis. Latency to fall (60-sec cut-off), time spent in motion, and distance traveled were measured and recorded. From the later 2 components of this data, the walking speed was calculated. Two trials per session, interspersed by a 10-min inter-trial period, were performed 24 h after hemorrhage induction.

Statistical analysis

Quantitative data are expressed as the mean ± SEM. The *t*-test or Mann–Whitney rank sum tests were used when appropriate. Chi-squared was used for mortality measurements. Statistical significance was considered $p < 0.05$.

Results

The hematoma observed in the right cerebellum was accompanied by brain edema in a dose-related fashion ($p < 0.05$ compared to sham; Table 1). Neurological deficits assessed by both beam walking ability and the inclined plane were significantly increased compared to sham ($p < 0.05$; Student *t*-test) at 0.4 and 0.6 U in females, but only at 0.6 units for the males. Wire-hang showed dose-dependent trends, but was significantly different compared to sham, only at the highest dose for both sexes ($p < 0.05$; Student *t*-test; Table 1).

When comparing sexes, both the hemorrhagic volume and neurologic disability score were significantly increased in females compared to their male counterparts ($p < 0.05$; Student *t*-test; Figs. 1 and 2). Furthermore, females experienced a mortality of 16%, while there was no mortality in the male groups. However, this difference was not significant ($p > 0.05$; Chi-square).

Discussion

ICH has been less-studied than ischemic strokes, and hindbrain hemorrhages have been even less-studied compared to forebrain-based hemorrhages [1]. Cossu *et al.* [3] created an animal model of cerebellar hemorrhage in rats, where they performed an occipital craniectomy to expose the posterior cerebellum, and then injected autologous blood into the right side. However, their model led to dissipation of intracranial pressure (ICP), providing limited clinical relevance.

Clinically, after cerebellar hemorrhage, the resultant obstructive hydrocephalus and brainstem compression are major determinants of patient outcome [7, 9]. Therefore, any experimental model of cerebellar hemorrhage must approximate these compressive and obstructive ef-

Table 1. *Effects of increasing collagenase dose on edema and neurological outcomes*

Collagenase dose	Male				Female			
	0 µL	1 µL	2 µL	3 µL	0 µL	1 µL	2 µL	3 µL
Brain water content (percentage)	78.95 ± 0.21	79.15 ± 0.62 ($p = 0.686$)	80.08 ± 0.40 ($p = 0.001$)	81.05 ± 0.38 ($p \leq 0.001$)	79.28 ± 0.30	80.20 ± 0.61 ($p = 0.034$)	80.95 ± 0.37 ($p \leq 0.001$)	81.18 ± 0.10 ($p \leq 0.001$)
Wire suspension (sec)	15.00 ± 5.76	13.50 ± 3.32 ($p = 0.668$)	9.80 ± 4.27 ($p = 0.162$)	7.38 ± 3.62 ($p = 0.017$)	13.13 ± 4.07	10.13 ± 4.80 ($p = 0.377$)	7.25 ± 3.78 ($p = 0.079$)	5.20 ± 3.26 ($p = 0.002$)
Inclined plane (angle of inclination)	56.13 ± 6.43	52.25 ± 2.33 ($p = 0.301$)	43.00 ± 3.02 ($p = 0.005$)	42.00 ± 2.14 ($p < 0.001$)	57.5 ± 4.34	47.50 ± 2.67 ($p = 0.008$)	42.00 ± 2.27 ($p \leq 0.001$)	39.70 ± 4.87 ($p \leq 0.001$)
Beam walking time (sec)	57.75 ± 4.50	53.38 ± 4.59 ($p = 0.222$)	44.80 ± 24.77 ($p = 0.556$)	23.06 ± 22.84 ($p = 0.015$)	60.00 ± 0.00	60.00 ± 0.00 ($p = 1.000$)	20.50 ± 25.14 ($p = 0.029$)	10.55 ± 10.22 ($p = 0.006$)
Beam walking distance (cm)	98.13 ± 48.45	46.25 ± 48.20 ($p = 0.787$)	49.00 ± 33.05 ($p = 0.113$)	4.50 ± 9.90 ($p = 0.008$)	168.8 ± 8.08	120.88 ± 24.69 ($p = 0.180$)	21.25 ± 42.50 ($p = 0.006$)	7.75 ± 16.43 ($p = 0.006$)
Beam walking speed (cm/sec)	12.26 ± 4.45	9.44 ± 7.07 ($p = 0.523$)	5.93 ± 6.44 ($p = 0.140$)	0.33 ± 0.77 ($p = 0.004$)	25.28 ± 0.06	12.76 ± 2.72 ($p \leq 0.001$)	1.37 ± 2.74 ($p \leq 0.001$)	0.61 ± 1.28 ($p \leq 0.006$)

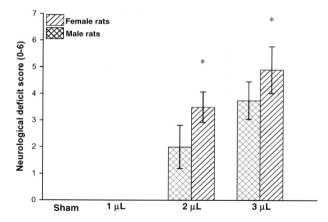

Fig. 1. Bar graph showing dose-response of collagenase (0.2 units per µL) and neurological deficit scores 24 h post-ICH ($n = 4$ per group), comparing male to female rats. Values expressed as mean ± standard deviation. $^{*}p < 0.05$

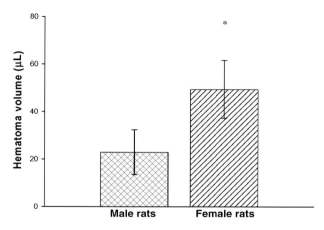

Fig. 2. Bar graph comparing male to female hematoma volumes, right cerebellums, 24 h post-ICH, $n = 4$ per group. Values expressed as mean ± standard deviation ($p = 0.012$). $^{*}p < 0.05$

fects from brain edema. However, these factors were eliminated by Cossu *et al.* [3], who exposed the convexity of the right cerebellar hemisphere and then injected autologous blood. Contrary to this method, we created a closed pressure system in our model by using a sealed 1-mm burr-hole after injecting collagenase, resulting in conserved hindbrain pressures.

Bacterial collagenase causes disruption of the basal lamina in cerebral blood vessels, thereby causing leakage of blood into the surrounding brain tissue [8]. Compared to the blood injection model, collagenase is believed to be a simpler method, creating more consistent hemorrhage volumes and allowing investigators to study different mechanisms of hemorrhage [10]. Taken together, this cerebellar hemorrhage model provides additional facets in the study of the pathophysiology of cerebellar hemorrhage, and should be a very useful tool for investigators.

Our novel cerebellar hemorrhage rat model injected collagenase through a burr-hole, thereby preserving elevated ICP. We demonstrated dose- and sex-dependent changes in hemorrhagic volume, brain edema, and neurological deficits. This model could be used to further test treatments and pathophysiological mechanisms of cerebellar hemorrhage.

Acknowledgement

Funding provided by National Institutes of Health Grants NS52492 (JT) and NS53407 (JHZ).

References

1. Chung Y, Haines SJ (1993) Experimental brain stem surgery. Neurosurg Clin N Am 4: 405–414
2. Colombel C, Lalonde R, Caston J (2002) The effects of unilateral removal of the cerebellar hemispheres on motor functions and weight gain in rats. Brain Res 950: 231–238
3. Cossu M, Pau A, Siccardi D, Viale GL (1994) Infratentorial ischaemia following experimental cerebellar haemorrhage in the rat. Acta Neurochir (Wien) 131: 146–150
4. Fernandez AM, de la Vega AG, Torres-Aleman I (1998) Insulin-like growth factor I restores motor coordination in a rat model of cerebellar ataxia. Proc Natl Acad Sci USA 95: 1253–1258
5. Henninger N, Eberius KH, Sicard KM, Kollmar R, Sommer C, Schwab S, Schäbitz WR (2006) A new model of thromboembolic stroke in the posterior circulation of the rat. J Neurosci Meth 156: 1–9
6. Hill MD, Silver FL, Austin PC, Tu JV (2000) Rate of stroke recurrence in patients with primary intracerebral hemorrhage. Stroke 31: 123–127
7. Qureshi AI, Tuhrim S, Broderick JP, Batjer HH, Hondo H, Hanley DF (2001) Spontaneous intracerebral hemorrhage. N Engl J Med 344: 1450–1460
8. Rosenberg GA, Mun-Bryce S, Wesley M, Kornfeld M (1990) Collagenase-induced intracerebral hemorrhage in rats. Stroke 21: 801–807
9. Sutherland GR, Auer RN (2006) Primary intracerebral hemorrhage. J Clin Neurosci 13: 511–517
10. Tang J, Liu J, Zhou C, Ostanin D, Grisham MB, Neil Granger D, Zhang JH (2005) Role of NADPH oxidase in the brain injury of intracerebral hemorrhage. J Neurochem 94: 1342–1350
11. Voetsch B, DeWitt LD, Pessin MS, Caplan LR (2004) Basilar artery occlusive disease in the New England Medical Center Posterior Circulation Registry. Arch Neurol 61: 496–504

Acta Neurochir Suppl (2008) 105: 135–137
© Springer-Verlag 2008
Printed in Austria

A rat model of pontine hemorrhage

T. Lekic[1], J. Tang[1], J. H. Zhang[1,2,3]

[1] Department of Physiology and Pharmacology, Loma Linda University, Loma Linda, CA, USA
[2] Department of Neurosurgery, Loma Linda University, Loma Linda, CA, USA
[3] Department of Anesthesiology, Loma Linda University, Loma Linda, CA, USA

Summary

Approximately 15% of all strokes are due to intracerebral hemorrhage, and of these, 5 to 9% will occur in the pons, with mortality approximately 60% of the time. However, there is not an adequate animal model to fully address this important clinical problem.

To this end, pontine hemorrhage was induced in rats using stereotaxic injection of 0.15 units of collagenase. At 24, 48, and 72 h ($n = 4$ per group), the hemorrhagic volume, brain water content, body temperature, and neurological function (corner turn, inclined plane, and neurological deficit score) were assessed. All tested parameters were significantly increased, compared to sham, without any differences between time points. Furthermore, the extent of brainstem edema was highly correlated with neurological score, inclined plane, and body temperature. This new pontine hemorrhage rat model demonstrated brain edema and neurological deficits, and can be used to test treatment strategies for pontine hemorrhage.

Keywords: Pons; brainstem; collagenase; stroke; pontine hemorrhage.

Introduction

Approximately 15% of strokes are due to intracerebral hemorrhage (ICH) [7], and 5 to 9% of these occur in the pons, with an associated rate of mortality around 60% [9]. Occhiogrosso *et al.* [6] demonstrated the safety of a placing a stereotactic cannula into the rat brainstem without any residual neurological deficits. Previously, a cat brainstem hemorrhage model using autologous blood injection was described, but it required complex surgical procedures [1]. Herein we describe the first experimental model of pontine hemorrhage (IPonH) in rodents.

Materials and methods

All procedures used for these studies were in compliance with the *Guide for the Care and Use of Laboratory Animals* and approved by the Animal Care and Use Committee at Loma Linda University. Aseptic

technique was used for all surgeries, and rats were allowed free access to food and water.

Experimental design

A total of 24 male Sprague-Dawley rats (300 to 395 g; Harlan, Indianapolis, IN, USA) were used in this study. IPonH was induced in rats using stereotaxic injection of 0.7 units of collagenase. Brain water content and neurological functions were assessed at 24, 48, and 72 h after IPonH. Then, a separate cohort was used for hemorrhagic volume measurements at 24 h ($n = 4$ per group). Animals were euthanized after neurological testing, and then samples were collected for either hemoglobin assay or brain edema measurements.

IPonH induction

Briefly, rats were anesthetized with isoflurane and placed prone in a stereotaxic head frame (Kopf Instruments, Tujunga, CA, USA). Then, using a collagenase injection ICH model with methods similar to those described previously [8], we used the following stereotactic coordinates to localize the brainstem: 9 mm posterior, 7 mm ventral, and 1.4 mm lateral to the bregma. A posterior cranial burr-hole (1 mm) was drilled, and a 27-gauge needle was inserted at a rate of 1 mm/min. A micro-infusion pump (Harvard Apparatus, Holliston, MA, USA) infused the bacterial collagenase (0.2 U in 1 μL saline; VII-S, Sigma-Aldrich, St. Louis, MO, USA) through a Hamilton syringe at a rate of 0.1 μL/min. The needle remained in place for an additional 10 min after injection to prevent potential "back-leakage". Upon needle removal, the burr-hole was sealed with bone wax, the incision sutured closed, and the animals were allowed to recover. Sham surgeries consisted of needle insertion alone.

Neurological deficit scoring

Neurological testing was performed at 24, 48, and 72 h after IPonH. The scoring system consisted of 14 tests with possible scores of 0 to 3 for each test (0 = worst; 3 = best). We used this system with modifications, as follows: (a) spontaneous activity; (b) alertness; (c) symmetry in the movement of head and neck; (d) symmetry in the movement of forelimbs; (e) forepaw outstretching; (f) climbing; (g) beam balance; (h) body proprioception; (i) corneal reflex; (j) lethargy; (k) circling; and response to (l) vibrissae touch, (m) pin to body, (n) pinching ears. The score given to each rat at the completion of the evaluation was the summation of all 14 individual test scores. The minimum total neurological score was 0 and the maximum total score was 42; this scoring method

Correspondence: John H. Zhang, Department of Physiology and Pharmacology, Loma Linda University School of Medicine, Loma Linda, CA 92354, USA. e-mail: Johnzhang3910@yahoo.com

has been described in greater detail elsewhere [4]. The examiner had no specific knowledge as to the extent of neurological injury in each rat.

Inclined plane paradigm

Used previously by others [3] as an indirect measure of overall muscular strength and integrated motor-proprioceptive abilities, this test consisted of a 20 cm (width) × 70 cm (length) × 10 cm (height) box, with a hinge attached to a heavy wooden base in such a way that one end of the box could be lifted to establish an inclined plane. Angle was recorded by an analog protractor attached to the side of the device. Rats were placed right side up and left side up, toward the side of board to be raised. Plane was raised from 10 to 90° at 5° intervals until the animal began to slip backward. The highest angle achieved was recorded for the 2 trials, which included a 1-hour inter-trial period. The average angle across 2 body positions for both trials was recorded as the final value.

Hemorrhagic volume

At 24 h after induction of IPonH, hemoglobin assay was performed, as described elsewhere [10]. Briefly, rats were killed by an overdose of isoflurane and perfused transcardially with 300 mL of ice-cold (4 °C) phosphate-buffered saline (PBS). The brainstem was extracted and dissected free of the cerebellum and cerebral hemispheres. This tissue was homogenized (Tissuemiser homogenizer; Fisher Scientific, Pittsburgh, PA, USA) for 60 sec in a test tube with distilled water (total volume, 3 mL). After the centrifugation phase (15 800 g for 30 min; Eppendorf Microcentrifuge model 5417R, Hamburg, Germany), Drabkin's reagent (400 μL; Sigma-Aldrich) was added into the 100 μL aliquots of supernatant (4 samples per brain) and allowed to react for 15 min. The solution's absorbance was read using a spectrophotometer (540 nm;

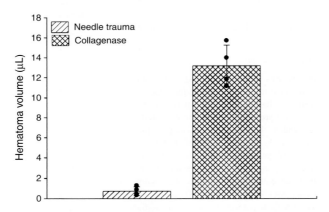

Fig. 1. Hemorrhagic volume was measured spectrophotometrically at 24 h after IPonH induction. Significant amount of bleeding with 0.15 units of collagenase compared to needle trauma (13.153 μL ± 2.070 vs. 0.733 μL ± 0.426; $p > 0.001$, Student t-test, mean ± SEM).

Spectronic Genesis 5, Thermo Electron Corp., Waltham, MA, USA), and the amount of blood in each brain was calculated using a curve generated previously using known blood volumes from the same brain region.

Brain water content

Brain edema was measured using methods described previously [10–12]. Briefly, under deep anesthesia, rats were decapitated, and brains were immediately removed and divided into 4 parts: brainstem, cerebellum, and right and left cerebral hemispheres. The cerebral hemispheres were used as internal controls. These tissue samples were weighed on an electronic analytical balance (APX-60, Denver Instrument, Denver, CO, USA) to the nearest 0.01 mg to obtain the wet weight (WW), and the tissue was then dried at 100 °C for 24 h to determine dry weight (DW). Finally, brain water content (%) was calculated as $(WW - DW)/WW \times 100$.

Statistical analysis

Quantitative data are expressed as mean ± SEM. Statistical significance was verified by Student t-test, ANOVA, and Scheffé tests. Statistical significance was considered $p < 0.05$.

Results

All parameters tested were significantly increased, compared to shams, at 24, 48, and 72 h after IPonH. Parameters included brain water content, body temperature, neurological deficit score, corner turn (percent left turning), and inclined plane angles, ($p < 0.01$ versus sham, Student t-test, mean ± SEM; Table 1). However, there were no statistical differences between any of the time-points for the parameters tested ($p > 0.05$, ANOVA, mean ± SEM; Table 1).

The hemoglobin assay demonstrated spectrophotometrically significant amounts of bleeding with 0.15 units of collagenase compared to needle trauma (13.153 μL ± 2.070 vs. 0.733 μL ± 0.426; $p > 0.001$, Student t-test, mean ± SEM). Furthermore, the range of bleeding between animals was fairly narrow (min: 11.150, max: 15.690, median: 12.885), suggesting good reproducibility of the bleeding amount.

Additionally, the extent of brainstem edema was highly correlated with degree of neurological deficit scoring, inclined plane angle, and body temperature (data not shown). Nonetheless, mortality was 0% among all groups.

Table 1. *Changes in brain edema, neurological function, and temperature at 24, 48, and 72 h after induction of pontine hemorrhage*

	Sham	24 h	48 h	72 h
Brain water content (% brainstem)	73.200 ± 0.283	75.150 ± 0.300#	75.175 ± 0.991*	75.225 ± 0.171#
Neurological deficit score	37.500 ± 1.291	24.033 ± 4.930#	22.563 ± 8.728*	22.875 ± 3.351#
Inclined plane (angle of inclination)	52.750 ± 2.754	43.933 ± 5.688*	45.875 ± 4.970*	45.000 ± 2.708*
Corner turning (percent to left)	55.000 ± 17.321	90.000 ± 13.540#	82.000 ± 16.432*	100.00 ± 0.000*
Rectal temperature (°C)	36.873 ± 0.377	38.445 ± 0.291#	38.688 ± 0.452#	38.675 ± 0.310#

* $p < 0.01$ and # $p < 0.001$ versus sham, ANOVA, mean ± SEM.

Discussion

ICH has been less-studied than ischemic stroke, and hindbrain hemorrhage has been even less-studied compared to forebrain-based hemorrhage [1, 2]. Several animal studies have delineated the neurophysiologic and anatomic structures of the hindbrain, which in turn, guided studies of posterior fossa mass lesion removal and cerebellopontine angle manipulations [1]. However, the effects of intraparenchymal hemorrhage of the pons/brainstem had only been previously studied by Chung *et al.* [1], who created an autologous blood injection model using an invasive transtentorial technique. However, the severity of the surgery dramatically limited the study of functional outcomes, which diminishes the utility of that model.

In this study, we describe a novel IPonH model using rats, which demonstrates brain edema and neurological deficits. This model can be applied toward testing treatment strategies and pathophysiological mechanisms. Also, the observed sustained temperature elevation was consistent with the hyperthermia described in several human clinical case reports of brainstem hemorrhage [5], and needs to be explored further. Finally, future studies are needed to elucidate the molecular mechanisms involved with the corresponding neurological deficits, brain edema, hemorrhagic volume, and temperature elevations.

Acknowledgements

Funding provided by National Institutes of Health grants NS52492 (JT) and NS53407 (JHZ).

References

1. Chung Y, Haines SJ (1993) Experimental brain stem surgery. Neurosurg Clin N Am 4: 405–414
2. Cossu M, Pau A, Siccardi D, Viale GL (1994) Infratentorial ischaemia following experimental cerebellar haemorrhage in the rat. Acta Neurochir (Wien) 131: 146–150
3. Fernandez AM, de la Vega AG, Torres-Aleman I (1998) Insulin-like growth factor I restores motor coordination in a rat model of cerebellar ataxia. Proc Natl Acad Sci USA 95: 1253–1258
4. Garcia JH, Wagner S, Liu KF, Hu XJ (1995) Neurological deficit and extent of neuronal necrosis attributable to middle cerebral artery occlusion in rats. Statistical validation. Stroke 26: 627–635
5. Kitanaka C, Inoh Y, Toyoda T, Sasaki T, Eguchi T (1994) Malignant brain stem hyperthermia caused by brain stem hemorrhage. Stroke 25: 518–520
6. Occhiogrosso G, Edgar MA, Sandberg DI, Souweidane MM (2003) Prolonged convection-enhanced delivery into the rat brainstem. Neurosurgery 52: 388–394
7. Qureshi AI, Tuhrim S, Broderick JP, Batjer HH, Hondo H, Hanley DF (2001) Spontaneous intracerebral hemorrhage. N Engl J Med 344: 1450–1460
8. Rosenberg GA, Mun-Bryce S, Wesley M, Kornfeld M (1990) Collagenase-induced intracerebral hemorrhage in rats. Stroke 21: 801–807
9. Sutherland GR, Auer RN (2006) Primary intracerebral hemorrhage. J Clin Neurosci 13: 511–517
10. Tang J, Liu J, Zhou C, Alexander JS, Nanda A, Granger DN, Zhang JH (2004) MMP-9 deficiency enhances collagenase-induced intracerebral hemorrhage and brain injury in mutant mice. J Cereb Blood Flow Metab 24: 1133–1145
11. Tang J, Liu J, Zhou C, Ostanin D, Grisham MB, Neil Granger D, Zhang JH (2005) Role of NADPH oxidase in the brain injury of intracerebral hemorrhage. J Neurochem 94: 1342–1350
12. Xi G, Hua Y, Keep RF, Younger JG, Hoff JT (2002) Brain edema after intracerebral hemorrhage: the effects of systemic complement depletion. Acta Neurochir Suppl 81: 253–256

Human intracerebral hemorrhage

Acta Neurochir Suppl (2008) 105: 141–145
© Springer-Verlag 2008
Printed in Austria

The optimal time-window for surgical treatment of spontaneous intracerebral hemorrhage: result of prospective randomized controlled trial of 500 cases

Y. F. Wang, J. S. Wu, Y. Mao, X. C. Chen, L. F. Zhou, Y. Zhang

Department of Neurosurgery, Huashan Hospital, Shanghai Medical College, Fudan University, Shanghai, China

Summary

The aim of this clinical study was to determine the optimal time-window for surgical treatment of spontaneous intracerebral hemorrhage (ICH). From January 1998 to September 2000, 17 hospitals in Shanghai participated in a prospective randomized controlled trial. Among a consecutive series of 500 patients with spontaneous ICH, 234 underwent medical treatment and 266 patients received surgical treatment. According to the interval from initial onset to treatment, they were divided into 3 stages: *ultra-early* (≤ 7 h), *early* (7–24 h), and *delayed* (> 24 h). Perioperative evaluation (Glasgow Outcome Score), long-term outcome (the activities of daily living [ADL] score), mortality, as well as incidence of associated complications were compared respectively. We found that: a) in the *ultra-early* and *early* stages, both the perioperative and long-term outcome of surgical treatment was definitely better than medical treatment; b) for the outcome of surgical treatment, there was no significant difference between *ultra-early* and *early* stages; c) in *ultra-early* stage, risk of postoperative rebleeding was significantly higher, and decreased henceforth; d) in *delayed* stage, incidence of associated respiratory, urinary, and gastrointestinal system complications was higher in surgery group than in medication group. In summary, our study yielded conclusive evidence that the *early* stage (within 7–24 h) was the optimal time-window for surgical intervention of spontaneous ICH.

Keywords: Intracerebral hemorrhage; hypertension; surgery; time-window.

Introduction

Spontaneous intracerebral hemorrhage (ICH) most commonly results from hypertensive damage to vessel walls. It is the leading cause of death in the aged population in China. Currently, advanced minimally-invasive surgical techniques have led to improved outcome from surgery, according to various published data of clinical observations. Nevertheless, firm conclusions are still lacking with regard to the role of operative treatment.

Therefore from January 1998 to December 2000, a randomized prospective controlled trial was undertaken in 17 Shanghai hospitals to compare the outcome of operative treatment and conservative treatment for patients with spontaneous ICH. When analyzing the therapeutic effects, careful attention was paid to calibrate the differences in the constituent ratio of the key prognostic factors. Our findings revealed that operative treatment was associated with a better outcome than conservative treatment for patients with spontaneous ICH [2, 11]. Timing of surgical intervention is an important prognostic factor in patients being treated surgically for spontaneous ICH. But the optimal time-window for surgical evacuation of the hematoma continues to be controversial. In this study, the therapeutic effect and follow-up outcomes were assessed and compared between surgically and conservatively treated groups at different stages, and an optimal time-window for surgical intervention in patients with ICH is proposed.

Materials and methods

Patient population

The inclusion and exclusion criteria for patients are listed in Table 1. The executants in each hospital were required to randomize eligible patients into surgical group (those receiving operative treatment) or medication group (those receiving conservative treatment) by referring to a unified random digits table. Operative or conservative treatment was offered to each enrolled patient in accordance with the standard protocol set up by the research center. All patients were eligible based on clinical aspects and computed tomography (CT) imaging evaluations, and who complied with the protocol after being provided informed consent. The clinical trial was approved by the local ethics committee before commencing.

Correspondence: Ying Mao, M.D., Ph.D., Shanghai Neurosurgical Center, Department of Neurosurgery, Huashan Hospital, Shanghai Medical School, Fudan University, 12# Wulumuqi Zhong Road, Shanghai 200040, P.R. China. e-mail: yingmao168@hotmail.com

Table 1. *Study inclusion and exclusion criteria for patients*

	Criteria for inclusion	Criteria for exclusion
Cause	History of hypertension or blood pressure increases at time of onset and spontaneous ICH excluding other reasons (aneurysm, arteriovenous malformation, Moyamoya, traumatic)	>180/110 mmHg
Location	Emergency CT scanning displays hematoma in cortex, subcortical white matter, basal ganglia, capsula interna, thalamus, cerebellum, ICH ruptured into ventricles	ICH in brain stem
Volume*	Supratentorial ICH ≥30 mL; infratentorial ICH ≥10 mL	Supratentorial ICH <20 mL; infratentorial ICH <10 mL
Age	≤70 years	>70 years
Consciousness	Glasgow Coma Score ≥7	Glasgow Coma Score <7
Vital signs	Stable	Unstable, cerebral hernia
Body condition		Severe disease of heart and lung; coagulation disorders

CT Computed tomography; *ICH* intracerebral hemorrhage.

* Hematoma volume measure (mL) = length × width × height (layer thickness) × 1/2, Standard CT scanning is applied.

Prior to treatment, the ascending clinical scale was standardized as follow: *Severe*, coma (Glasgow Coma Score [GCS], 7–8); *Moderate*, semicoma (GCS, 9–12); *Mild*, mild conscious disturbance (GCS, 13–15). The patient would be scored one level upward if they possessed any of the following attributes: age ≥61 years; history of acute cerebral vascular accident; history of severe systematic disease related to heart, lung, liver, kidney, etc.; body temperature >38 °C; diabetes.

Treatment strategies

Therapeutics in the medication group consisted of administration of hemostatics, dehydration agents to release surrounding brain tissue edema and decrease the elevated intracranial pressure, symptomatic treatment, and supportive treatment. Treatment strategies in the surgical group included the following: 1) minimally-invasive approach with a keyhole of 2.5 cm in diameter for surgical evacuation of hematoma; 2) stereotaxic catheter insertion and hematoma evacuation; 3) endoscopic removal of hematoma; 4) lateral ventriculopuncture and catheter insertion for continuous drainage of hematoma ruptured into ventricle; 5) direct clot removal by craniotomy. Each kind of surgical method except craniotomy was incorporated with intracavity thrombolysis using 500,000 U of combined streptokinase (r-SK) in 5 mL saline per day. Drainage of the residual clot was continued for 72 h postoperatively. The accompanying standardized therapeutics in the surgical group were similar to those received by the medication group.

Perioperative assessment and long-term follow-up

All patents in both medication and surgical treatment groups were divided into 3 time-windows according to various stages from onset to treatment: *ultra-early* stage, ≤7 h; *early* stage, 7–24 h, *delayed* stage, >24 h. Therapeutic effect was compared between the surgical group and the medication group in the same stage, and among each of 3 stages. Perioperative therapeutic effect was assessed by Glasgow Outcome Scale (GOS): 5, good recovery; 4, moderate disability; 3, severe disability; 2, persistent vegetative; 1, death. Long-term activities of daily living (ADL) status was scored according to the Modified Rankin Scale (MRS) and the Barthel Index (BI): *Score 5*, patients with MRS 0 or 1, the BI cutoff score was 90. Excellent, patients did not require help from another person for everyday activities; *Score 4*, patients with MRS 2 or 3, the cutoff score on the BI was 60. Slight disability, able to be self-caring, partial independence; *Score 3*, patients with MRS 4 or 5, the BI <60. Severe disability, neither able to be self-caring, nor able to walk by oneself; *Score 2*, vegetative state; *Score 1*, death. Other evaluation criterion included: 1) mortality, including both perioperative mortality and long-term mortality; 2) excellent rehabilitation, sum of the constituent ratio in patients with ADL Score 5 and 4. One could decide to choose MRS 3 and BI 60 as cut-off scores for favorable outcome; (3) incidence of associated complications, with respect to all kinds of complications during the course of treatment.

Perioperative therapeutic effect was evaluated 1 month after treatment, primarily based on clinical observation by the attending neurosurgeons. Long-term follow-up continued up to 6 months after treatment. Follow-up data were based on patient and family responses on questionnaire forms, which were completed on-site (recommended to all patients at enrollment) or by telephone contact (in cases where an on-site visit was impossible) at each follow-up interval. Data regarding patient survival and functional status were recorded by 2 independent neurosurgeons who were not members of the treatment group and who were blinded to treatment strategies.

Statistical analysis

Due to their potential to impact outcome evaluation, the χ^2-test and independent sample *t*-test were used to estimate the initial baseline of qualitative data in both groups; cmh χ^2 was used to inspect the balance of qualitative data in order; rank-sum test was adopted to compare the therapeutic effect of either treatment. Stepwise regression method using multinomial logistic regression model was constructed to account for effects of prognostic factors (multivariate statistical analysis). All statistical analyses were conducted using SPSS software (Release 13.0; SPSS Inc., Chicago, IL).

Results

Patient population

A total of 500 cases were eligible in the trial, of which 234 were enrolled in the medication group and 266 were enrolled in the surgical group. There were 361 males and 139 females, aged 12 to 70 years (mean, 56.67 ± 10.53 yrs). Preoperative GCS varied from 7 to 15 (mean, 11.02 ± 2.60), and hematoma volume ranged from 12 to 130 mL (mean, 36.57 ± 18.23 mL). Perioperative assessment was conducted on all patients (100%), and long-term follow-up was achieved in 98.6% cases.

Table 2. *Results of stepwise multinomial logistic regression model*

Index	Perioperative evaluation (Glasgow Outcome Scale)		Long-term outcome (ADL score)		Mortality		Disability		Excellent rehabilitation	
Variables	OR value	p-value	OR value	p-value	OR value	p-value	OR value	p-value	OR value	p-value
Clinical scale	1.492	0.0278	1.658	0.0060	2.325	0.0001	2.131	0.0001	2.069	0.0001
Hematoma volume	0.510	0.0012	0.560	0.0058	0.344	0.0040	0.474	0.0017	0.582	0.0284
Conscious state	0.701	0.0223	0.714	0.0308	–	–	0.595	0.0002	0.653	0.0027
Glasgow Coma Score	1.168	0.0264	1.157	0.0373	–	–	–	–	–	–
Respiratory complication	2.079	0.0036	2.298	0.0008	2.160	0.0204	3.105	0.0001	1.987	0.0091
Cardiovascular complication	–	–	2.250	0.0488	2.795	0.0442	–	–	–	–
Urinary complication	2.881	0.0022	–	–	–	–	–	–	–	–

OR Odds ratio; *p* probability; "–" $p > 0.05$, no statistical difference.

Table 3. *Stratified comparison between surgical and medication groups in each stage of time-window*

Stages	Groups	Variables	Perioperative evaluation (Glasgow Outcome Scale)	Long-term outcome (ADL score)	Mortality	Excellent rehabilitation
Ultra-early stage, ≤7 h	Medication (n = 92) vs. surgery (n = 125)	cmh χ^2 p-value	14.047 0.001	17.033 0.001	12.222 0.001	19.161 0.001
Early stage, 7–24 h	Medication (n = 81) vs. surgery (n = 91)	cmh χ^2 p-value	13.929 0.001	10.400 0.001	11.396 0.001	8.303 0.004
Delayed stage >24 h	Medication (n = 61) vs. surgery (n = 50)	cmh χ^2 p-value	2.780 0.095	0.667 0.414	0.017 0.896	1.629 0.202

Initial baseline prerequisites in both groups

A stepwise regression analysis was conducted using the multinomial logistic regression model, showing that prognosis was affected by the following predictors: clinical scale, hematoma volume, state of consciousness, GCS, and associated complications in the respiratory, urinary, and cardiovascular systems (Table 2) [2]. Clinical scale is a comprehensive index derived from the state of consciousness and GCS; therefore, these 3 factors were all considered under clinical scale. A significant imbalance of 2 prognostic factors, which included both clinical scale and hematoma volume, was inspected. The mean clinical scale of patients in the surgical group was significantly lower than that of patients in the medication group, and the mean hematoma volume in the surgical group was significantly higher than that of the medication group ($p < 0.01$). As these 2 factors were calibrated using the stepwise multinomial logistic regression model, certain conclusions could still be effectively drawn in this controlled study regarding the role of operative treatment as well as optimal time-window of surgery. The results of statistical analysis are shown in Table 3.

Perioperative assessment

For patients in the *ultra-early* stage (≤7 h), the mean GOS score of patients in the surgical group was sig-

nificantly higher than that in the medication group ($p < 0.01$). For patients in the *early* stage (7–24 h), the mean GOS score of patients in the surgical group was also significantly higher than that in the medication group ($p < 0.01$). Conversely, for patients in the *delayed* stage (>24 h), there was no significant difference in the mean GOS score between the 2 groups.

Long-term follow-up

For patients in the *ultra-early* stage (≤7 h), the mean ADL score for patients in the surgical group was significantly higher than that in the medication group ($p < 0.01$). For patients in the *early* stage (7–24 h), the mean ADL score for patients in the surgical group was also significantly higher than in the medication group ($p < 0.01$). Nevertheless, for patients in the *delayed* stage (>24 h), there was no significant difference in mean ADL score between the 2 groups.

Mortality

In the *ultra-early* stage (≤7 h), mortality in the surgical group was 15.8% (19 cases; perioperative death in 17 cases, 13.6%), compared to 30.0% (27 cases) in the medication group (perioperative death in 22 cases, 24.4%) ($p < 0.01$). In the *early* stage (7–24 h), mortality

Table 4. *Stratified comparison of associated complications between surgical and medication groups in each stage of time-window*

Stages	Index and variables	Associated complications (%)					
		ICH enlarged or rebleeding	Respiratory apparatus	Cardio-vascular system	Urinary system	Digestive system	Blood pressure uncontrolled
Ultra-early stage, ≤ 7 h	Medication ($n = 92$)	4.3	10.9	2.2	6.5	10.9	0
	Surgery ($n = 125$)	14.4	15.2	7.2	7.2	9.6	0.8
	χ^2-value	5.878	0.858	2.782	0.038	0.094	0.758
	p-value	0.015	0.354	0.123	0.846	0.759	1.000
Early stage, 7–24 h	Medication ($n = 81$)	2.5	18.5	4.9	3.7	9.9	0
	Surgery ($n = 91$)	5.5	19.8	3.3	8.8	17.6	0
	χ^2-value	1.005	0.044	1.444	1.853	2.119	–
	p-value	0.449	0.834	0.486	0.173	0.145	
Delayed stage, >24 h	Medication ($n = 61$)	0	8.2	3.3	4.9	4.9	0
	Surgery ($n = 50$)	6.0	24.0	6.0	20.0	16.0	0
	χ^2-value	3.762	5.291	0.473	6.045	3.780	–
	p-value	0.088	0.021	0.656	0.014	0.050	

ICH Intra cerebral hemorrhage.

in the surgical group was 8.9% (8 cases; perioperative death in 6 cases, 6.7%), compared to 17.5% (14 cases) in the medication group (perioperative death in 10 cases, 12.5%) ($p < 0.01$). In the *delayed* stage (>24 h), mortality in the surgical group and in the medication group were 8.0% (4 cases; perioperative death in 3 cases, 6.0%) and 3.3% (2 cases; perioperative death in 1 case, 1.7%) respectively; this was not a statistically significant difference.

Excellent rehabilitation

In the *ultra-early* stage (≤ 7 h), the ratio of patients with excellent rehabilitation in the surgical group was 68.3%, compared to 46.7% in the medication group ($p < 0.01$). In the *early* stage (7–24 h), the ratio of patients with excellent rehabilitation in the surgical group was 67.7% compared to 65.0% in the medication group ($p < 0.01$). There was no significant difference between the 2 groups for patients in the *delayed* stage (>24 h).

Associated complications

As shown in Table 4, in the *ultra-early* stage (≤ 7 h), the risk of a rebleeding in the surgical group was higher than in the medication group ($p < 0.05$). In the *delayed* stage (>24 h), occurrence of complications of respiratory, urinary, and digestive systems was higher in the surgical group than in the medication group ($p < 0.05$).

Comparison of surgical outcome between stages

The prognostic factors of all patients who underwent operative treatment in 3 stages were well balanced besides "clinical scale" and "hematoma volume" ($p > 0.05$). Incidence of rebleeding for patients in the *ultra-early* stage (≤ 7 h), *early* stage (7–24 h), and *delayed* stage (>24 h) was 14.4%, 5.5%, and 6.0%, respectively ($p < 0.05$). The result of rank-sum test showed that the risk of rebleeding was much higher in the *ultra-early* stage (≤ 7 h) than in the other 2 stages. Furthermore, there was no statistically significant difference in risk of rebleeding between the *early* stage (7–24 h) and *delayed* stage (>24 h). There was no statistically significant difference in postoperative complication incidence among the 3 stages ($p > 0.05$). There was no statistically significant difference in either GOS or ADL scores among the 3 stages ($p > 0.05$). Mortality for operative cases in *ultra-early* stage (≤ 7 h), *early* stage (7–24 h), and *delayed* stage (>24 h) was 15.8, 8.9 and 8.0%, respectively. The difference among the 3 stages was not statistically significant ($p > 0.05$).

Discussion

The accumulation of knowledge about the occurrence and development of ICH and its pathological and physiological mechanisms has made timing of surgery more of a theoretical issue than an empirical judgment. In 1961, Fisher proposed that ICH was formed by one hemorrhage, rather than continuous bleeding in small amounts. Juvela *et al.*'s [4] prospective randomized controlled study of surgical and conservative treatment showed that if time to treatment exceeded 24 h, operation was not a better option than medication. In 1977, Kaneko *et al.* [5] introduced the concept of ultra-early operation for ICH, which meant an operation within 7 h after the onset of hemorrhage. They believed that clinical symptoms would worsen due to the intensifying of cerebral edema, and that it was advisable to remove the hematoma before surrounding brain tissue (penumbra) was severely damaged, which was helpful for function recovery and mortality reduction.

Some scholars supported this opinion and suggested ultra-early operation to remove the hematoma within 6 h after onset of ICH [5, 6] to eliminate oppression of the hematoma on surrounding brain tissue as early as possible to improve perfusion in the penumbra. Secondly, early removal of hematoma decreases secondary brain edema related to presence of thrombin and some other possible inflammatory mediators [3, 8–10]. However, other scholars argued that in the ultra-early stage of ICH, formation of hematoma is not stable enough, and it is difficult to arrest rebleeding effectively under direct visualization in the course of minimally-invasive surgery and, therefore, the risk of rebleeding is quite high. Kazui et al. [7], by analyzing the CT images of 204 patients with ICH, found that in 30% of cases, hematoma continued to expand 3 h after initial onset, in 17% cases 6 h after initial onset, but in no cases 24 h after initial onset. They concluded that hematoma expansion mostly took place 3 to 6 h after initial onset, and if the surgery was performed within 3 h after initial onset, a second hemorrhage was likely to occur after the hematoma cavity was decompressed. Surgery performed 6 h after initial onset would be safer. As rebleeding is the main complication leading to postoperative mortality or severe disability [1], ultra-early operative intervention is not recommended.

In our clinical trial, the comparison of therapeutic effect between surgical group and medication group demonstrated that patients who underwent operative intervention less than 7 h (ultra-early stage) after initial onset had a higher risk of rebleeding than those receiving medication. Secondly, surgery performed within 24 h (ultra-early and early stages) after initial onset was related to a better outcome and less mortality than with medication. Thirdly, there was no significant difference, regarding perioperative evaluation, long-term outcome, and mortality, between patients receiving surgery more than 24 h after initial onset (delayed stage) and patients receiving medication in the same stage. Moreover, delayed surgery was associated with higher incidence of complications of the respiratory, urinary, and digestive systems. Further comparison of therapeutic

effect among surgical cases in different time-windows showed no significant difference regarding perioperative evaluation, long-term outcome, and mortality, except the definitely higher risk of rebleeding for patients who underwent operative intervention less than 7 h after initial onset.

In conclusion, this multicenter clinical study has provided conclusive evidence that the early stage (7–24 h) is the optimal time-window for surgical evacuation of hematoma in patients with spontaneous ICH. It is associated with a favorable outcome, less risk of postoperative rebleeding, and fewer associated complications.

References

1. Broderick JP, Brott TG, Tomsick T, Barsan W, Spilker J (1990) Ultra-early evaluation of intracerebral hemorrhage. J Neurosurg 72: 195–199
2. Chen XC, Wu JS, Zhou XP, Zhang Y, Wang ZQ, Qin ZY, Pang L (2001) The randomized multicentric prospective controlled trial in the standardized treatment of hypertensive intracerebral hematomas: the comparison of surgical therapeutic outcomes with conservative therapy. Chin J Clin Neurosci 9: 365–368
3. Gong C, Hoff JT, Keep RF (2000) Acute inflammatory reaction following experimental intracerebral hemorrhage in rat. Brain Res 871: 57–65
4. Juvela S, Heiskanen O, Poranen A, Valtonen S, Kuurne T, Kaste M, Troupp H (1989) The treatment of spontaneous intracerebral hemorrhage. A prospective randomized trial of surgical and conservative treatment. J Neurosurg 70: 755–758
5. Kaneko M, Tanaka K, Shimada T, Sato K, Uemura K (1983) Long-term evaluation of ultra-early operation for hypertensive intracerebral hemorrhage in 100 cases. J Neurosurg 58: 838–842
6. Kanno T, Nagata J, Hoshino M, Nakagawa T, Chaudhari M, Sano H, Katada K (1986) Evaluation of the hypertensive intracerebral hematoma based on the study of long-term outcome – Part II. A role of surgery in putaminal hemorrhage [Japanese]. No Shinkei Geka 14: 1307–1311
7. Kazui S, Naritomi H, Yamamoto H, Sawada T, Yamaguchi T (1996) Enlargement of spontaneous intracerebral hemorrhage. Incidence and time course. Stroke 27: 1783–1787
8. Xi G, Wagner KR, Keep RF, Hua Y, de Courten-Myers GM, Broderick JP, Brott TG, Hoff JT (1998) Role of blood clot formation on early edema development after experimental intracerebral hemorrhage. Stroke 29: 2580–2586
9. Xi G, Hua Y, Bhasin RR, Ennis SR, Keep RF, Hoff JT (2001) Mechanisms of edema formation after intracerebral hemorrhage: effects of extravasated red blood cells on blood flow and blood-brain barrier integrity. Stroke 32: 2932–2938
10. Yang GY, Betz AL, Hoff JT (1994) The effects of blood or plasma clot on brain edema in the rat with intracerebral hemorrhage. Acta Neurochir Suppl (Wien) 60: 555–557
11. Zhou LF, Pang L (2001) Minimally invasive surgery for hypertensive hematomas – a prospective randomized multiple centers trial. Chin J Clin Neurosci 9: 151–154

Acta Neurochir Suppl (2008) 105: 147–151
© Springer-Verlag 2008
Printed in Austria

Preliminary findings of the minimally-invasive surgery plus rtPA for intracerebral hemorrhage evacuation (MISTIE) clinical trial

T. Morgan[1], M. Zuccarello[2], R. Narayan[2], P. Keyl[3], K. Lane[1], D. Hanley[1]

[1] Johns Hopkins University, Baltimore, MD, USA
[2] University of Cincinnati, Cincinnati, OH, USA
[3] Keyl Associates, East Sandwich, MA, USA

Summary

Introduction. Compared to ischemic stroke, intracerebral hemorrhage (ICH) is easily and rapidly identified, occurs in younger patients, and produces relatively small initial injury to cerebral tissues – all factors suggesting that interventional amelioration is possible. Investigations from the last decade established that extent of ICH-mediated brain injury relates directly to blood clot volume and duration of blood exposure to brain tissue. Using minimally-invasive surgery plus recombinant tissue plasminogen activator (rtPA), MISTIE investigators explored aggressive avenues to treat ICH.

Methods. We investigated the difference between surgical intervention plus rtPA and standard medical management for ICH. Subjects in both groups were medically managed according to standard ICU protocols. Subjects randomized to surgery underwent stereotactic catheter placement and clot aspiration. Injections of rtPA were then given through hematoma catheter every 8 h, up to 9 doses, or until a clot-reduction endpoint. After each injection the system was flushed with sterile saline and closed for 60 min before opening to spontaneous drainage.

Results. Average aspiration of clots for all patients randomized to surgery plus rtPA was 20% of mean initial clot size. After acute treatment phase (aspiration plus rtPA), clot was reduced an average of 46%. Recorded adverse events were within safety limits, including 30-day mortality, 8%; symptomatic re-bleeding, 8%; and bacterial ventriculitis, 0%. Patients randomized to medical management showed 4% clot resolution in a similar time window. Preliminary analysis indicates that clot resolution rates are greatly dependent on catheter placement. Location of ICH also affects efficacy of aggressive treatment of ICH.

Conclusion. There is tentative indication that minimally-invasive surgery plus rtPA shows greater clot resolution than traditional medical management.

Keywords: Thrombolysis; recombinant tissue plasminogen activator; stereotaxis; aspiration; intracerebral hemorrhage.

Correspondence: Timothy Morgan, BSc, Johns Hopkins University, 1550 Orleans Street, CRB II 3M50 South, Baltimore, MD 21231, USA. e-mail: tmorga10@jhmi.edu

Introduction

Spontaneous intracerebral hemorrhage (ICH) affects thousands of adults in the United States every year [1, 5–7, 12, 20]. Although it is easily identified using computed tomography (CT), treatment of ICH presents many challenges. It has been shown that patients with smaller bleeds (< 20 cc) have a lower mortality and better clinical outcome [3, 4, 13]. This leads to the hypothesis that methods of removing ICH in stable patients could result in lowered risk of mortality and improved outcome. Unless presented with a severe unmitigated bleed, most physicians are reluctant to aggressively treat ICH. Conventional treatment of ICH consists of medical monitoring, and only in the most severe cases craniotomy [19]. Pilot data from several trials support minimally-invasive surgery (MIS) as a safe method of treating ICH [10, 11, 14, 15, 17, 18, 22, 25]. Positive results have been shown in several clinical trials using thrombolytic agents, specifically recombinant tissue plasminogen activator (rtPA) [2, 8, 9, 16, 21, 23, 24]. In summary, the following premises have led to the Minimally Invasive Surgery plus rtPA for Intracerebral Hemorrhage Evacuation (MISTIE) clinical trial: 1) evacuating blood clot in stable patients increases the chance of good outcome; 2) stereotactic MIS can safely and effectively provide a channel for clot aspiration, drug delivery, and clot drainage; 3) rtPA can safely and effectively lyse clot to accelerate drainage.

Background

The MISTIE clinical trial is a phase II, safety and efficacy study of ICH treatment, sponsored by the National

Institutes of Health/National Institute of Neurological Disorders and Stroke. The trial is a 2-arm study designed to observe the differences between patients randomized to MIS plus rtPA versus best practice medical management. The MISTIE trial enrolled 25 patients in the first of 3 stages of dose-finding of rtPA. A total of 60 enrolled patients will complete this phase of the study (each stage of dose finding will enroll 20 patients with a 3:1 MIS + rtPA to medical management randomization scheme). Each site will have one run-in patient as their first enrollment; this patient is automatically designated as a surgical patient. We present our preliminary analyses of the first 21 enrolled patients.

Methods

Inclusion criteria for the study are as follows. Patients must be between the ages of 18 and 80, with a Glasgow Coma Scale (GCS) score ≤14 or a National Institutes of Health Stroke Scale (NIHSS) score ≥6. The eligible patient's diagnostic CT must show evidence of ICH ≥25cc shown to be stable at least 6h later by a second CT scan (clot volume calculated using the $A \times B \times C/2$ method). The patient must have a historical Rankin score of 0 or 1 and a negative pregnancy test.

Exclusion criteria are: any infratentorial hemorrhage, intraventricular hemorrhage requiring external ventricular drainage, coagulopathy (patients with platelet count ≤100,000, international normalized ratio ≥1.7, abnormal prothrombin time, or an elevated activated partial thromboplastin time. Reversal of warfarin is permitted). Magnetic resonance angiography or computed tomographic angiography must be obtained prior to enrollment to rule out aneurysm, arteriovenous malformation, or any other vascular anomaly.

For enrolled patients randomized to surgery, a 14-French cannula is stereotactically placed into the center of the parenchymal clot two-thirds the length of the long axis, and within the middle one-third of the clot. Directly after catheter placement, an initial aspiration of clot is conducted using a 10cc syringe until the surgeon notes the first resistance to free-hand suction. This is the only aspiration in the treatment. Following completion of hematoma aspiration, a soft ventriculostomy catheter is then passed through the rigid cannula and the rigid cannula is removed leaving the soft catheter in the center of the residual hematoma. A postoperative CT scan is taken to confirm accurate placement and check for any instance of new bleeding. After CT, the patient begins a dosing regimen of 0.3 mg rtPA followed by a sterile flush. After each dose, the system is closed for 1h to allow drug/clot interaction. After 1h, the system is opened for gravitational drainage. Subsequent doses are given every 8h, up to 9 doses, or until a clinical endpoint is reached. Clinical endpoints include: 1) reduction of clot to 80% of original size (measured on the scan that shows clot stability prior to enrollment), or 2) clot size is reduced to 15cc or less. Additional endpoints include any bleeding events involving a new hemorrhage, or extension of exiting hemorrhage by 5cc or more (treatment failures). CT scans are taken once every 24h to evaluate drainage, or as clinically indicated.

Results

Patients responded favorably to the surgery plus rtPA treatment compared to the 2 patients in the group randomized to medical management. On average, 20% of the clot was removed through surgical aspiration alone.

Table 1. *Mean clot size in surgical patients versus medically-managed patients at critical points during acute-treatment phase*

Treatment	Starting volume (cc)	Post-surgery volume (cc)	End-of-treatment volume (cc)	7-day follow-up volume (cc)
Minimally-invasive surgery plus rtPA ($n = 19$)	48.07	37.02	25.21	19.37
Medical management ($n = 2$)	38.97	N/A	N/A	36.65

rtPA Recombinant tissue plasminogen activator.

After treatment, average clot size was reduced by nearly 50% of starting volume, whereas patients randomized to medical management showed only a 6% reduction of clot through a 7-day period (Table 1).

Surgical patients received an average of 4 doses of rtPA, with 4 patients receiving no doses (clot reduction endpoint was met through aspiration alone) and 3 patients receiving 9 doses (Table 2). Recorded adverse events were within safety limits, including 30-day mortality, 8%; symptomatic re-bleeding, 8%; and bacterial ventriculitis, 0%.

Table 2. *Patient demographics and treatment*

Patient no.	Age (years)/sex	GCS score	ICH size at stability on CT (cm³)	Treatment	No. of doses
1	73/M	11	23.02	MIS + rtPA	0
2	51/M	12	39.64	MIS + rtPA	6
3	70/F	14	56.43	MIS + rtPA	3
4	54/M	11	28.12	MIS + rtPA	8
5	49/M	11	20.00	medical management	0
6	66/F	11	28.38	MIS + rtPA	2
7	59/M	7	31.76	MIS + rtPA	6
8	65/M	9	55.59	MIS + rtPA	9
9	71/M	15	74.22	MIS + rtPA	4
10	60/M	6	59.76	MIS + rtPA	9
11	79/F	14	42.40	MIS + rtPA	0
12	77/M	8	51.25	MIS + rtPA	0
13	62/F	13	23.33	MIS + rtPA	3
14	64/M	15	30.69	MIS + rtPA	1
15	50/F	8	29.27	MIS + rtPA	3
16	47/F	8	37.18	MIS + rtPA	5
17	71/F	10	28.42	MIS + rtPA	6
18	56/M	13	43.87	MIS + rtPA	1
19	65/F	10	44.52	MIS + rtPA	0
20	75/F	14	57.94	medical management	0
21	74/F	14	185.42	MIS + rtPA	9
Mean	64/11M:10F	11	47.20	19:2	4

CT Computed tomography; *F* female; *GCS* Glasgow Coma Scale; *ICH* intracerebral hemorrhage; *M* male; *MIS* minimally-invasive surgery; *rtPA* recombinant tissue plasminogen activator.

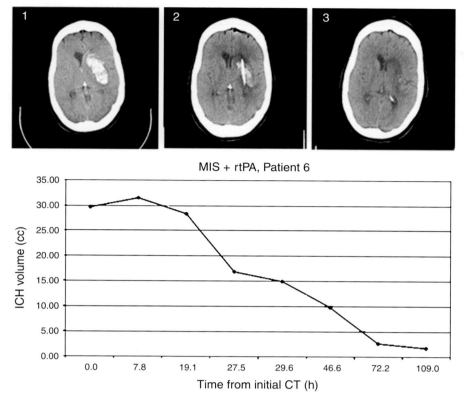

MIS + rtPA, Patient 6

Fig. 1. Patient randomized to treatment (surgery plus rtPA). During initial surgical aspiration, 11.54 cc of clot was removed. Two doses of rtPA were given before patient reached clot reduction endpoint. Image *1* taken at 0 h, image *2* taken at 30 h (directly after aspiration and catheter placement), and image *3* taken at 72 h (end of treatment)

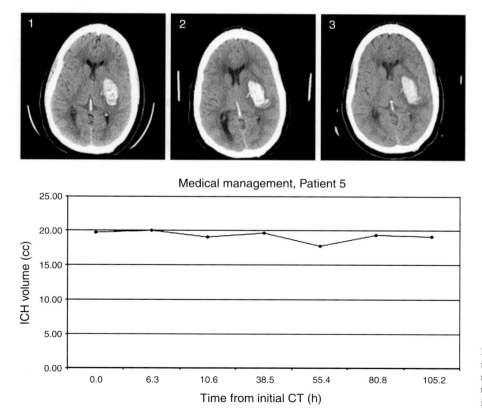

Medical management, Patient 5

Fig. 2. Patient randomized to medical management. Clot volume remained relatively stable over time. Image *1* taken at 0 h, image *2* taken at 38.5 h, image *3* taken at 81 h

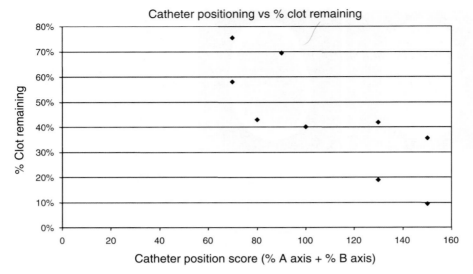

Fig. 3. Catheter position versus % clot
remaining at the end of treatment

Discussion

Clot resolution rate for surgical patients appears to be
highly correlated with catheter placement. A comparative
look at catheter placements performed during the trial focused on 3 criteria: 1) catheter goes through the center of
the clot; 2) catheter runs through the long axis of the clot;
and 3) catheter spans at least two-thirds the length of the
long axis of the clot. Using this scoring rubric, CT scans of
all surgical patients were graded for catheter placement
efficiency. This scoring (a score of 0 being lowest and
150 representing optimal catheter placement) was related
to overall clot resolution through the treatment period.
An appreciable trend toward optimal catheter placement
leading to greater clot resolution is seen in Fig. 3.

Conclusions

It has been shown that the methods used for stereotactic
catheter placement for hematoma aspiration and intracranial thrombolytic therapy are safe, and appear to be
effective when compared to current medical management of large intracerebral hematomas. Early analysis
indicates that catheter positioning plays an important
role in the effectiveness of treatment following the
MISTIE surgical protocol. Further analyses of additional
patients enrolled in the study will be forthcoming.

References

1. Abdul-Ghaffar NU, el-Sonbaty MR, el-Din Abdul-Baky MS,
   Marafie AA, al-Said AM (1997) Stroke in Kuwait: a three-year
   prospective study. Neuroepidemiology 16: 40–47
2. Akdemir H, Selçuklu A, Paşaoğlu A, Oktem IS, Kavuncu I (1995)
   Treatment of severe intraventricular hemorrhage by intraventricular
   infusion of urokinase. Neurosurg Rev 18: 95–100
3. Becker KJ, Baxter AB, Bybee HM, Tirschwell DL, Abouelsaad T,
   Cohen WA (1999) Extravasation of radiographic contrast is an
   independent predictor of death in primary intracerebral hemorrhage. Stroke 30: 2025–2032
4. Broderick JP, Brott T, Tomsick T, Miller R, Huster G (1993)
   Intracerebral hemorrhage more than twice as common as subarachnoid hemorrhage. J Neurosurg 78: 188–191
5. Brown RD Jr, Ransom J, Hass S, Petty GW, O'Fallon WM,
   Whisnant JP, Leibson CL (1999) Use of nursing home after stroke
   and dependence on stroke severity: a population-based analysis.
   Stroke 30: 924–929
6. Caplan LR (1992) Intracerebral hemorrhage. Lancet 339: 656–658
7. Daverat P, Castel JP, Dartigues JF, Orgogozo JM (1991) Death and
   functional outcome after spontaneous intracerebral hemorrhage. A
   prospective study of 166 cases using multivariate analysis. Stroke
   22: 1–6
8. Findlay JM, Weir BK, Kassell NF, Disney LB, Grace MG
   (1991) Intracisternal recombinant tissue plasminogen activator after aneurysmal subarachnoid hemorrhage. J Neurosurg 75:
   181–188
9. Findlay JM, Grace MG, Weir BK (1993) Treatment of intraventricular hemorrhage with tissue plasminogen activator. Neurosurgery
   32: 941–947
10. Hondo H, Uno M, Sasaki K Ebisudani D, Shichijo F, Tóth Z,
    Matsumoto K (1990) Computed tomography controlled aspira-
    tion surgery for hypertensive intracerebral hemorrhage. Experi-
    ence of more than 400 cases. Stereotact Funct Neurosurg 54–55:
    432–437
11. Kandel EI, Peresedov VV (1985) Stereotaxic evacuation of spon-
    taneous intracerebral hematomas. J Neurosurg 62: 206–213
12. Kumral E, Ozkaya B, Sagduyu A, Sirin H, Vardarli E, Pehlivan M
    (1998) The EGE stroke registry: a hospital-based study in the
    Aegean region, Izmir, Turkey. Analysis of 2000 stroke patients.
    Cerebrovasc Dis 8: 278–288
13. Lampl Y, Gilad R, Eshel Y, Sarova-Pinhas I (1995) Neurological
    and functional outcome in patients with supratentorial hemor-
    rhages. A prospective study. Stroke 26: 2249–2253
14. Lippitz BE, Mayfrank L, Spetzger U, Warnke JP, Bertalanffy H,
    Gilsbach JM (1994) Lysis of basal ganglia haematoma with recom-
    binant tissue plasminogen activator (rtPA) after stereotactic aspira-
    tion: initial results. Acta Neurochir (Wien) 127: 157–160
15. Matsumoto K, Hondo H (1984) CT-guided stereotaxic evacua-
    tion of hypertensive intracerebral hematomas. J Neurosurg 61:
    440–448

16. Mayfrank L, Lippitz B, Groth M, Bertalanffy H, Gilsbach JM (1993) Effect of recombinant tissue plasminogen activator on clot lysis and ventricular dilatation in the treatment of severe intraventricular haemorrhage. Acta Neurochir (Wien) 122: 32–38

17. Miller DW, Barnett GH, Kormos DW, Steiner CP (1993) Stereotactically guided thrombolysis of deep cerebral hemorrhage: preliminary results. Cleve Clin J Med 60: 321–324

18. Mohadjer M, Braus DF, Myers A, Scheremet R, Krauss JK (1992) CT-stereotactic fibrinolysis of spontaneous intracerebral hematomas. Neurosurg Rev 15: 105–110

19. Morgenstern LB, Frankowski RF, Shedden P, Pasteur W, Grotta JC (1998) Surgical treatment for intracerebral hemorrhage (STICH): a single-center, randomized clinical trial. Neurology 51: 1359–1363

20. Ojemann RG, Heros RC (1983) Spontaneous brain hemorrhage. Stroke 14: 468–475

21. Rohde V, Schaller C, Hassler WE (1995) Intraventricular recombinant tissue plasminogen activator for lysis of intraventricular haemorrhage. J Neurol Neurosurg Psychiatry 58: 447–451

22. Schaller C, Rohde V, Meyer B, Hassler W (1995) Stereotactic puncture and lysis of spontaneous intracerebral hemorrhage using recombinant tissue-plasminogen activator. Neurosurgery 36: 328–335

23. Shen PH, Matsuoka Y, Kawajiri K, Kanai M, Hoda K, Yamamoto S, Nishimura S (1990) Treatment of intraventricular hemorrhage using urokinase. Neurol Med Chir (Tokyo) 30: 329–333

24. Todo T, Usui M, Takakura K (1991) Treatment of severe intraventricular hemorrhage by intraventricular infusion of urokinase. J Neurosurg 74: 81–86

25. Tzaan WC, Lee ST, Lui TN (1997) Combined use of stereotactic aspiration and intracerebral streptokinase infusion in the surgical treatment of hypertensive intracerebral hemorrhage. J Formos Med Assoc 96: 962–967

Acta Neurochir Suppl (2008) 105: 153–159
© Springer-Verlag 2008
Printed in Austria

Pediatric cerebrovascular diseases: report of 204 cases

C. Y. Xia, R. Zhang, Y. Mao, L. F. Zhou

Department of Neurosurgery, Huashan Hospital, Shanghai Medical College, Fu Dan University, Shanghai, China

Summary

Objective. To investigate the epidemiology of pediatric cerebrovascular diseases.

Methods. Retrospective review of clinical data for 204 pediatric patients under the age of 18 treated for cerebrovascular disease at Huashan Hospital within the past 13 years.

Results. Mean age was 12.7 years and male-to-female ratio was 1.91:1. Onset of symptoms was acute or subacute in 73.5% (150/204). Main clinical manifestations include: headaches (70.6%), vomiting (50.0%), loss of consciousness (22.5%), convulsions (21.6%), and focal neurological deficits (13.2%). The most common etiologies were: arteriovenous malformations (42.2%; 86/204), cavernomas (16.2%; 33/204), aneurysms (8.8%; 18/204), and Moyamoya disease (5.9%; 12/204). The cause remained unknown in 21% (43/204).

Conclusions. As the main neurological medical center in the southern part of China, the statistics of Huashan Hospital could be representative. The epidemiology of pediatric cerebrovascular diseases has its own specificity. Pediatric cerebrovascular disease must be diagnosed in a timely manner and treated urgently, according to the distinct clinical features of the pediatric patient.

Keywords: Cerebrovascular disease; pediatric; epidemiology; etiology; clinical presentation.

Introduction

Children are not true miniature versions of adults because of their physiological features during development [12]. Characteristics of pediatric cerebrovascular disease differ from adults in etiology, clinical features, diagnosis, and treatment. Cerebrovascular disease must be diagnosed timely and treated urgently or it will endanger the lives of children; furthermore, survivors often have sequelae of the nervous system. Most of the current reports of pediatric cerebrovascular disease are sporadic case analyses or introductory experiences, and few large series have yet been reported. Thus, to investigate the

clinical characteristics of cerebrovascular disease, we performed a retrospective analysis of clinical epidemiology (including age distribution, etiology, clinical presentations, diagnosis, and treatment) in 204 children under the age of 18 treated at our hospital during the period 1993–2006.

Materials and methods

Patients

Included in this retrospective study were patients younger than 18 years of age who had been diagnosed with cerebrovascular disease at our hospital during the period 1993–2006. Patients with traumatic bleeds or abnormal hematological findings were excluded from the study.

Methods

The following information was collected during review of the medical records: neuro-imaging investigations, current age, age at time of onset, sex, underlying etiologies, initial clinical presentation, neurological signs at admission, diagnostic procedures, anatomic location, therapy, and neurological outcome at time of discharge. Most instances of cerebrovascular disease were diagnosed by cerebral digital subtraction angiography (DSA) or pathology; only a few were obtained by clinical presentation and/or other corresponding neuro-imaging findings (computed tomography [CT] and/or magnetic resonance imaging [MRI]). Etiologies were all based on cerebral DSA or pathology. We performed χ^2 test or Fisher exact probability test ($p < 0.05$) using Stata 7.0 software (StataCorp LP, College Station, TX).

Results

Age and sex

The study group consisted of 204 patients, 134 boys and 70 girls. Sex ratio was m:f = 1.91:1. Ages ranged from 32 days to 17.9 years, with a mean age of 12.7 years. Mean ages were 12.4 and 13.1 years for boys and girls, respectively. The age distribution of all patients and ma-

Correspondence: Rong Zhang, M.D., #12 Wulumuqi Zhong Road, Shanghai 200040, China. e-mail: rong.z.zhang@gmail.com

Table 1. *Age distribution and major etiologies of 204 pediatric patients*

Age group (years)	Number of patients with arteriovenous malformation		Number of patients with cavernoma		Number of patients with aneurysm		Number of patients with Moyamoya disease		Total	
	Male	Female	Male	Female	Male	Female	Male	Female	Male (%)	Female (%)
0–3	1	0	1	0	0	0	0	0	3 (1.5)	0 (0)
3–6	3	3	0	0	1	0	0	0	5 (2.5)	6 (2.9)
6–9	6	2	2	1	1	3	3	0	21 (10.3)	6 (2.9)
9–12	12	6	3	4	2	1	1	0	32 (15.7)	14 (6.9)
12–15	20	9	9	4	6	1	3	3	47 (23.0)	27 (13.2)
15–18	15	9	5	4	2	1	2	0	26 (12.7)	17 (8.3)
Total	57	29	20	13	12	6	9	3	134 (65.7)	70 (34.3)

jor etiologies is summarized in Table 1. We found that patients aged between 9 and 15 years had greater likelihood for the disease (58.8%; 120/204), and boys were more likely than girls to have the 4 major etiologies.

Clinical presentation

Symptoms included headaches (70.6%; 144/204), vomiting (50.0%; 102/204), impaired consciousness (22.5%; 46/204), convulsions (21.6%; 44/204), and focal neurological deficits (13.2%; 27/204), as well as accidental discovery without symptoms (4.9%; 10/204). Onset of symptoms was acute and subacute in 73.5% (150/204) of patients. Subacute is defined as a prolonged and protracted course over a period of several hours up to a few days that did not lead to immediate hospitalization. Acute is defined as a sudden onset of symptoms (e.g., epileptic seizure, abrupt unconsciousness, splitting headache, etc.) that resulted in immediate hospitalization.

Etiologies

The following etiologies were found: arteriovenous malformation (AVM) 42.2% (86/204); cavernomas 16.2% (33/204); aneurysms 8.8% (18/204); Moyamoya disease 5.9% (12/204); complex vascular malformations 2.0% (4/204, aneurysm + AVM); arteriovenous fistula (AVF) 1.0% (2/204); venous malformations 1.0% (2/204); meningioangiomatosis 1.0% (2/204); telangiectasia 0.5% (1/204); and dural AVF (DAVF) 0.5% (1/204). The causes were unknown in 21.1% (43/204), which included 16 (7.8%) patients with negative DSA and 27 (13.3%) patients without DSA examinations. In the 16 patients with negative DSA, there were 3 patients whose lesions may have been resected in emergency operations because of acute hemorrhage, and the other

13 patients underwent conservative treatment owing to mild hemorrhage in deep brain or functional area. Etiologies for 27 patients without DSA examinations were not available because either parents/guardians gave up treatment or patients died soon after onset of the disease.

The first etiology was AVM in female, male, and entire group, respectively. There was no obvious variation ($p = 0.835$) between boys and girls in the percentage of the first 4 known causes (Table 2).

Location

Lesions in 181 cases were supratentorial (88.7%); 23 cases were infratentorial (11.3%); 7.8% percent of the lesions occurred midline, and 6.9% bilaterally. Hemorrhage occurred in 182 cases (89.2%): intracerebral hemorrhage 144 (79.1%), intraventricular 26 (14.3%), and subarachnoid 12 (6.6%). AVMs were located mainly supratentor-

Table 2. *Etiologies of 204 cases of pediatric cerebrovascular disease*

Etiology	Number of male patients (%)	Number of female patients (%)	Total (%)
Arteriovenous malformation	57 (42.5)	29 (41.4)	86 (42.2)
Cavernoma	20 (14.9)	13 (18.6)	33 (16.2)
Unknown	17 (12.7)	10 (14.3)	27 (13.2)
Aneurysm	12 (9.0)	6 (8.6)	18 (8.8)
Digital subtraction angiography (negative)	11 (8.2)	5 (7.1)	16 (7.8)
Moyamoya disease	9 (6.7)	3 (4.3)	12 (5.9)
Arteriovenous malformation + aneurysm	4 (3.0)	0	4 (2.0)
Arteriovenous fistula	2 (1.5)	0	2 (1.0)
Venous malformations	0	2 (2.9)	2 (1.0)
Meningioangiomatosis	1 (0.7)	1 (1.4)	2 (1.0)
Telangiectasia	0	1 (1.4)	1 (0.5)
Dural arteriovenous fistula	1 (0.7)	0	1 (0.5)
Total	134 (100)	70 (100)	204 (100)

Table 3. *Locations of pediatric intracranial lesions*

Location	Number of patients with arteriovenous malformation	Number of patients with cavernoma
Frontal lobe	21	7
Temporal lobe	10	11
Parietal lobe	7	4
Occipital lobe	13	1
Temporo-parietal lobe	3	–
Lateral fissure	3	–
Corpus callosum	6	1
Lateral ventricle	5	1
Cerebellum	11	1
Brainstem	2	4 (all in pons)
Others	5 (1 basilar ganglion; 1 fronto-temporal lobe; 1 fronto-parietal lobe; 2 parieto-occipital lobe)	3 (2 with multiple lesions in frontal lobe; 1 in frontal lobe and cerebellum, respectively)
Total	86	33

Table 4. *Locations of aneurysms in 18 pediatric patients*

Location	Number of patients
Anterior cerebral artery	2 (A3)
Anterior communicating artery	1
Internal carotid artery	3 (2 in C1; 1 in C5)
Middle cerebral artery	6 (1 in M1; 1 in M2 multiple; 2 in M3; 1 in M3–4; 1 in M4)
Posterior cerebral artery	3 (1 in occipital ramification; 1 in posterior choroidal artery; 1 in tentorial hiatus)
Posterior communicating artery	1
Multiple locations	2 (1 in C1 and bifurcate of M1–2; 1 distal of middle and posterior cerebral arteries)
Total	18

ial (73.3%; 63/86) and frequently in frontal or occipital lobe, while infratentorial AVMs were found mainly in cerebellum (see Table 3). Cavernomas were also mainly located supratentorial (84.8%; 28/33) and more frequently in frontal or temporal lobe; occasionally in infratentorial but 4/5 in pons (Table 3). Aneurysms in 6 cases were located in the middle cerebral artery (MCA), 10 in distal arteries, and 5 around the circle of Willis (Table 4). Moyamoya disease occurred bilaterally in 10 cases and unilaterally in only 2 ($p = 0.03$).

Diagnosis

To confirm intracranial hemorrhage, CT was performed for 195/204 children, and etiology was chiefly based on DSA in 130/204 children or pathology in 78/204 chil-

dren. To screen the etiologies, MRI/magnetic resonance angiography (MRA) was performed on 66 children and computed tomographic angiography (CTA) on 25 children. MRI was mainly performed on 31 children suspected of cavernoma, of which 29 cases were treated surgically and the imaging diagnoses of 28 cases (96.6%; 28/29) were consistent with pathological diagnosis. Only 1 child with cavernoma was misdiagnosed preoperatively because of atypical MRI signal due to repeating hemorrhage. MRI/MRA was also used for 8 children with Moyamoya disease (100% diagnostically consistent with DSA). CTA had a diagnostic coincidence of 78.9% (15/19), and was performed on children highly suspected of AVM or aneurysm but who couldn't tolerate DSA examination.

Therapeutic management and outcome

Treatment was chiefly based on the individual cause as determined by DSA or/and MRI/MRA. According to the location and size of AVMs confirmed by DSA, we performed microscopic resection of the AVMs in 48.8% (42/86) of children, embolization in 12.8% (11/86), stereotactic radiotherapy in 9.3% (8/86), and stereotactic radiotherapy after embolization in 1 child. Other methods included microscopic resection of cavernomas in 87.9% (29/33), clipping aneurysm in 50% (9/18), embolization of aneurysm in 5.6% (1/18), and EDAMS (encephalo-duro-arterio-myo-synangiosis) operations in 75% (9/12) of children with Moyamoya disease. In 32.4% (66/204) of patients, no invasive treatment such surgery or an endovascular intervention was performed after negative DSA findings; 8 of these 66 children died, and the survivors were advised to follow-up with DSA. Nineteen (9.3%, 19/204) children required ventricular drainage because of hydrocephalus or severe intraventricular hemorrhage, of which 7 (3.4%; 7/204) required a permanent ventriculo-peritoneal shunt.

The outcome of survivors was assessed by their condition at time of hospital discharge, and included cure (no obvious neurological deficits) in 61.3%, improving (symptoms or signs improving, but with diverse neurological deficits) in 21.1%, ineffective treatment (no improvement of symptoms or signs) in 13.7%, and death in 3.9% (Table 5). Of all etiologies, the group with highest cure rate was cavernoma (84.8%; 28/33); the others in turn were AVM (66.3%; 57/86), negative DSA (56.3%; 9/16), and Moyamoya disease (41.7%; 5/12). The unknown etiologies group had severe mortality (22.2%; 6/27), and the AVM group had 2 deaths (2.3%; 2/86).

Table 5. *Outcome of 204 cases of pediatric cerebrovascular disease*

Etiology	Number of patients cured (%)	Number of patients improving (%)	Number of patients receiving ineffective treatment (%)	Number of deaths (%)	Total
Arteriovenous malformation	57 (66.3)	14 (16.3)	13 (15.1)	2 (2.3)	86
Cavernoma	28 (84.8)	2 (6.1)	3 (9.1)	0	33
Unknown	13 (48.1)	8 (29.6)	0	6 (22.2)	27
Aneurysm	6 (33.3)	5 (27.8)	7 (38.9)	0	18
Digital subtraction angiography (negative)	9 (56.3)	7 (43.8)	0	0	16
Moyamoya disease	5 (41.7)	4 (33.3)	3 (25.0)	0	12
Arteriovenous malformation + aneurysm	3 (75.0)	1 (25.0)	0	0	4
Arteriovenous fistula	1 (50.0)	1 (50.0)	0	0	2
Venous malformations	1 (50.0)	0	1 (50.0)	0	2
Meningioangiomatosis	2 (100.0)	0	0	0	2
Telangiectasia	0	1 (100.0)	0	0	1
Dural arteriovenous fistula	0	0	1 (100.0)	0	1
Total	125 (61.3%)	43 (21.1%)	28 (13.7%)	8 (3.9%)	204

All 8 children died (overall mortality, 3.9%) of acute massive intracranial hemorrhage aggravated too rapidly to be effectively rescued (Table 5).

Discussion

Pediatric cerebrovascular disease has characteristic features that differ from the adult form of the disease: 1) male predominance; 2) chief etiology was AVMs, and more occurred in the 9–18 year age group in our series; 3) infratentorial cavernomas mainly occurred in the pons; 4) intracranial aneurysms were generally found in distal arteries as opposed to the circle of Willis; 5) ischemic presentation was more often seen in pediatric Moyamoya disease.

Etiologies and age distribution

The chief etiologies of cerebrovascular disease in adults are cerebral infarction and intracerebral hemorrhage caused by hypertension or atherosclerosis, rather than intracerebral vascular abnormality. In the latter, aneurysms are more common than AVMs in adults. The etiologies of cerebrovascular disease in children are obviously different than those of adults. The major cause was AVMs, accounting for 30–60% of cerebrovascular disease in children, and other vascular abnormalities such as cavernoma, Moyamoya disease, and aneurysm were relatively uncommon, and there were some unknown causes as well [7, 14, 15, 17, 19]. In our series, AVMs (42.2%) were the most common and occurred mostly in the age group from 9 to 18 years (82.6%; 71/86). Cavernoma (16.2%) and aneurysm (8.8%) were fairly uncommon. These findings are consistent with the study done by Liu *et al.* [11], who reported 9 cases

(18%) with cavernoma and 3 cases (6%) with aneurysm in a series of 50 children with non-traumatic stroke. Cavernoma may be more common because MRI is more frequently used in the diagnosis of intracerebral hemorrhage, and the increasing vigilance for angiogram-negative cavernoma. In our series, there were still 17 cases with unknown etiology on DSA and other neuro-imaging examinations.

The sex ratio (m:f = 1.91:1) of our patients and the fact that pediatric cerebrovascular disease occurred more frequently in boys is consistent with the literature by Al-Jarallah *et al.* [1] (sex ratio, m:f = 1.72:1). The etiologies of pediatric cerebrovascular disease are different according to age group [1]: hematological disease is seen more in newborns, latent vitamin K deficiency is seen more at 0–6 months and especially under 3 months, and AVM seen more in children aged greater than 5 years. Our series with only 3 patients under 3 years did not show this characteristic, perhaps because of the lack of a pediatric department in our hospital. We did find that the highest incidence of AVM was in the age group from 9 to 15 years (54.6%; 47/86), and a similar trait was seen in cavernoma, aneurysm, Moyamoya disease, and other etiologies.

Clinical presentation and diagnosis

Onset of symptoms was acute and subacute in 73.5% of the children in our series (83% in the series by May Llanas *et al.* [13]), and the symptoms were caused mainly by hemorrhage (89.2%; 182/204) and clinical presentations included increased intracranial pressure, sudden loss of consciousness, seizures, local neurological deficits, and others. In our series, there were different features associated with the different causes of pediatric cerebrovascular disease: children's aneurysms were more common near the distal arteries (10/18) than near the circle of Willis (5/18), which is contrary in adults; infratentorial cavernomas mainly occurred in the pons (80%; 4/5); in cases of Moyamoya disease, ischemic presentation (9 cases) such as dizziness and fatigue of the limbs was more often seen than hemorrhagic (3 cases, all were intraventricular hemorrhage) ($p = 0.039$), while the hemorrhagic type was common in adults [6]. Clinical presentation also differed with the age groups of children. Older children who were able to describe their complaints did not differ from adults, except for their higher incidence rate of seizures. In our series, the first highest incidence rate was in cavernomas (30.3%; 10/33), the second highest was in AVMs (18.6%; 16/86), and the total was 21.6% (44/204). Younger patients who could not describe their complaints had nonspecific presentation, of which the most common [16] were increased tension in fontanel, vomiting, refusing feeding of milk, screaming, progressive facial paleness, tics, crying and disquiet, faintness, change in pupil size, unconsciousness, and others.

According to the above presentations, further neuroimaging examinations are necessary to confirm suspected intracranial hemorrhage. CT is the examination of first choice, but B-mode ultrasonography could be combined with CT in infants with unclosed fontanel, especially for follow-up of the evolving intracerebral hemorrhage already confirmed by CT in conservative treatment. It can be safely, easily performed at bedside for dynamic follow-up with highly positive findings in intracerebral hemorrhage but without radiation and trauma [10]. As CT is easily available nowadays, examination of cerebrospinal fluid by lumbar puncture is seldom performed to confirm intracerebral hemorrhage. This procedure is not only traumatic for the patient and unhelpful for making the treatment plan, but may also precipitate cerebral herniation in the acute phase.

To determine disease causes, CTA, MRI/MRA, and DSA are selected according to the disease conditions, the degree of the child's ability to cooperate, and suspected etiologies. CTA has great value in the diagnosis of cerebrovascular disease. Wu *et al.* [18] reported that 3D-CTA had the same sensitivity and specificity of 100% as that of DSA in AVM, AVF, and venous malformations, and the sensitivity of 3D-CTA for aneurysm and Moyamoya was 90.9% and 84.6%, respectively. The advantages of CTA are as follows [3]: 1) It can be performed safely, quickly, less expensively, and at any moment. 2) CTA compared with DSA provides more complete anatomic information (unlimited viewing angles, 3-dimensional views, virtual endoscopy, and information on bony and adjacent vessel relationships, true neck-to-dome relationships in aneurysms, and the presence of calcium or atheromas). 3) CTA can be performed easily and expeditiously after spontaneous intracranial hemorrhage has been confirmed while the patient is still on the CT table, thus saving time for rescue of the patient. CTA is suitable for younger children who cannot cooperate, and is especially attractive for evaluation of critically ill patients who cannot tolerate DSA examination, or at centers where urgent DSA may be difficult to obtain. MRI/MRA has special advantages for children because there is no radiation or trauma involved. It is especially suitable for the children who are suspected of cavernomas or ischemic cerebrovascular diseases (e.g., Moyamoya disease), are in relatively stable condition, and for differential diagnosis with the apoplexy of brain tumor. MRI can provide effective complementary information for cases with negative DSA findings (e.g., cavernomas). In our series, MRI/MRA were chiefly performed on children suspected of cavernomas and Moyamoya disease, and the preoperative diagnostic coincidence rates were 96.6% (28/29) in cavernomas and 100% (8/8) in Moyamoya disease. DSA is still the gold standard for the diagnosis of cerebrovascular disease [5]. It can provide correct imaging information about the dynamic supply and drainage of blood in abnormal blood vessels (especially in AVMs and DAVF), and can provide details for further management options. In our experience, the techniques of DSA were not obviously different between children and adults, and the microcatheter was no more difficult to insert into the target vessels of children and had less distortion than in adults. General anesthesia is commonly required for children, but local anesthesia can be undertaken for older children who can cooperate. With the development of imaging and microcatheter techniques, the safety of cerebral DSA in children has been obviously improved. Burger *et al.* [2] reported the rate of intraprocedural complications was 0.0% (95% CI, 0.0–1.4%), and only one 7-year-old girl with a type IV DAVF of the right transverse sinus died of a ruptured posterior fossa varix 3 h after completion of an uneventful cerebral angiogram (0.4%; 95% CI, 0.01–2.29%). It is possible that the rupture of the varicose vein may have been coincidental or precipitated by the straining induced by the sudden vomiting approximately 3 h after angiography, when the patient awoke from anesthesia without deficit but with slight nausea. Most patients tolerate emergency DSA examinations, whereas only a few cannot tolerate it because cerebral herniation had occurred or would occur in the children with decreasing consciousness after sudden onset (5.4% in our series).

According to the clinical features of cerebrovascular disease, definite diagnoses can be acquired with appropriate neuro-imaging examinations or by combining with the above methods. Of major concern are younger children who cannot depict their complaints, have no specific presentations, and have delayed or inconspicuous intracranial pressure. Such patients require special attention.

Treatment and outcome

Cerebrovascular disease is treated by medication and surgical methods. Medications included those for osmotic dehydration, prophylactic anti-convulsion, hemostatic administration, and others. These were applicable to all cases. Surgical methods were selected based on the cause of the individual's symptoms and condition at admission. In our experience, it is very important to determine the specific cause as soon as possible and then select active measures (surgical operation, endovascular intervention, stereotactic radiotherapy, or combined application of methods) based on the cause, thereby lowering mortality, decreasing sequelae, and improving quality-of-life for our patients. For children with AVM or cavernoma who can tolerate craniotomy, we generally performed microscopic resection of the lesions. In the case of aneurysm, we performed surgical clipping or embolization according to cerebral DSA. For AVMs located in important functional areas or deep in the brain for which total resection or complete embolization was not possible, we suggested stereotactic radiotherapy. In cases of symptomatic Moyamoya disease, we performed EDAMS operations. In children with cerebral hemorrhage with cause undetermined by DSA and/or other neuro-imaging examinations, we provided guidance for close clinical follow-up including another DSA examination.

In some cases, DSA is not able to detect underlying lesions, for the following reasons [4]: the blood supply of the anomaly is compressed by the hematoma around it; spasm of supplying artery; thrombosis in the vascular malformation; destruction of vascular malformation during bleeding; slow flow and high coagulative state in the abnormal vessels. It is very important to 1) establish intravenous access in children prior to surgery, 2) enforce careful administration of anesthesia during the operation, 3) apply microscopic techniques during the operation, 4) correctly estimate and supply the bleeding volume in a timely manner, and 5) pay attention to prophylactic anti-convulsion therapy after the operation. General postoperative nursing should also attach importance to caring for younger children, especially avoiding too much or too rapid transfusion that can induce heart failure.

The prognosis of pediatric cerebrovascular disease is better than in adults, partly owing to better reconstruction of cerebral function after intracerebral hemorrhage. In our series, the total rate of cure and improving was 82.4% (168/204), and mortality was 3.9% (8/204). Death occurred in the AVM (2 patients) and unknown etiology (6 patients) groups, and all had acute massive hemorrhage and were unable to be rescued. In the 17 articles on pediatric hemorrhagic stroke reviewed by Jordan *et al.* [8], mortality was from 7% to 52%, and mean mortality was 24%. Thus, the mortality in our series was lower than that of the literature. Children with Moyamoya disease can also have good outcomes after EDAMS operations, especially for the ischemic type for which neurological functions can be obviously improved [9]. In the 9 children in our study who underwent surgery, the preoperative ischemic symptoms and signs disappeared in 5 patients and obviously improved in 4 patients.

In summary, better prognosis and treatment efficacy can be attained if we can recognize the clinical features of pediatric cerebrovascular disease, make a timely diagnosis, acquire an etiology as soon as possible, and then actively take effective measures to deal with the etiology. The high rate of cure and improvement (82.4%; 168/204) in our series are attributed to all of the above.

References

1. Al-Jarallah A, Al-Rifai MT, Riela AR, Roach ES (2000) Nontraumatic brain hemorrhage in children: etiology and presentation. J Child Neurol 15: 284–289
2. Burger IM, Murphy KJ, Jordan LC, Tamargo RJ, Gailloud P (2006) Safety of cerebral digital subtraction angiography in children: complication rate analysis in 241 consecutive diagnostic angiograms. Stroke 37: 2535–2539
3. Chappell ET, Moure FC, Good MC (2003) Comparison of computed tomographic angiography with digital subtraction angiography in the diagnosis of cerebral aneurysms: a meta-analysis. Neurosurgery 52: 624–631
4. el-Gohary EG, Tomita T, Gutierrez FA, McLone DG (1987) Angiographically occult vascular malformations in childhood. Neurosurgery 20: 759–766

5. Gandhi D (2004) Computed tomography and magnetic resonance angiography in cervicocranial vascular disease. J Neuroophthalmol 24: 306–314

6. Han DH, Kwon OK, Byun BJ, Choi BY, Choi CW, Choi JU, Choi SG, Doh JO, Han JW, Jung S, Kang SD, Kim DJ, Kim HI, Kim HD, Kim MC, Kim SC, Kim SC, Kim Y, Kwun BD, Lee BG, Lim YJ, Moon JG, Park HS, Shin MS, Song JH, Suk JS, Yim MB (2000) A co-operative study: clinical characteristics of 334 Korean patients with moyamoya disease treated at neurosurgical institutes (1976–1994). Acta Neurochir (Wien) 142: 1263–1274

7. Ji Y, Zheng N, Guo JQ et al. (2004) Clinical analysis of spontaneous intracerebral hemorrhage in 30 children. J Appl Clin Pediatr 19: 704–705

8. Jordan LC, Hillis AE (2007) Hemorrhagic stroke in children. Pediatr Neurol 36: 73–80

9. Kim DS, Kang SG, Yoo DS, Huh PW, Cho KS, Park CK (2007) Surgical results in pediatric moyamoya disease: angiographic revascularization and the clinical results. Clin Neurol Neurosurg 109: 125–131

10. Leijser LM, de Vries LS, Cowan FM (2006) Using cerebral ultrasound effectively in the newborn infant. Early Hum Dev 82: 827–835

11. Liu AC, Segaren N, Cox TS, Hayward RD, Chong WK, Ganesan V, Saunders DE (2006) Is there a role for magnetic resonance imaging in the evaluation of non-traumatic intraparenchymal haemorrhage in children? Pediatr Radiol 36: 940–946

12. Luo SQ, Zhang YQ (2002) Work hard to improve the level of pediatric neurosurgery in China. Chin J Neurosurg 18: 345–346

13. May Llanas ME, Alcover Bloch E, Cambra Lasaosa FJ, Campistol Plana J, Palomeque Rico A (1999) Non-traumatic cerebral hemorrhage in childhood: etiology, clinical manifestations and management [Spanish]. An Esp Pediatr 51: 257–261

14. Meyer-Heim AD, Boltshauser E (2003) Spontaneous intracranial haemorrhage in children: aetiology, presentation and outcome. Brain Dev 25: 416–421

15. Tian DF, Zou Y, Chen QX, Liu RZ, Wang GA (2005) Spontaneous intracranial hemorrhage in children: a report of 29 cases. Pediatr Emerg Med 12: 138–139

16. Wang W, Li BR, Ao LM (2002) Intracranial hemorrhage in different age groups of children : a report of 100 cases. J Clin Pediatr 20: 83–84

17. Wang Y, Ma WL (2000) Spontaneous intracranial hemorrhage in childhood: a report of 44 cases. Chin J Pediatr Surg 21: 28–29

18. Wu JS, Chen S, Mao Y, Zhou LF, Chen XC, Zuo CJ (2001) The role of 3D-CT/3D-CTA technique in the field of neurological surgery. Chin J Min Invas Neurosurg 6: 222–226

19. Zhou F, Qiu JB, Guo JQ (2005) The etiology and diagnosis of spontaneous intracerebral hemorrhage in children. Chin J Clin Neurosurg 10: 301–302

Acta Neurochir Suppl (2008) 105: 161–164
© Springer-Verlag 2008
Printed in Austria

Xenon-CT study of regional cerebral blood flow around hematoma in patients with basal ganglia hemorrhage

H. Y. Ding, X. Han, C. Z. Lv, Q. Dong

Department of Neurology, Huashan Hospital, Fudan University, Shanghai, China

Summary

Background. Xenon-CT is a quantitive technique for estimating cerebral blood flow. To investigate whether penumbra exists around hematoma, regional cerebral blood flow (rCBF) was measured by Xenon-CT in patients with intracerebral hemorrhage (ICH).

Methods. Xenon-CT was performed on 15 patients with basal ganglia hemorrhage and hematoma volume <50 mL. rCBF was measured within 36 h of onset and an average of 13 days later by 27-pixel rings in perihematomal area and its enantiomorph in contralateral hemisphere. Penumbra was defined as rCBF $8-20 \, \text{mL} \cdot 100 \, \text{g}^{-1} \cdot \text{min}^{-1}$.

Results. Average ICH volume was 13 ± 7 mL (6.4–23.7 mL). First rCBF examination was conducted at 21.7 ± 9.4 h (5–37 h), second rCBF examination was conducted at 13.4 ± 1.8 days (11–18 days) after onset. Within 36 h of onset, mean perihematomal rCBF was $28.4 \pm 7.8 \, \text{mL} \cdot 100 \, \text{g}^{-1} \cdot \text{min}^{-1}$; contralateral region was $34.2 \pm 12.2 \, \text{mL} \cdot 100 \, \text{g}^{-1} \cdot \text{min}^{-1}$ ($p = 0.11$). Average 13 days after onset, mean rCBF close to hematoma was $19.4 \pm 8.1 \, \text{mL} \cdot 100 \, \text{g}^{-1} \cdot \text{min}^{-1}$; rCBF in contralateral region was $40.1 \pm 11.3 \, \text{mL} \cdot 100 \, \text{g}^{-1} \cdot \text{min}^{-1}$ ($p < 0.0001$). rCBF in distal perihematomal region was $27.8 \pm 9.5 \, \text{mL} \cdot 100 \, \text{g}^{-1} \cdot \text{min}^{-1}$; the difference was significant compared to contralateral region ($p = 0.0003$). One patient's rCBF in area of edema around hematoma was less than $20 \, \text{mL} \cdot 100 \, \text{g}^{-1} \cdot \text{min}^{-1}$ at first examination. At second examination, 6 patients had same occurrence in region adjacent to hematoma and 2 patients experienced it in distal perihematomal region.

Conclusions. Reduced perihematomal rCBF was shown after ICH; this phenomenon lasted at least 14 days. A number of ICH patients experienced penumbra around hematoma.

Keywords: Intracerebral hemorrhage; regional cerebral blood flow; penumbra; Xenon-CT.

Introduction

The incidence of intracerebral hemorrhage (ICH) among the Asian population is 55 per 100,000 – twice that of the Caucasian race. Prospective observational studies in

---

Correspondence: Qiang Dong, Department of Neurology, Fudan University, Huashan Hospital, 14F ward, Wulumuqi Middle Road No. 12, Shanghai, China. e-mail: qiang_dong@hotmail.com

both animals and human beings [3, 4] have dispelled the concept of major ischemia in the edematous tissue surrounding the hemorrhage. Nevertheless, some controversy persists based on human magnetic resonance imaging (MRI) apparent diffusion coefficient (ADC) studies of the perihemorrhagic region [2], which indicate a rim of tissue at risk for secondary ischemia in large hematomas with elevated intracranial pressure (ICP). Xenon-enhanced computed tomography (XeCT) cerebral blood flow (CBF) study is an emerging real-time, high-resolution technique for quantifying CBF. We report our CBF measurement results on 20 spontaneous ICH patients with small to moderately sized hematomas who underwent XeCT during a 20-month study period.

Materials and methods

Patients

This prospective study began in June 2002 and lasted 20 months. Twenty patients with spontaneous single basal ganglia hemorrhage underwent XeCT examination. Inclusion criteria for our study was as follows: 1) age >18 years; 2) diagnosis of intraparenchymal hemorrhage confirmed by CT images; 3) patient was conscious or had slightly lethargy for a good technical quality XeCT CBF study; 4) first XeCT scans were able to be performed within 48 h of ictus; 5) hemorrhage volume was ≤50 mL. Exclusion criteria included: 1) head trauma; 2) radiographic evidence of subarachnoid hemorrhage or intraventricular hemorrhage; 3) an underlying mass lesion or vascular malformation; 4) infratentorial ICH. Clinical data included demographic information, ICH onset time, time to XeCT CBF study. Radiological data included hematoma volume. Five subjects were excluded from this study because of poor technical quality XeCT studies related to motion artifact.

XeCT CBF study

In order to investigate changes in regional CBF (rCBF) around the hematoma during acute and subacute phases, each patient underwent 2 XeCT CBF examinations: the first within 48 h of ictus, the second about

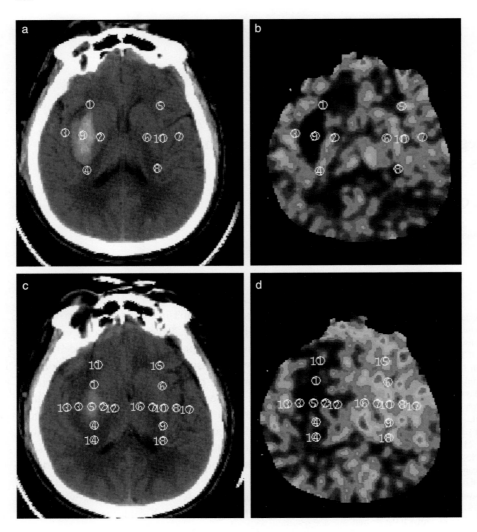

Fig. 1. Panel (a) First CT image of head: ①②③④ edema region; ⑤⑥⑦⑧ their mirror region at contralateral hemisphere; ⑨ hematoma; ⑩ hematoma's mirror region. Panel (b) Corresponding CBF map. Panel (c) Second CT image of head: ①②③④ edema region adjacent to hematoma; 11,12,13,14 edema region adjacent to normal tissue. Panel (d) Corresponding CBF map

13 days later. We used a computer-generated template that is part of the XeCT computer software (Diversified Diagnostic Products Inc., Houston, TX). Four contiguous CT-defined levels of 1-cm slice thickness were obtained along the orbitomeatal line. Voxels ($1 \times 1 \times 10$ mm) corresponded to CBF in cubic centimeters per 100 g per minute and were color-coded according to an ordinal scale of CBF values. A color-coded, quantitative CBF map was produced and displayed with individual CT images. XeCT computer software calculated the mean CBF within regions of interest. Our analysis included hematoma and perihematomal edema. In the first CBF examination, we found that the width of perihematomal edema in most patients was equivalent to 27 pixels; that is, mean diameter of edema was about 6 mm, so we decided to use a 27-pixel ring to measure CBF. One 27-pixel ring was placed at the center of hematoma in each slice, and the average CBF for the 4 rings was defined as the CBF of hematoma.

In the first examination, the 4 27-pixel rings were placed in region of edema on respective slices at up, down, right, and left positions. The mean CBF was the CBF of edema in these slices. However, the width of edema was increased by time of the second examination, so we divided the region of edema into 2 parts: "Region 1" was adjacent to hematoma; "Region 2" was distal of edema and was adjacent to normal tissue. Again, we used 27-pixel rings to measure CBF. Perihematomal edema CBF was defined as [(CBF of Region 1 + CBF of Region 2)/2] (Fig. 1).

Statistical analysis

Data management and analysis were performed using Statistical Package for the Social Science (SPSS) version 10.0 (SPSS, Inc., Chicago, IL). Hematoma volumes and CBF values were summarized as average and standard deviation. Changes in CBF between the 2 examinations were analyzed with Student *t*-test.

Results

A total of 15 patients performed a total of twenty one XeCT examinations; 9 of these patients were male. Average age was 55.8 ± 9.2 years (40–75 years). We obtained CBF results for 10 patients in the acute phase (within 48 h of the ictus), and 11 patients in the subacute phase (average 13 days after onset). Among these cases, 6 patient had results in both CBF studies. We defined penumbra range as CBF between 8 and $20 \, \text{mL} \cdot 100 \, \text{g}^{-1} \cdot \text{min}^{-1}$.

The results for 10 patients who underwent acute phase studies are presented in Table 1. Mean hematoma vol-

Table 1. *Cerebral blood flow (mL · 100 g^{-1} · min^{-1}) data for 10 patients recorded within 48 h (acute phase) of ictus*

Patient no.	Age (years)	Hematoma volume (mL)	Study time (h)	Hematoma CBF	Mirror of hematoma CBF	Edema CBF	Mirror of edema CBF
1	63	16.72	19	11.15	33.5	26.68	39.62
2	75	16.45	22	6.38	28.75	20.62	18.39
3	57	24.00	26	6.55	23.18	37.63	17.74
4	57	5.08	34	20.43	43.23	29.46	38.88
5	54	11.85	37	10.93	47.20	27.44	35.31
6	40	13.30	13	6.20	31.45	31.07	33.93
7	54	6.04	19	6.73	47.07	29.21	42.37
8	54	9.44	18	26.3	53.68	42.29	58.59
9	49	8.97	24	11.10	37.30	24.64	32.61
10	65	42.48	5	2.30	24.43	15.16	24.58
Mean	56.80	15.43	21.70	10.81	36.98	28.42	34.20
SD	9.45	11.05	9.38	7.31	10.45	7.75	12.16

CBF Cerebral blood flow; *SD* standard deviation.

Table 2. *Cerebral blood flow (mL · 100 g^{-1} · min^{-1}) data for 11 patients recorded during subacute phase*

Patient no.	Age (years)	Hematoma volume (mL)	Study time (days)	Hematoma CBF	Edema Region 1 CBF	Edema Region 2 CBF	Mirror of edema CBF
1	63	16.72	13	5.88	8.30	14.30	29.33
2	75	16.45	12	4.43	8.58	17.28	28.18
3	41	23.25	14	1.20	13.73	24.58	37.39
4	57	5.08	13	10.80	25.35	38.80	52.34
5	53	18.64	18	9.50	16.76	25.63	41.55
6	40	13.30	14	13.70	29.13	23.72	47.88
7	52	10.83	11	5.93	23.13	23.13	43.62
8	56	12.19	14	6.88	18.79	33.11	28.08
9	54	9.44	13	14.45	33.91	47.64	63.86
10	67	22.81	12	10.68	20.91	31.65	34.35
11	49	8.97	13	16.50	14.66	25.42	34.23
Mean	55.2	14.33	13.36	9.09	19.39	27.75	40.07
SD	10.4	5.80	1.80	4.69	8.12	9.54	11.26

CBF Cerebral blood flow; *SD* standard deviation.

ume was 15.4 mL (5.1–42.5 mL). Mean studied time was 21.7 h (5–37 h) after onset. CBF of hematoma was 10.8 mL · 100 g^{-1} · min^{-1} (2.3–26.3 mL · 100 g^{-1} · min^{-1}), CBF of its mirror region at contralateral hemisphere was 37 mL · 100 g^{-1} · min^{-1} (23.2–53.7 mL · 100 g^{-1} · min^{-1}; $p < 0.0001$). Mean perihematomal edema CBF was 28.4 mL · 100 g^{-1} · min^{-1}, was not within penumbra range, and was 9% lower than its mirror region CBF of 34.2 mL · 100 g^{-1} · min^{-1} (17.7–58.6 mL · 100 g^{-1} · min^{-1}; $p = 0.11$). Only 1 patient's edema CBF fell below penumbra range. This patient also had the largest hematoma volume, which exceeded 40 mL. All other hematoma volumes fell below 30 mL, and had perihematomal region CBF greater than 20 mL · 100 g^{-1} · min^{-1}.

Results for 11 patients who underwent subacute phase studies are presented in Table 2. Studies were performed between 11 and 18 days after onset and the mean CBF of edema adjacent to hematoma (Region 1) was 19.4 mL · 100 g^{-1} · min^{-1} (8.3–33.9 mL · 100 g^{-1} · min^{-1}), just within penumbra range; CBF of its mirror region was 40.1 mL · 100 g^{-1} · min^{-1} ($p < 0.0001$). However, CBF of edema adjacent to normal tissue (Region 2) was 27.8 mL · 100 g^{-1} · min^{-1} (14.3–47.6 mL · 100 g^{-1} · min^{-1}), higher than penumbra range, and differed from its mirror region ($p = 0.0003$). Mean of perihematomal region CBF [(Region 1 CBF + Region 2 CBF)/2] was about 41% of mirror region in contralateral hemisphere. When comparing acute and subacute studies, CBF of perihematomal region decreased, and the percentage of difference between perihematomal region and its mirror region [(mirror CBF – edema CBF)/mirror CBF × 100%] was also apparently reduced ($p = 0.033$). On the other hand, CBF of perihematomal mirror region was unchanged ($p = 0.265$), and so avoided the influence of different examination times to CBF absolute value.

Discussion

Whether or not significant perihematomal ischemia exists in patients with spontaneous ICH continues to be debated. Ours is the first study to describe changes in perihematomal CBF from up to 48 h of onset to 2 weeks later. As found in the results of other studies, neither ischemia nor penumbra was found in the acute phase; however, with time, ischemic penumbra emerge around the hematoma.

According to Kaufmann's study [1], XeCT CBF defines penumbra as $8\text{--}20\,\text{mL} \cdot 100\,\text{g}^{-1} \cdot \text{min}^{-1}$ tissue surrounding hematoma. Our study found perihematomal CBF within 48 h of onset decreased slightly, no more than 9% of mirror region. At subacute phase about 2 weeks later, CBF surrounding hematoma reduced 41% compared with mirror region. Fifty-five percent (6/11) of patients had penumbra-level perihematomal CBF in region adjacent to hematoma; 2 patients (18%) even had it in distal region adjacent to normal tissue.

Most studies selected patients within 6 h of onset, and came to the conclusion that ischemia did not exist in that time window; however, signs of ischemia still could not be ignored in some special patients, especially in cases of greater hematoma volume. For example, in the prospective trial reported by Schellinger *et al.* [5], MRI within 6 h of onset in 32 spontaneous ICH patients with small to moderately sized hematomas found no significant mean transit time or ADC changes within a 1-cm radius of the clot. However, subgroup analysis showed there were 4 patients in which mean transit time was delayed more than 2 sec compared to mirror region in contralateral hemisphere, and there were 7 patients with relatively prolonged ADC. These phenomena suggested ischemia or penumbra exists in perihematomal region. Eleven patients with acute spontaneous ICH underwent 2 technetium-99 hexamethylporpyenenamine oxime single-photon emission CT (Tc-^{99}HMPAO SPECT) scans within 2 days of ictus and subsequently at 4–7 days [6]. The authors found diminished perihematomal perfusion, which improved after surgical clot evacuation. Therefore, according to our study results and that of

other authors, we surmise that perihematomal CBF decreases with time.

Data pertaining to perihematomal CBF in the subacute phase has been scarce. Animal studies have shown that CBF around hematoma is restored during acute phase [7], but this phenomenon is transient, and was found to decline once again after 48 h from onset. Yonezawa *et al.* [8] observed a rat model of ICH for 30 days, and found not only injured hemisphere, but also healthy hemisphere CBF declined within 4 h of onset, but at 24 h after onset, frontal lobe and basal ganglia region of injured hemisphere was restored, even to normal levels. However, after 24 h, CBF then decreased once again for up to 30 days after onset. This study supports our results.

References

1. Kaufmann AM, Firlik AD, Fukui MB, Wechsler LR, Jungries CA, Yonas H (1999) Ischemic core and penumbra in human stroke. Stroke 30: 93–99
2. Kidwell CS, Saver JL, Mattiello J, Warach S, Liebeskind DS, Starkman S, Vespa PM, Villablanca JP, Martin NA, Frazee J, Alger JR (2001) Diffusion-perfusion MR evaluation of perihematomal injury in hyperacute intracerebral hemorrhage. Neurology 57: 1611–1617
3. Powers WJ, Zazulia AR, Videen TO, Adams RE, Yundt KD, Aiyagari V, Grubb RL Jr, Diringer MN (2001) Autoregulation of cerebral blood flow surrounding acute (6 to 22 h) intracerebral hemorrhage. Neurology 57: 18–24
4. Qureshi AI, Wilson DA, Hanley DF, Traystman RJ (1999) Pharmacologic reduction of mean arterial pressure does not adversely affect regional cerebral blood flow and intracranial pressure in experimental intracerebral hemorrhage. Crit Care Med 27: 965–971
5. Schellinger PD, Fiebach JB, Hoffmann K, Becker K, Orakcioglu B, Kollmar R, Jüttler E, Schramm P, Schwab S, Sartor K, Hacke W (2003) Stroke MRI in intracerebral hemorrhage: is there a perihemorrhagic penumbra? Stroke 34: 1674–1680
6. Siddique MS, Fernandes HM, Wooldridge TD, Fenwick JD, Slomka P, Mendelow AD (2002) Reversible ischemia around intracerebral hemorrhage: a single-photon emission computerized tomography study. J Neurosurg 96: 736–741
7. Yang GY, Betz AL, Chenevert TL, Brunberg JA, Hoff JT (1994) Experimental intracerebral hemorrhage: relationship between brain edema, blood flow, and blood-brain barrier permeability in rats. J Neurosurg 81: 93–102
8. Yonezawa T, Hashimoto H, Sakaki T (1999) Serial change of cerebral blood flow after collagenase induced intracerebral hemorrhage in rats [Japanese]. No Shinkei Geka 27: 419–425

Acta Neurochir Suppl (2008) 105: 165–170
© Springer-Verlag 2008
Printed in Austria

Preliminary application of pyramidal tractography in evaluating prognosis of patients with hypertensive intracerebral hemorrhage

T. M. Qiu, Y. Zhang, J. S. Wu

Department of Neurosurgery, Huashan Hospital, Fudan University, and Shanghai Neurosurgical Center, Shanghai, China

Summary

Objective. To discover the practical value of pyramidal tractography in evaluating the prognosis of hypertensive intracerebral hemorrhage (ICH) patients.

Methods. Eight acute-stage patients with hypertensive ICH were studied. We used magnetic resonance diffusion tensor imaging (DTI), applied white matter fiber tracking to deal with the raw DTI data, and thereafter obtained tractography data. The form, conformation, and spatial position of pyramidal tracts were observed, and the extent of injury assessed by measurement of continuity, integrity, and spatial displacement. Meanwhile, a 6-month follow-up survey was conducted to obtain patient neurological function index in order to analyze potential correlations with the tractography data.

Results. Tractography accurately identified the number of white matter fiber tracts, which showed a positive correlation with neurological function outcomes.

Conclusions. Pyramidal tractography is able to clearly identify form, conformation, and spatial displacement range of pyramidal tracts, and therefore can effectively predict long-term neurological function outcomes for hypertensive ICH patients.

Keywords: Pyramidal tract; hypertensive intracerebral hemorrhage; prognosis.

Introduction

White matter fiber tracking, or tractography, is an important imaging technology developed from magnetic resonance diffusion tensor imaging (DTI). It is a non-invasive imaging method used to show the white matter fiber tracts in living brain [4]. At the end of 20th century, researchers such as Mori *et al.* [11] first released a DTI study on white matter fiber tracts of animal and human brains.

The pyramidal tract (PT) is one of the most important white matter fiber tracts in human brain. Composed of corticospinal and corticonuclear tracts, it is the major projection tract dominating limb movements. Diseases such as intracranial tumors, inflammation, congenital white matter pathologies, and vascular disorders can all lead to PT disorganization or limb function impairment. In previous DTI studies related to PT in brain tumors, white matter pathology, and ischemic stroke, results have shown that such technology has practical value for guiding therapy, pathology analysis, and determining prognosis [13, 16, 17].

We applied white matter fiber tracking technology to hypertensive intracerebral hemorrhage (ICH) patients to obtain their pyramidal tractography. Our goal was to analyze the correlation between the imaging data and the patient outcome in terms of limb function, and to discover the technology's practical value for assessing prognosis for neurological function in hypertensive ICH patients.

Patients and methods

Patients

From June to September 2006, our emergency room treated 8 ICH patients; 4 males and 4 females ranging in age from 30 to 59 years (average age, 47 ± 11 years) (Table 1). Upon admission to the hospital, all showed symptoms of cranial hypertension, including sudden headache and vomiting, together with hemiplegia of differing levels. Emergency head computed tomography (CT) images revealed a hematoma at the internal capsule of the basal ganglia in each case. DTI scans were performed within the first 5 days after ICH. Each patient and their family were informed of the purpose of the scan and possible DTI risks, and consent was received to proceed. We used Chin-Sang Chung's ICH classification methods for cerebral hemorrhage at the internal capsule of basal ganglia [1].

DTI scan and image post-processing

We used a GE 3T Signa Horizon magnetic resonance scanner (GE Healthcare, Fairfield, CT) with standard head coil. DTI parameters were

Correspondence: Yi Zhang and Tian-Ming Qiu, Department of Neurosurgery, Huashan Hospital, Fudan University, Shanghai 200040, China. e-mails: zhangtang1218@vip.sina.com, tianming2100@sohu.com

Table 1. *Patient demographics and tractography data*

Pt. no.	Gender	Age (years)	Classification of intracerebral hemorrhage	Normal side		Affected side		KPS score after 6 months
				Seed points	EPT	Seed points	EPT	
1	Male	59	left posterior lateral	180	142	180	9	70
2	Female	56	left lateral	180	156	180	107	90
3	Female	44	left posterior lateral and medial	180	178	180	60	70
4	Male	40	left lateral	180	133	180	0	30
5	Female	50	left posterior lateral	180	175	180	0	30
6	Female	30	right posterior lateral	180	173	180	0	50
7	Male	58	left posterior lateral	180	161	180	7	50
8	Male	43	left lateral	180	173	180	154	90

EPT Effective pyramidal tracts; *KPS* Karnofsky Performance Scale.

as follows: pulse sequence of single shot spin-echo EPI (SE EPI); repeat time/echo time (TR/TE) = 8000/84 msec; seam height = 5 mm; no interval; matrix = 128 × 128 pixels; field of vision (FOV) = 240 mm × 240 mm; number of excitation (NEX) = 1; 25 diffusion gradient directions on each layer, 29 layers. The scan scope was, in general, from pontomedullary sulcus to calvaria, no contrast media, scan time 5.1 min. On the platform of workstation SUN ADW 4.0_05 (SUN Microsystems Inc., Santa Clara, CA), using diffusion tensor module of FuncTool 2.6.6i software (GE Healthcare) to post-process the generated DTI images.

Pyramidal tractography

Original DTI images in DICOM 3.0 format were imported into a personal computer post-process with the application software Volume-One version 1.72 (VOLUME-ONE Developers Group, http://volume-one.org/main.htm) and dTV.II (Image Process and Analysis Laboratory, The University of Tokyo, Japan) to obtain separate maps of fractional anisotropy (FA) and directionally encoded color (DEC). In DEC map, red represents fiber tracts of left-right course (*x*-axis), green represents front-back course (*y*-axis), and blue represents upper-lower course (*z*-axis).

Our study focuses mainly on the PT injury following hypertensive ICH. Therefore, we used tractography on PTs, as follows. A FA horizontal position map was taken through the internal capsule for reference, and seed points put at the bilateral posterior limbs of the internal capsule (the blue parts on DEC map), and the radius set at 3.5 mm, so that all selected seed points at imaging were guaranteed constant (seed points to be 180 after calculation). Meanwhile, the central lobule cortex area was set as the target area. A computer was used to separately auto-trace, define those PTs reaching central cortex area as effective pyramidal tracts (EPT), and to show the results on map. The end-trace condition of this study was FA <0.18, or until 160 steps. This method resulted in a 3-dimensional PT tractography.

Follow-up survey

All patients received expected standard of care, and follow-up surveys were performed 6 months after initial treatment. Karnofsky Performance Scale (KPS) was used to evaluate long-term quality of life for each patient.

Statistics and analysis

We used dTV.II software to separately calculate bilateral EPT drawn lines for each patient. STATA 8.0 statistics software package (StataCorp LP, College Station, TX) was used for self-paired *t*-test of chased EPT drawn lines on the normal and affected sides of patient brain. We used effective fiber tract drawn lines for the affected sides and patient KPS data to carry out Spearman's rank correlation analysis (α = 0.05).

Results

For all 8 patients, we obtained a DTI scan, post-processed images on a personal computer, and obtained satisfactory FA (e.g. Figs. 1B and 2B), DEC maps (e.g. Figs. 1C and 2C), and 3-dimensional pyramidal tractography (e.g. Figs. 1D–G and 2D–G). On the DEC map axial image, the posterior limb structure of internal capsule and the hematoma-induced injury were obvious. The anterior limb of internal capsule on the normal side was marked in green and contained mainly front-back frontopontine tract and anterior thalamic radiations. The posterior limb of the internal capsule was marked in blue and included mainly upper-lower corticospinal tract and corticonuclear tract. On the affected side, the structure of the posterior limb of the internal capsule was unclear, obviously affected by hematoma injury (Figs. 1B–C and 2B–C). The PT structure changes for all directions were clearer when shown on 3-dimensional pyramidal tractography. Also, PT hematoma injury was obvious on the affected side (Figs. 1D–E and 2D–E), and EPT much sparser than on the normal side. Therefore, PT on normal and affected side are in sharp contrast (Figs. 1F–G and 2F–G).

After to computer calculation of effective fiber tract drawn lines on each patient's normal and affected side, self-paired *t*-test was conducted. We found that EPT drawn lines traced from the posterior limb of the internal capsule on the normal side to the central motion layer were far more evident than the ones traced on the posterior limb of internal capsule on the affected side. These results were statistically significant ($t = 5.9401$; $p = 0.0006 < 0.005$).

All patients received a follow-up survey 6 months after initial treatment to evaluate their long-term quality of life. Because EPT and KPS data were spread in a non-normal distribution, Spearman's rank correlation analysis was used to analyze the 2 data groups. The data

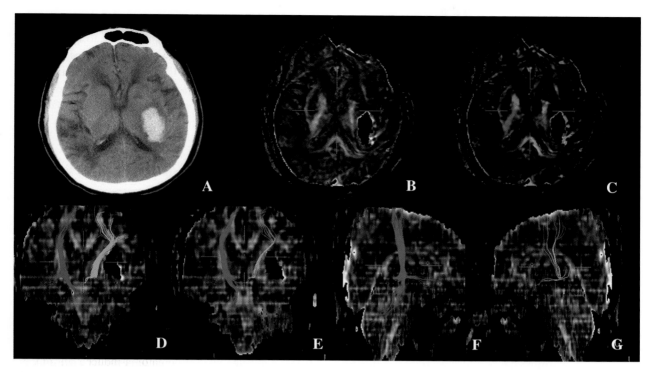

Fig. 1. Case 1: 59-year-old male with a 3-h history of conscious disturbance, Glasgow Coma Scale score of 11, muscle strength grade 0. Panels B and C show FA image and DEC image; panels D through G show PTs after tractography. The calculation resulted in few effective fiber tracts. KPS score 6 months after ICH was 70

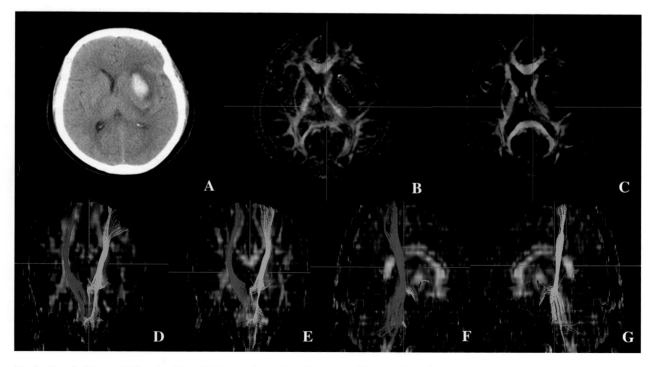

Fig. 2. Case 2: 56-year-old female with a 4-h history of conscious disturbance, Glasgow Coma Scale score of 10, muscle strength grade 0. Panels B and C show FA image and DEC image; panels D through G show PTs after tractography. PT was only pressed by hematoma. KPS score 6 months after ICH was 90

showed positive correlation (rank-correlation coefficient: $r_s = 0.95$; $p = 0.0003$) (Table 1).

Discussion

Basic principles of pyramidal tractography

Diffusion refers to the random movement of water molecules. It has two basic forms; isotropic and anisotropic. Isotropy means the free diffusion of water molecules in a non-obstacle space, while anisotropy refers to the restricted diffusion of water molecules in a with-obstacle space. In human brain PT, water molecule diffusion has the barrier of axolemma and myelin sheath and, therefore, diffusion is quicker in the direction of PT fibers than in the direction of vertical fibers [6]. The anisotropic characteristic of water molecule diffusion in brain is basic to PT DTI. DTI can fully describe water molecule movements in all directions and the relevance between different directions. Three mutually perpendicular feature vectors determine the partial fiber frame of the diffusion tensor. Every fiber frame, like a 3-dimensional ellipsoidal, is named a voxel. The size of 3 feature vectors is called diffusion coefficient (high diffusion coefficient $\lambda 1$, middle $\lambda 2$, and low $\lambda 3$). Pierpaoli *et al.*'s [15] diffusion character classification of intracerebral white matter fiber has shown that white matter fiber tracts generally follow $\lambda 1 > \lambda 2 > \lambda 3$. The vector corresponding to high diffusion coefficient is called high eigenvector. Its direction is regarded the same as with the partial PT fiber direction where such voxels locate. FA can be calculated by diffusion coefficient [10]. Of all tissues, FA scope lies between 0 and 1; 0 for highest isotropic diffusion and 1 for highest anisotropic diffusion.

White matter fiber tracking, or tractography, is an important new imaging technology developed from DTI. Based on color coding of DTI and neuroanatomy descriptions, fiber tractography is an imaging method where the initial area of interest is marked with seeds, and then from the seeded area, the effective diffusion tensor directions of voxels are continuously chased. For example, the procedure for pyramidal tractography would be as follows: on a FA map of DTI, set the posterior limb of internal capsule region as seed area, calculate each voxel diffusion tensor from the selected seed area, and chase along the diffusion tensor direction to the 2 adjoining up and down voxels. Repeat the above process of a 2-way chase. A continuous track is therefore established until all tracks reach the last voxel with threshold value for the diffusion tensor. The generated series of tracks in sheaf arrangement are pyramidal tractography. Pyramidal tractography is able to vividly show the 3-dimensional configuration, spatial structure, and extension trend of PTs. If further setting a target on motion layer according to the somatosensory homunculus of Penfield and Rasmussen, projection fibers of each motion unit can be accurately displayed [12].

Clinical application of pyramidal tractography in hypertensive ICH

Currently, the technology of white matter fiber tractography has already been applied to diseases such as brain tumors, acute ischemic cerebral apoplexy, dysplasia of corpus callosum, etc. [10]. However, there have been no reports of its application in hypertensive ICH. After hypertensive ICH, the destruction, extrusion, and displacement due to the hematoma lead to changes in integrity or spatial structure of fiber tracts in axolemma or myelin sheath. It also damages the diffusion barrier of water molecules, making their descent its diffusion anisotropy, and finally causing a fall in the DTI FA value. Therefore, we set the lower limit of FA as the end-chase point for pyramidal tractography. On FA and DEC maps, the posterior limb structure of the internal capsule become less clear and are obviously affected by the hematoma. Effective fiber tracts, in this study, are not necessarily those FA-fit tracts during tracing. Effective fiber tracts, in this study, are not necessarily those FA-fit tracts during tracing. They are limited to projection fiber tracts chased from posterior limb of internal capsule to central brain motion layer, excluding those starting from posterior limb of the internal capsule but broken or displaced before reaching parietal cortex area. Fig. 1D and E shows, for one patient, tracts from the seed area of internal capsule posterior limb, the PT configuration, structure and projection fiber tract number from the set area and those from there finally reaching the central motion layer. These photographs clearly show that, although many PTs start from posterior limb of internal capsule, they are either broken or extruded by the hematoma before reaching the central motion layer. Chased by pyramidal tractography, the PTs finally reaching the central motion layer are effective projection fiber tracts relevant to the patient's clinical prognosis.

Two typical cases are presented in this report. Images of case 1 (Fig. 1) indicate PTs, with involvement of hematoma, had obvious fragmentation and displacement. Calculations showed few effective fiber tracts, equating to poor prognosis. In case 2 (Fig. 2), images show that PTs were only pressed by hematoma and slightly displaced from the original dissection position. Calculations showed more effective fiber tracts, equating to good prognosis. We first carried out self-paired *t*-test on effective fiber tract drawn lines on normal and affected sides of each patient, finding that the drawn lines on normal side were far more than the number on the affected side, thus proving our hypothesis. Furthermore, our study adopted Spearman's rank correlation to analyze effective fiber tract drawn lines, and followed up with the patient KPS score 6 months later. This method showed a clear relationship between EPT on the affected side and patient prognosis. Such results suggest that by the effective fiber tract drawn lines on the affected side, we could deduce an ICH patient's long-term motor function.

Potential application of pyramidal tractography in hypertensive ICH

Current pyramidal tractography technology is not yet mature, and lacks a unified and standardized method for setting of tractography parameters. Regarding PT DTI of white matter fiber tracts, different researchers choose various tracer methods and termination conditions [2, 8, 18]. Meanwhile, their set FA termination figures vary from 0.12 to 0.24, and methods of choosing target areas differ. Various tractography parameters and tracer methods lead to different pyramidal tractographies. As a result, neurological prognosis based on imaging can have different conclusions. Therefore, a large sample size for prospective contrast study is required to evaluate and standardize various parameters in pyramidal tractography. In our study, the FA tracer termination figure is set at the default of dTV application software, and target area was determined using basic principles of neuroanatomy of brain motor pathways.

In recent years, more and more researchers have adopted pyramidal tractography to study PT structure in normal or diseased human brain [7, 8, 17]. Hypertensive ICH patients usually suffer muscle injury at different levels, which is related to hematoma-involved PTs. Our study has a correlation analysis between EPT drawn lines and patient prognosis. The results indicate that EPT drawn lines can help predict the patient's future motor function and quality of life. Due to the limited sample size, no regression analysis was carried out. Therefore, exact criteria to deduce long-term quality of life using EPT drawn lines is not yet available. We anticipate that through prospective contrast study of a larger sample

size, we could predict the outcome of hypertensive ICH patients via imaging foundations.

Many studies have proven pyramidal tractography useful to improve effects of PT-involved tumor surgery [3, 5, 9, 14, 19]. The imaging findings in our study show that hematoma affects PT involvement differently in each patient. Some PTs were fragmented by hematoma, some became sparse by infiltration inside hematoma, and some became displaced by hematoma extrusion. Two cases from this study fully demonstrate this. Case 1 showed PT fragmentation by hematoma, while in case 2, hematoma caused only minor PT extrusion. Although both patients appeared to be hemiplegic at first, after a period of recovery, the prognosis in case 2 became much better than in case 1. Therefore, further study is necessary to determine whether pyramidal tractography can distinguish PT damage in different hematoma patients, help identify indication for early operation, and provide support for the preoperative plan, ultimately avoiding iatrogenic PT injury from improper operative approaches.

Acknowledgments

Funding of this project was provided by Key Project of Shanghai Science and Technology Commission (No. 054119615).

References

1. Chung CS, Caplan LR, Yamamoto Y, Chang HM, Lee SJ, Song HJ, Lee HS, Shin HK, Yoo KM (2000) Striatocapsular haemorrhage. Brain 123: 1850–1862
2. Clark CA, Barrick TR, Murphy MM, Bell BA (2003) White matter fiber tracking in patients with space-occupying lesions of the brain: a new technique for neurosurgical planning? Neuroimage 20: 1601–1608
3. Coenen VA, Krings T, Axer H, Weidemann J, Kränzlein H, Hans FJ, Thron A, Gilsbach JM, Rohde V (2003) Intraoperative three-dimensional visualization of the pyramidal tract in a neuronavigation system (PTV) reliably predicts true position of principal motor pathways. Surg Neurol 60: 381–390
4. Conturo TE, Lori NF, Cull TS, Akbudak E, Snyder AZ, Shimony JS, McKinstry RC, Burton H, Raichle ME (1999) Tracking neuronal fiber pathways in the living human brain. Proc Natl Acad Sci USA 96: 10422–10427
5. Krings T, Reinges MH, Thiex R, Gilsbach JM, Thron A (2001) Functional and diffusion-weighted magnetic resonance images of space-occupying lesions affecting the motor system: imaging the motor cortex and pyramidal tracts. J Neurosurg 95: 816–824
6. Le Bihan D, Mangin JF, Poupon C, Clark CA, Pappata S, Molko N, Chabriat H (2001) Diffusion tensor imaging: concepts and applications. J Magn Reson Imaging 13: 534–546
7. Lee JS, Han MK, Kim SH, Kwon OK, Kim JH (2005) Fiber tracking by diffusion tensor imaging in corticospinal tract stroke: topographical correlation with clinical symptoms. Neuroimage 26: 771–776
8. Lehéricy S, Ducros M, Van de Moortele PF, Francois C, Thivard L, Poupon C, Swindale N, Ugurbil K, Kim DS (2004) Diffusion tensor

fiber tracking shows distinct corticostriatal circuits in humans. Ann Neurol 55: 522–529

9. Li ZX, Dai JP, Jiang T, Li SW, Sun YL, Liang XL, Gao PY (2005) Diffusion tensor tractography in patients with brain gliomas involving pyramidal tracts: clinical application and outcome. Chin J Med Imaging Technol 21: 1802–1805

10. Masutani Y, Aoki S, Abe O, Hayashi N, Otomo K (2003) MR diffusion tensor imaging: recent advance and new techniques for diffusion tensor visualization. Eur J Radiol 46: 53–66

11. Mori S, Crain BJ, Chacko VP, van Zijl PC (1999) Three-dimensional tracking of axonal projections in the brain by magnetic resonance imaging. Ann Neurol 45: 265–269

12. Nakamura A, Yamada T, Goto A, Kato T, Ito K, Abe Y, Kachi T, Kakigi R (1998) Somatosensory homunculus as drawn by MEG. Neuroimage 7: 377–386

13. Niizuma K, Fujimura M, Kumabe T, Higano S, Tominaga T (2006) Surgical treatment of paraventricular cavernous angioma: fibre tracking for visualizing the corticospinal tract and determining surgical approach. J Clin Neurosci 13: 1028–1032

14. Nimsky C, Ganslandt O, Merhof D, Sorensen AG, Fahlbusch R (2006) Intraoperative visualization of the pyramidal tract by diffusion-tensor-imaging-based fiber tracking. Neuroimage 30: 1219–1229

15. Pierpaoli C, Jezzard P, Basser PJ, Barnett A, Di Chiro G (1996) Diffusion tensor MR imaging of the human brain. Radiology 201: 637–648

16. Reich DS, Smith SA, Jones CK, Zackowski KM, van Zijl PC, Calabresi PA, Mori S (2006) Quantitative characterization of the corticospinal tract at 3T. Am J Neuroradiol 27: 2168–2178

17. Werring DJ, Toosy AT, Clark CA, Parker GJ, Barker GJ, Miller DH, Thompson AJ (2000) Diffusion tensor imaging can detect and quantify corticospinal tract degeneration after stroke. J Neurol Neurosurg Psychiatry 69: 269–272

18. Witwer BP, Moftakhar R, Hasan KM, Deshmukh P, Haughton V, Field A, Arfanakis K, Noyes J, Moritz CH, Meyerand ME, Rowley HA, Alexander AL, Badie B (2002) Diffusion-tensor imaging of white matter tracts in patients with cerebral neoplasm. J Neurosurg 97: 568–575

19. Wu JS, Zhou LF, Hong XN, Mao Y, Du GH (2003) Role of diffusion tensor imaging in neuronavigation surgery of brain tumors involving pyramidal tracts [Chinese]. Chin J Surg 41: 662–666

Experimental intracranial hemorrhage (non-intracerebral hemorrhage)

Acta Neurochir Suppl (2008) 105: 173–178
© Springer-Verlag 2008
Printed in Austria

Mechanisms and markers for hemorrhagic transformation after stroke

A. Rosell, C. Foerch, Y. Murata, E. H. Lo

Neuroprotection Research Laboratory, Departments of Radiology and Neurology, Massachusetts General Hospital,
and Program in Neuroscience, Harvard Medical School, Boston, MA, USA

Summary

Intracerebral hemorrhagic transformation is a multifactorial phenomenon in which ischemic brain tissue converts into a hemorrhagic lesion with blood vessel leakage. Hemorrhagic transformation can significantly contribute to additional brain injury after stroke. Especially threatening are the thrombolytic-induced hemorrhages after reperfusion therapy with tissue plasminogen activator (tPA), the only treatment available for ischemic stroke. In this context, it is important to understand its underlying mechanisms and identify early markers of hemorrhagic transformation, so that we can both search for new treatments as well as predict clinical outcomes in patients. In this review, we discuss the emerging mechanisms for hemorrhagic transformation after stroke, and briefly survey potential molecular, genetic, and neuroimaging markers that might be used for early detection of this challenging clinical problem.

Keywords: Intracerebral hemorrhage; tissue plasminogen activator; hemorrhagic transformation; *blood–brain barrier.*

Introduction

Stroke is a primary cause of death and disability worldwide. Ischemic stroke can lead to large infarct areas with a complex pathophysiology that includes excitotoxicity, apoptosis, oxidative stress, and neurovascular matrix proteolysis. These overlapping pathways may be connected by a common neuroinflammatory response, which perturbs homeostasis within the so-called neurovascular unit [54]. Further breakdown of the blood–brain barrier (BBB) after vessel reperfusion can thus lead to hemorrhagic transformation (HT). In some patients, a large and symptomatic intracranial hemorrhage (ICH) can occur, significantly worsening neurological outcome and increasing mortality rate up to 40%.

Of special interest is thrombolytic-associated hemorrhage. Thrombolysis can be accomplished with tissue plasminogen activator (tPA), the only Food and Drug Administration (FDA)-approved drug for acute ischemic stroke. The rationale is straight-forward, i.e., to reestablish cerebral blood flow in the occluded artery [38]. Although it is an effective therapy, tPA can only be administered within the first 3 h of ischemic onset due to the increased risk of hemorrhagic conversion beyond this narrow time-window. Hence, only a small percentage of all ischemic stroke patients benefit from thrombolytic therapy.

In this scenario, it is imperative that we dissect the underlying mechanisms involved in this difficult phenomenon and further identify early markers of risk. An increased emphasis on neurovascular mechanisms and targets has emerged that may eventually reveal novel combination therapies. Different diagnostic approaches have also been explored as potential biomarkers, including blood molecular markers, genetic individual background, and neuroimaging techniques.

In this short review, we briefly discuss the triggering mechanisms of HT in the ischemic brain, and survey the potential biological and radiological tools that could guide clinicians to manage HT, and select the best candidates for thrombolytic therapies after stroke.

Mechanisms of HT

Fundamentally, HT in cerebral ischemia occurs after an increase in permeability within the BBB. Further rupture damages the entire neurovascular unit, which comprises the extracellular matrix, endothelial cells, astrocytes, neurons, and pericytes. Thus, neurovascular injury in this context can significantly extend parenchymal injury into irreversible infarction and pan-necrosis [30]. The underlying pathways of ischemia, HT, and neurovascular

Correspondence: Eng H. Lo, MGH East 149-2401, Charlestown, MA 02129, USA. e-mail: Lo@helix.mgh.harvard.edu compromise are highly complex and diverse. Here, we will focus on what we believe might be rate-limiting mechanisms triggered by proteolysis, oxidative stress, and leukocyte infiltration.

At the neurovascular interface, proteolysis of the matrix is a major contributor to intracranial hemorrhage. Degradation of essential components such as laminin, fibronectin, collagens, or proteoglycans, destabilizes structural support for the BBB, producing leakage and breakdown. Although many proteases are expressed in the brain under normal and ischemic conditions, both animal and human studies suggest that the matrix metalloproteinase (MMP) family and the tPA system play a central role. In the past decade, many groups have demonstrated that MMPs such as MMP-2, MMP-3, and MMP-9, are rapidly increased in the ischemic brain, and these responses are closely related to infarct extension, neurological outcome, or hemorrhagic conversion [40, 42, 44, 46]. In particular, a specific role has been proposed for MMP-9 as a triggering protease for HT. Animal models have demonstrated that MMP-9 and MMP-3 increase after thrombolysis [48, 51], and pharmacological or genetic inhibition of MMP-9 significantly decreases the risk of hemorrhagic complications after thrombolysis [1, 47]. Furthermore, microvascular basal lamina injury and loss of collagen type IV can be reversed with hypothermic treatments that reduce enzymatic activity of MMP-2 and MMP-9 in ischemia-reperfusion rat models [22]. These results are consistent with human studies showing that MMP-9 peaks in areas that undergo hemorrhagic conversion, correlating with enhanced erythrocyte extravasation, neutrophil infiltration, and severe collagen IV degradation in the basal lamina [43].

Within the plasminogen activator family, tPA, urokinase-type plasminogen activator (uPA), and plasminogen activator inhibitors (PAIs) have been studied. In the context of stroke therapy, tPA is a serine protease that catalyses the conversion of plasminogen to plasmin, which then is intended to lyse the clot in ischemic stroke. In the properly selected set of patients, thrombolysis with tPA rescues brain tissue. But in addition to its intended role in clot lysis, tPA might be potentially neurotoxic and may also trigger important protease actions on the neurovascular unit, some of which would be responsible for mediating HT in the ischemic brain [25]. Animal models attribute BBB injury to protease effects of pleiotropic actions of tPA, including activation of apoptosis [32], cleavage of the N-methyl-D-aspartate (NMDA) NR1 subunit [37], or activation of other extracellular proteases such as MMP-9 [53].

Deep cerebral tissue oxygenation changes occur after cerebral ischemia and reperfusion, providing oxygen as a substrate for numerous enzymatic oxidation reactions. Oxygen radicals, the products of these biochemical and physiological reactions, can accumulate and damage cellular lipids, proteins, and nucleic acids, and initiate cell signaling pathways after cerebral ischemia [8]. In fact, free radical production and oxidative stress-associated BBB disruption after transient focal cerebral ischemia have been identified as major triggering mechanisms for HT [20]. Related to the previous proteolytic mechanisms described, two interesting investigations on murine models of cerebral ischemia-reperfusion suggest that oxidative stress mediates BBB disruption through metalloproteinase activation in mice lacking copper/zinc-superoxide dismutase [17], and that treatment with the free radical scavenger, α-phenyl-tert-butyl nitrone (α-PBN), significantly reduces tPA-induced cerebral hemorrhage in embolic focal ischemia [1].

Ultimately, protease dysfunction and oxidative stress might contribute to a larger integrated inflammatory response in stroke. Leukocyte recruitment, activation, and infiltration are likely to play a critical role in HT. Interaction of inflammatory leukocytes with cerebral endothelial cells thorough adhesion molecules such as V-CAM and/or I-CAM might underlie endothelial dysfunction and cell injury [3]. The recruitment of neutrophils to the area of ischemia can occur rapidly (within hours) as a first step to inflammation, involving the expression of multiple proteins (selectins, cytokines, integrins, MMPs). A late response includes the activation of resident microglial cells and peripheral macrophages. Because these events are highly correlated, blockade of this molecular inflammatory cascade has become a potential therapeutic target for reducing HT in stroke. These targets may also serve to extend the therapeutic time-window for tPA. An embolic stroke model in rats have shown that early administration of proteasome inhibitor PS-519 or minocycline reduces inflammation [55] and MMP-9 levels [35] respectively, and, thus, can extend the time-window for tPA to 6 h without increasing the incidence of HT.

Molecular markers

The mechanistic findings of HT can be also confirmed by molecular measurements in human stroke that might guide clinicians in diagnosis and prognosis of ICH. Ideal molecular markers would be those available to measure at bedside within minutes in biological fluids such as urine or blood. Using this approach, some groups have identified different biomarkers of HT after cerebral ischemia related to BBB proteolysis, oxidative stress, or hemostasis.

As markers of proteolysis, MMPs are good candidates and, to date, MMP-9 has been the most-studied MMP in the bloodstream related to hemorrhagic conversions. Consistent with the hypothesis of deleterious MMP roles during ischemic stroke, hyperacute MMP-9 plasma level appears to be a powerful predictor of further hemorrhagic complication after tPA thrombolysis [33], since stroke patients treated with tPA present increased levels of MMP-9 compared to untreated patients [39].

The ability to detect early alterations in BBB integrity would be a precious tool for the management of ischemic stroke. As specific a marker of vascular damage, elevated plasma levels of cellular fibronectin have been associated with HT after thrombolysis [6]. Together with the cerebral endothelium, astrocyte end-feet comprise crucial elements that give biochemical and structural support to the BBB. In this regard, serum level of a calcium binding protein (S100B), an astroglial cytoplasmic protein, has been related to HT after ischemic stroke. Interestingly, a high S100B level before thrombolytic therapy predicts further parenchymal hemorrhages and becomes an independent risk factor for HT [16]. Another astrocytic protein marker of brain damage is glial fibrillary acidic protein (GFAP). The same authors reported elevated serum levels in hemorrhagic versus ischemic strokes, suggesting its potential role as a marker for intracerebral bleeding [15]. Whether GFAP might also serve as a marker for hemorrhagic conversions after ischemic stroke still needs to be determined.

Endogenous hemostatic status might also be a decisive factor for the risk of bleeding, especially after thrombolytic therapy, depending on the individual patient's coagulation and fibrinolysis balance. Two relevant investigations reported differing results when evaluating blood levels of fibrinolysis inhibitors, such as PAI-1 or the thrombin-activated fibrinolysis inhibitor (TAFI) before thrombolysis. Whereas the first study showed that baseline PAI-1 and TAFI levels predicted further symptomatic intracranial hemorrhage [41], the second study failed to detect a difference in levels for PAI-1, TAFI, and other hemostatic markers between patients that developed HT and patients that did not [10]. Perhaps larger investigations may be required to resolve these confounding results and validate the utility of these potential markers in the clinic.

The measurement of free radical levels in stroke would be incredibly important, given the large body of literature supporting the importance of this central pathophysiology in stroke; however, technically, this is extremely challenging. Therefore, other molecules, such as products of lipid peroxidation (malondialdehyde, 4-hydroxynonenal, isoprostane, etc.) or indirect measurements such as enzymatic and non-enzymatic antioxidants (vitamins, uric acid, superoxide dismutase, etc.), have been used as surrogate markers of oxidative stress after stroke [9]. Although the importance of oxidative stress as a triggering mechanism for HT is unquestionable, there are currently not many fully quantitative studies to test the use of oxidative stress molecular markers for predicting hemorrhagic conversions that follow ischemic stroke. Recently, plasma level of F2-isoprostanes (free radical-induced products of neuronal arachidonic acid peroxidation) has been found elevated in acute ischemic stroke compared to controls [26]. Hence, the authors present a potential valid plasma biomarker for oxidative stress after stroke. Whether F2-isoprostanes could become markers of HT needs to be determined.

Genetic markers

Apart from monogenic disorders associated with stroke, such as Fabry disease or CADASIL, the cause of ischemic stroke is complex and will involve a combination of environmental and genetic risk factors. Certain genetic mutations or single nucleotide polymorphisms might determine our predisposition to stroke, response to pharmacotherapy, and outcome-response.

Increasingly, the influence of several polymorphisms has been the focus of many investigations. The question is whether there are any markers that can be used to define high-risk populations for HT after thrombolytic therapies. Early studies were conducted to determine the risk of ischemic stroke or a primary ICH. More recently, studies have been directed to predict the safety (potential development of an HT) and efficacy (achieving vessel recanalization) of thrombolysis. In this regard, two studies investigating the influence of relevant molecules such as MMP-9 and Apo-E in ischemic strokes that received thrombolytic therapy showed negative results. According to these studies, polymorphism of the promoter region of the MMP-9 gene (C-1562T) was not associated with HT events, despite increased levels of plasma MMP-9 [34]. Furthermore, the NINDS tPA Stroke Study Group could not detect a relationship between ApoE4 phenotype and clinical outcome, including adverse events such as symptomatic ICH [5].

The coagulation/fibrinolysis system has also been the focus of a search for functional polymorphisms that could predict the risk of bleeding. The well-studied coagulation factor XIII functional polymorphism V34L (a single G-to-T mutation) is known to be associated with the development of primary ICH [7] and recently, the GENOtPA study group has shown that patients carrying the L34 variant presented with severe ICH compared to patients with the V/V genotype in a cohort of ischemic strokes treated with tPA [18]. Another interesting polymorphism that may influence vessel recanalization after thrombolytic therapy may lie in the promoter region of the PAI-1 (4G/5G), in the coding region of the TAFI gene (C1040T), and an insertion/deletion (I/D) in the intron 16 of the angiotensin converting enzyme (ACE) gene [12, 13]. However, these studies failed to establish a correlation between functional mutations and rates of HT in stroke.

In spite of the challenge, it is likely that multiple genes might yet influence the development of intracranial bleeding, especially after tPA administration. A single mutation would be ideal. But some combination may ultimately help us select the best candidates for thrombolysis.

Neuroimaging markers

Early ischemic alterations in brain tissue on pre-treatment computed tomography (CT) scans, such as blurring of the gray matter–white matter distinction and the putaminal border as well as sulcal effacement, were among the first neuroimaging parameters reported to be predictors of HT after thrombolytic therapy [23]. However, widespread use was limited due to difficulties in reliably defining the true areas of interest [19]. Currently, the development of more advanced CT technologies allows direct monitoring of BBB function [4, 31]. Using dynamic perfusion CT, Lin and colleagues [31] reported as many as 88% of ischemic stroke patients to reveal increased microvascular permeability measures in ischemic areas within the first 3 h after stroke onset. Microvascular permeability was found to be significantly higher in patients developing subsequent HT and thus, may qualify as a predictor of HT in both tPA and non-tPA patients.

Magnetic resonance imaging (MRI)-based studies reported an early parenchymal contrast enhancement on T1-weighted images after the application of gadolinium-containing contrast agents, which may be indicative of BBB disruption and impending HT in the acute phase of stroke. In the experimental setting, such enhancement was first observed in rats subjected to transient middle cerebral artery occlusion that subsequently developed petechial hemorrhage [11, 28, 36]. The pathophysiological correlate is most likely a loss of basal lamina in cerebral microvessels, which allows the extravasation of contrast medium molecules into the extravascular space [21]. MRI-based studies in humans confirmed the occurrence of an early leptomeningeal, parenchymal, and cerebrospinal fluid contrast enhancement in ischemic stroke and underlined its association with acute BBB disruption and the development of subsequent hemorrhage [29, 52].

Kassner and colleagues [24] used dynamic MR permeability imaging to quantify defects in the BBB in a small series of patients with acute ischemic stroke who did not undergo thrombolytic therapy, and reported an association between hemorrhagic conversion and elevated permeability parameters. Very recently, using permeability images derived from a pretreatment standard perfusion MRI, Bang and colleagues [2] showed an association between hemorrhage and permeability image abnormalities in patients with acute stroke undergoing recanalization therapy.

Other MR parameters that may serve as hemorrhage predictors include lower apparent diffusion coefficient values [49, 50] and a persistently delayed perfusion [50] in ischemic areas. The size of the lesion on diffusion-weighted imaging was recently reported to predict symptomatic ICH after thrombolytic therapy [45]. However, it is unclear whether these MRI changes represent mechanistically-related events or are only related to non-specific severity of overall tissue damage. Some studies have pointed out that silent microbleeds, a possible indicator of pre-existing severe microangiopathy, may also be a predictor of an increased risk of hemorrhagic conversion after thrombolytic treatment [27], but other groups found contrary results [14]. In the end, systematic MRI studies utilizing consistent protocols for quantitation might be required to resolve inter-site differences.

Conclusions

Ischemic stroke is a devastating event involving activation of multiple pathological mechanisms in the ischemic brain and leads to cell death, edema, inflammation, and BBB rupture. Especially threatening is the development of HT, which may be further enhanced by tPA administration, the only FDA-approved stroke drug for dissolving the obstructing clot. Advances in research on many fronts are now beginning to provide multiple potential tools such as biological markers, genetic risk factors, or neuroimaging assays, which might eventually be used to guide clinicians to predict, and hopefully prevent, hemorrhagic complications. Correlating these surrogate markers with the underlying mechanisms would be best. Ultimately, a combination of new targets for therapy, together with novel biomarkers, may even help extend the narrow 3-hour time-window for tPA administration to provide therapeutic benefit without increasing the incidence of HT.

Acknowledgements

Supported in part by National Institutes of Health grants R01-NS37074, R01-NS48422, R01-NS53560, R01-NS56458, P50-NS10828, and P01-NS55104.

References

1. Asahi M, Asahi K, Wang X, Lo EH (2000) Reduction of tissue plasminogen activator-induced hemorrhage and brain injury by free radical spin trapping after embolic focal cerebral ischemia in rats. J Cereb Blood Flow Metab 20: 452–457

2. Bang OY, Buck BH, Saver JL, Alger JR, Yoon SR, Starkman S, Ovbiagele B, Kim D, Ali LK, Sanossian N, Jahan R, Duckwiler GR, Viñuela F, Salamon N, Villablanca JP, Liebeskind DS (2007) Prediction of hemorrhagic transformation after recanalization therapy using T2*-permeability magnetic resonance imaging. Ann Neurol 62: 170–176

3. Bevilacqua MP (1993) Endothelial-leukocyte adhesion molecules. Annu Rev Immunol 11: 767–804

4. Bisdas S, Hartel M, Cheong LH, Koh TS, Vogl TJ (2007) Prediction of subsequent hemorrhage in acute ischemic stroke using permeability CT imaging and a distributed parameter tracer kinetic model. J Neuroradiol 34: 101–108

5. Broderick J, Lu M, Jackson C, Pancioli A, Tilley BC, Fagan SC, Kothari R, Levine SR, Marler JR, Lyden PD, Haley EC Jr, Brott T, Grotta JC; NINDS t-PA Stroke Study Group (2001) Apolipoprotein E phenotype and the efficacy of intravenous tissue plasminogen activator in acute ischemic stroke. Ann Neurol 49: 736–744

6. Castellanos M, Leira R, Serena J, Blanco M, Pedraza S, Castillo J, Dávalos A (2004) Plasma cellular-fibronectin concentration predicts hemorrhagic transformation after thrombolytic therapy in acute ischemic stroke. Stroke 35: 1671–1676

7. Catto AJ, Kohler HP, Bannan S, Stickland M, Carter A, Grant PJ (1998) Factor XIII Val 34 Leu: a novel association with primary intracerebral hemorrhage. Stroke 29: 813–816

8. Chan PH (1996) Role of oxidants in ischemic brain damage. Stroke 27: 1124–1129

9. Cherubini A, Ruggiero C, Polidori MC, Mecocci P (2005) Potential markers of oxidative stress in stroke. Free Radic Biol Med 39: 841–852

10. Cocho D, Borrell M, Marti-Fàbregas J, Montaner J, Castellanos M, Bravo Y, Molina-Porcel L, Belvis R, Diaz-Manera JA, Martinez-Domeño A, Martinez-Lage M, Millán M, Fontcuberta J, Marti-
Vilalta JL (2006) Pretreatment hemostatic markers of symptomatic intracerebral hemorrhage in patients treated with tissue plasminogen activator. Stroke 37: 996–999

11. Dijkhuizen RM, Asahi M, Wu O, Rosen BR, Lo EH (2001) Delayed rt-PA treatment in a rat embolic stroke model: diagnosis and prognosis of ischemic injury and hemorrhagic transformation with magnetic resonance imaging. J Cereb Blood Flow Metab 21: 964–971

12. Fernández-Cadenas I, Molina CA, Alvarez-Sabín J, Ribó M, Penalba A, Ortega-Torres L, Delgado P, Quintana M, Rosell A, Montaner J (2006) ACE gene polymorphisms influence t-PA-induced brain vessel reopening following ischemic stroke. Neurosci Lett 398: 167–171

13. Fernandez-Cadenas I, Alvarez-Sabin J, Ribo M, Rubiera M, Mendioroz M, Molina CA, Rosell A, Montaner J (2007) Influence of thrombin-activatable fibrinolysis inhibitor and plasminogen activator inhibitor-1 gene polymorphisms on tissue-type plasminogen activator-induced recanalization in ischemic stroke patients. J Thromb Haemost 5: 1862–1868

14. Fiehler J, Albers GW, Boulanger JM, Derex L, Gass A, Hjort N, Kim JS, Liebeskind DS, Neumann-Haefelin T, Pedraza S, Rother J, Rothwell P, Rovira A, Schellinger PD, Trenkler J; MR STROKE Group (2007) Bleeding risk analysis in stroke imaging before thromboLysis (BRASIL): pooled analysis of T2*-weighted magnetic resonance imaging data from 570 patients. Stroke 38: 2738–2744

15. Foerch C, Curdt I, Yan B, Dvorak F, Hermans M, Berkefeld J, Raabe A, Neumann-Haefelin T, Steinmetz H, Sitzer M (2006) Serum glial fibrillary acidic protein as a biomarker for intracerebral haemorrhage in patients with acute stroke. J Neurol Neurosurg Psychiatry 77: 181–184

16. Foerch C, Wunderlich MT, Dvorak F, Humpich M, Kahles T, Goertler M, Alvarez-Sabín J, Wallesch CW, Molina CA, Steinmetz H, Sitzer M, Montaner J (2007) Elevated serum S100B levels indicate a higher risk of hemorrhagic transformation after thrombolytic therapy in acute stroke. Stroke 38: 2491–2495

17. Gasche Y, Copin JC, Sugawara T, Fujimura M, Chan PH (2001) Matrix metalloproteinase inhibition prevents oxidative stress-associated blood–brain barrier disruption after transient focal cerebral ischemia. J Cereb Blood Flow Metab 21: 1393–1400

18. González-Conejero R, Fernández-Cadenas I, Iniesta JA, Marti-Fabregas J, Obach V, Alvarez-Sabín J, Vicente V, Corral J, Montaner J; Proyecto Ictus Research Group (2006) Role of fibrinogen levels and factor XIII V34L polymorphism in thrombolytic therapy in stroke patients. Stroke 37: 2288–2293

19. Grotta JC, Chiu D, Lu M, Patel S, Levine SR, Tilley BC, Brott TG, Haley EC Jr, Lyden PD, Kothari R, Frankel M, Lewandowski CA, Libman R, Kwiatkowski T, Broderick JP, Marler JR, Corrigan J, Huff S, Mitsias P, Talati S, Tanne D (1999) Agreement and variability in the interpretation of early CT changes in stroke patients qualifying for intravenous rtPA therapy. Stroke 30: 1528–1533

20. Gürsoy-Ozdemir Y, Can A, Dalkara T (2004) Reperfusion-induced oxidative/nitrative injury to neurovascular unit after focal cerebral ischemia. Stroke 35: 1449–1453

21. Hamann GF, del Zoppo GJ, von Kummer R (1999) Hemorrhagic transformation of cerebral infarction-possible mechanisms. Thromb Haemost 82: 92–94

22. Hamann GF, Burggraf D, Martens HK, Liebetrau M, Jäger G, Wunderlich N, DeGeorgia M, Krieger DW (2004) Mild to moderate hypothermia prevents microvascular basal lamina antigen loss in experimental focal cerebral ischemia. Stroke 35: 764–769

23. Jaillard A, Cornu C, Durieux A, Moulin T, Boutitie F, Lees KR, Hommel M (1999) Hemorrhagic transformation in acute ischemic stroke: The MAST-E study. MAST-E group. Stroke 30: 1326–1332

24. Kassner A, Roberts T, Taylor K, Silver F, Mikulis D (2005) Prediction of hemorrhage in acute ischemic stroke using permeability MR imaging. Am J Neuroradiol 26: 2213–2217

25. Kaur J, Zhao Z, Klein GM, Lo EH, Buchan AM (2004) The neurotoxicity of tissue plasminogen activator? J Cereb Blood Flow Metab 24: 945–963

26. Kelly PJ, Morrow JD, Ning M, Koroshetz W, Lo EH, Terry E, Milne GL, Hubbard J, Lee H, Stevenson E, Lederer M, Furie KL (2008) Oxidative stress and matrix metalloproteinase-9 in acute ischemic stroke: the Biomarker Evaluation for Antioxidant Therapies in Stroke (BEAT-Stroke) study. Stroke 39: 100–104

27. Kidwell CS, Saver JL, Villablanca JP, Duckwiler G, Fredieu A, Gough K, Leary MC, Starkman S, Gobin YP, Jahan R, Vespa P, Liebeskind DS, Alger JR, Vinuela F (2002) Magnetic resonance imaging detection of microbleeds before thrombolysis: an emerging application. Stroke 33: 95–98

28. Knight RA, Barker PB, Fagan SC, Li Y, Jacobs MA, Welch KM (1998) Prediction of impending hemorrhagic transformation in ischemic stroke using magnetic resonance imaging in rats. Stroke 29: 144–151

29. Latour LL, Kang DW, Ezzeddine MA, Chalela JA, Warach S (2004) Early blood–brain barrier disruption in human focal brain ischemia. Ann Neurol 56: 468–477

30. Lee SR, Wang X, Tsuji K, Lo EH (2004) Extracellular proteolytic pathophysiology in the neurovascular unit after stroke. Neurol Res 26: 854–861

31. Lin K, Kazmi KS, Law M, Babb J, Peccerelli N, Pramanik BK (2007) Measuring elevated microvascular permeability and predicting hemorrhagic transformation in acute ischemic stroke using first-pass dynamic perfusion CT imaging. Am J Neuroradiol 28: 1292–1298

32. Liu D, Cheng T, Guo H, Fernández JA, Griffin JH, Song X, Zlokovic BV (2004) Tissue plasminogen activator neurovascular toxicity is controlled by activated protein C. Nat Med 10: 1379–1383

33. Montaner J, Molina CA, Monasterio J, Abilleira S, Arenillas JF, Ribó M, Quintana M, Alvarez-Sabin J (2003) Matrix metalloproteinase-9 pretreatment level predicts intracranial hemorrhagic complications after thrombolysis in human stroke. Circulation 107: 598–603

34. Montaner J, Fernández-Cadenas I, Molina CA, Monasterio J, Arenillas JF, Ribó M, Quintana M, Chacón P, Andreu AL, Alvarez-Sabín J (2003) Safety profile of tissue plasminogen activator treatment among stroke patients carrying a common polymorphism (C-1562T) in the promoter region of the matrix metalloproteinase-9 gene. Stroke 34: 2851–2855

35. Murata Y, Rosell A, Scannevin RH, Rhodes KJ, Wang X, Lo EH (2008) Extension of the thrombolytic time window with minocycline in experimental stroke. Stroke (in press)

36. Neumann-Haefelin C, Brinker G, Uhlenküken U, Pillekamp F, Hossmann KA, Hoehn M (2002) Prediction of hemorrhagic transformation after thrombolytic therapy of clot embolism: an MRI investigation in rat brain. Stroke 33: 1392–1398

37. Nicole O, Docagne F, Ali C, Margaill I, Carmeliet P, MacKenzie ET, Vivien D, Buisson A (2001) The proteolytic activity of tissue-plasminogen activator enhances NMDA receptor-mediated signaling. Nat Med 7: 59–64

38. NINDS rt-PA Stroke Study Group (1995) Tissue plasminogen activator for acute ischemic stroke. N Engl J Med 333: 1581–1587

39. Ning M, Furie KL, Koroshetz WJ, Lee H, Barron M, Lederer M, Wang X, Zhu M, Sorensen AG, Lo EH, Kelly PJ (2006) Association between tPA therapy and raised early matrix metalloproteinase-9 in acute stroke. Neurology 66: 1550–1555

40. Planas AM, Solé S, Justicia C (2001) Expression and activation of matrix metalloproteinase-2 and -9 in rat brain after transient focal cerebral ischemia. Neurobiol Dis 8: 834–846

41. Ribo M, Montaner J, Molina CA, Arenillas JF, Santamarina E, Quintana M, Alvarez-Sabin J (2004) Admission fibrinolytic profile is associated with symptomatic hemorrhagic transformation in stroke patients treated with tissue plasminogen activator. Stroke 35: 2123–2127

42. Rosell A, Ortega-Aznar A, Alvarez-Sabín J, Fernández-Cadenas I, Ribó M, Molina CA, Lo EH, Montaner J (2006) Increased brain expression of matrix metalloproteinase-9 after ischemic and hemorrhagic human stroke. Stroke 37: 1399–1406

43. Rosell A, Cuadrado E, Ortega-Aznar A, Hernández-Guillamon M, Lo EH, Montaner J (2007) MMP-9-positive neutrophil infiltration is associated to blood–brain barrier breakdown and basal lamina type IV collagen degradation during hemorrhagic transformation after human ischemic stroke. Stroke (in press)

44. Rosenberg GA, Navratil M, Barone F, Feuerstein G (1996) Proteolytic cascade enzymes increase in focal cerebral ischemia in rat. J Cereb Blood Flow Metab 16: 360–366

45. Singer OC, Humpich MC, Fiehler J, Albers GW, Lansberg MG, Kastrup A, Rovira A, Liebeskind DS, Gass A, Rosso C, Derex L, Kim JS, Neumann-Haefelin T; MR Stroke Study Group Investigators (2008) Risk for symptomatic intracerebral hemorrhage after thrombolysis assessed by diffusion-weighted magnetic resonance imaging. Ann Neurol 63:52–60

46. Solé S, Petegnief V, Gorina R, Chamorro A, Planas AM (2004) Activation of matrix metalloproteinase-3 and agrin cleavage in cerebral ischemia/reperfusion. J Neuropathol Exp Neurol 63: 338–349

47. Sumii T, Lo EH (2002) Involvement of matrix metalloproteinase in thrombolysis-associated hemorrhagic transformation after embolic focal ischemia in rats. Stroke 33: 831–836

48. Suzuki Y, Nagai N, Umemura K, Collen D, Lijnen HR (2007) Stromelysin-1 (MMP-3) is critical for intracranial bleeding after t-PA treatment of stroke in mice. J Thromb Haemost 5: 1732–1739

49. Tong DC, Adami A, Moseley ME, Marks MP (2000) Relationship between apparent diffusion coefficient and subsequent hemorrhagic transformation following acute ischemic stroke. Stroke 31: 2378–2384

50. Tong DC, Adami A, Moseley ME, Marks MP (2001) Prediction of hemorrhagic transformation following acute stroke: role of diffusion- and perfusion-weighted magnetic resonance imaging. Arch Neurol 58: 587–593

51. Tsuji K, Aoki T, Tejima E, Arai K, Lee SR, Atochin DN, Huang PL, Wang X, Montaner J, Lo EH (2005) Tissue plasminogen activator promotes matrix metalloproteinase-9 upregulation after focal cerebral ischemia. Stroke 36: 1954–1959

52. Vo KD, Santiago F, Lin W, Hsu CY, Lee Y, Lee JM (2003) MR imaging enhancement patterns as predictors of hemorrhagic transformation in acute ischemic stroke. Am J Neuroradiol 24: 674–679

53. Wang X, Lee SR, Arai K, Lee SR, Tsuji K, Rebeck GW, Lo EH (2003) Lipoprotein receptor-mediated induction of matrix metalloproteinase by tissue plasminogen activator. Nat Med 9: 1313–1317

54. Wang X, Lo EH (2003) Triggers and mediators of hemorrhagic transformation in cerebral ischemia. Mol Neurobiol 28: 229–244

55. Zhang L, Zhang ZG, Zhang RL, Lu M, Adams J, Elliott PJ, Chopp M (2001) Postischemic (6-h) treatment with recombinant human tissue plasminogen activator and proteasome inhibitor PS-519 reduces infarction in a rat model of embolic focal cerebral ischemia. Stroke 32: 2926–2931

Acta Neurochir Suppl (2008) 105: 179–184
© Springer-Verlag 2008
Printed in Austria

The clinical significance of acute brain injury in subarachnoid hemorrhage and opportunity for intervention

R. E. Ayer[1]**, J. H. Zhang**[1,2,3]

[1] Department of Physiology and Pharmacology, Loma Linda University Medical Center, Loma Linda, CA, USA
[2] Department of Neurosurgery, Loma Linda University Medical Center, Loma Linda, CA, USA
[3] Department of Anesthesiology, Loma Linda University Medical Center, Loma Linda, CA, USA

Summary

Aneurysmal subarachnoid hemorrhage (SAH) is a devastating neurological event that accounts for 3–7% of all strokes and carries a mortality rate as high as 40%. Delayed cerebral vasospasm has traditionally been recognized as the most treatable cause of morbidity and mortality from SAH. However, evidence is mounting that the physiological and cellular events of acute brain injury, which occur during the 24–72 h following aneurysm rupture, make significant contributions to patient outcomes, and may even be a more significant factor than delayed cerebral vasospasm. Acute brain injury in aneurysmal SAH is the result of physiological derangements such as increased intracranial pressure and decreased cerebral blood flow that result in global cerebral ischemia, and lead to the acute development of edema, oxidative stress, inflammation, apoptosis, and infarction. The consequence of these events is often death or significant neurological disability. In this study of acute brain injury, we elucidate some of the complex molecular signaling pathways responsible for these poor outcomes. Continued research in this area and the development of therapies to interrupt these cascades should be a major focus in the future as we continue to seek effective therapies for aneurysmal SAH.

Keywords: Subarachnoid hemorrhage; acute brain injury; blood–brain barrier; edema; apoptosis; infarction; oxidative stress; inflammation.

Introduction

Aneurysmal subarachnoid hemorrhage (SAH) has long been recognized as a devastating neurological event that accounts for 3–7% of all strokes [11, 54]. Although significant advances in the diagnosis and surgical treatment of SAH since the 1960s may have reduced mortality by as much as 15% and improved functional outcome [19], SAH still carries a mortality rate as high as 40% in some series [49]. For over a decade, the events following

Correspondence: J. H. Zhang, MD, Department of Neurosurgery, Loma Linda University Medical Center, 11234 Anderson Street, Room 2562B, Loma Linda, CA 92350, USA. e-mail: johnzhang3910@yahoo.com

the initial bleed after SAH have been recognized as the greatest contributor to mortality [4]; however, vasospasm has traditionally been recognized as the most treatable prognostic factor of poor outcome following SAH. More recently, the CONSCIOUS-1 clinical trial of clazosentan, an endothelin-1 receptor antagonist, demonstrated a 65% reduction in angiographic vasospasm that resulted in only mild reductions in delayed neurological deficits and failed to result in improved functional outcome [32, 33]. These surprising results have raised the practical question of drug side effects outweighing potential benefits, but preliminary evidence does not support this hypothesis [33]. Interestingly, this study spotlights the mounting evidence that early brain injury, which occurs in the hours immediately following SAH, is an important player in neurological outcomes [6]. Our review highlights the pathophysiology of early brain injury, provides evidence to suggest that early brain injury contributes to the neurological deterioration following SAH that has otherwise been solely attributed to cerebral vasospasm, and suggests potential avenues of investigation for the development of future therapies.

Blood–brain barrier disruption and edema

It has been established that an acute rise in intracranial pressure (ICP) occurs after aneurysmal SAH [59]. The mechanisms for this increased pressure are many: hemorrhage volume, impeded cerebrospinal fluid (CSF) drainage, cerebrovascular dysfunction resulting in vascular engorgement, and the formation of acute cerebral edema [6]. Elevated ICP in SAH is correlated with poor outcome, and therapies aimed at reducing the acute development of cerebral edema should prove to be ben-eficial [18, 59]. Edema after SAH has traditionally been overlooked, possibly due to the difficulty of its quantifi-cation on CT scans, but puncture models of SAH in animals confirm that global cerebral edema can occur within minutes to hours of aneurysm rupture, making it an important factor in the pathophysiology of acute brain injury [5, 23, 53].

A prospective cohort of 374 patients with spontaneous aneurysmal SAH found that CT scanning identified glob-al cerebral edema in 8% of SAH patients [7]. Other investigators have found similar incidences in other se-ries [25, 29], and cases of severe cerebral edema follow-ing SAH treated with craniectomy have also been reported [51]. The recognition of SAH patients with acute global cerebral edema has spurred further investi-gation into its significance. Claassen et al. [7] found that patients with global cerebral edema on CT had a 40% mortality at 3 months, compared to only an 18% mor-tality for patients without global cerebral edema. Kreiter et al. [26] found cerebral edema to be one of the major predictors of cognitive dysfunction following SAH. Global cerebral edema was also an independent predic-tor of mortality and morbidity following SAH, even after factors such as age, aneurysm size, and neurological grade at time of admission were considered. This edema developed independently of cerebral vasospasm and highlights the importance of early brain injury mecha-nisms in the development of edema.

The triggering event of global cerebral ischemia fol-lowing SAH is the circulatory arrest that occurs as ICP transiently reaches levels approximating arterial pres-sures [38]; this is supported clinically by the fact that one of the predictors of global cerebral edema at time of admission to the hospital includes the loss of conscious-ness [7]. This circulatory arrest creates a hypoxic state in the cerebral tissues and the resulting energy failure in the ischemic neurons and glia initiates the cascade of events leading to cellular swelling, or cytotoxic edema [41]. Apoptotic cascades are also initiated by the tran-sient ischemia following SAH, resulting in damage to neurons and the blood–brain barrier (BBB) [6, 7]. Apoptosis of the endothelial cells and perivascular astro-cytes that comprise the BBB cause the leakage of serum from the vascular lumen into cerebral tissues (vasogenic edema).

Numerous intracellular second messenger cascades have been implicated in initiating the apoptotic signal that disrupts the BBB [6, 42, 60]. Park et al. [42] dem-onstrated apoptosis in cerebral endothelial cells and an increased BBB permeability after experimental SAH that was reversed with caspase inhibition. Additionally, vascular endothelial growth factor (VEGF), a mitogen involved in angiogenesis and vascular permeability [36, 61, 62], is elevated following SAH [28, 60] and initiates cell death pathways in the neurovascular unit that com-prised the BBB [28]. Besides the initiation of apoptotic cascades, other mechanisms of BBB destruction exist. For example, matrix metalloproteinases (MMPs), which degrade the type IV collagen that makes up the base-ment membrane of the BBB, are known to be increased following experimental and human SAH [20, 37, 48, 52] and contribute to BBB breakdown [46, 47, 52]. The development of therapies that target these enzymes may have clinical efficacy, as Yatsushige et al. [60] found that decreased MMP-9 activity was associated with a preserved basement membrane and reduced cerebral edema 24 h after experimental SAH in rats. The devel-opment of therapies to reduce BBB disruption is com-plicated by the fact that the therapeutic window for these treatments may be limited. Already evidence exists that inhibiting factors may prove beneficial acutely, but if the inhibition is prolonged it may prove detrimental to re-covery, as in the case of VEGF [62] and MMPs [34].

Oxidative stress

Through their highly reactive unpaired electrons, free radicals are directly damaging to the neurovascular unit (endothelial cells, pericytes, astrocytes) and neurons through the promotion of lipid peroxidation, protein breakdown, and DNA damage [41]. The consequences of these events are neuronal apoptosis, endothelial inju-ry, and BBB breakdown (Fig. 1). Figueroa et al. [12] demonstrated that oxidative stress induced cortical neu-ron death through the mitochondrial pathway of apopto-sis as well as through necrosis. Endo et al. [9], through the use of transgenic rats, showed that reducing oxida-tive stress during acute brain injury reduced apoptosis, and promoted increased survival and neurological func-tion in experimental SAH. The administration of system-ic antioxidants in experimental SAH has also proven to reduce oxidative stress, protect the BBB, and improve neurological scores [14, 22, 58]. Free radical-mediated damage is non-specific and affects many cell types. The advantage of direct free radical scavenging, or the up regulation of native protective systems during acute in-jury, is the ability to prevent the initiation of multiple damaging cascades. This task seems less daunting than having to address each damaging cascade independent-

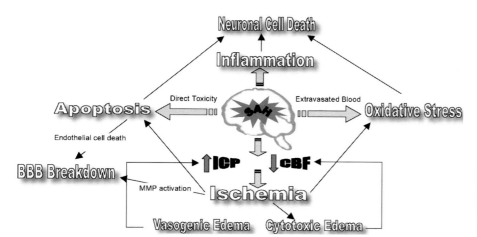

Fig. 1. Illustration of the simultaneous injurious pathways initiated during acute brain injury following SAH. Events that are initiated independently often make combined contributions to various outcomes

ly; however, identifying and utilizing an effective thera-peutic window may be the biggest challenge. By the time a patient is available to receive treatment, the dam-age caused by free radicals may have already been com-pleted or the second messenger signaling cascades leading to cell death may have already been activated. This issue may be a significant contributor to the poor performance of free radical scavengers in clinical trials [16, 24, 30, 31].

Inflammation

An inflammatory response occurs within the central ner-vous system (CNS) following SAH. Investigators have characterized the infiltration of lymphocytes and macro-phages into the CNS following SAH, indicating that SAH may illicit its own characteristic inflammatory re-action [27, 35]. It is interesting to note that neutrophil activation may not play a significant role in CNS in-flammation following SAH [40], and the CSF from SAH patients may be inhibitory to their activation [55]. Debate exists as to whether or not the infiltration of lymphocytes into the CNS is a neuroprotective part of the healing process, or a response that is detrimental to recovery; numerous conflicting reports are highly debat-ed [17]. Investigators have sought to resolve the conflict-ing evidence by examining the subpopulations of T-cells following various CNS injuries, particularly distinguish-ing between type 1 (Th1), type 2 (Th2), and type 3 (Th3) T helper cell subsets through the identification of their characteristic cytokines. Investigations of ischemic stroke models demonstrate potential for the development of a Th1 cellular response, resembling CNS autoimmune disease, that results from the exposure of CNS antigens to the immune system that are usually protected from recognition by an intact BBB [2]. The development of

immune tolerance to CNS antigens prior to experimental stroke has been found to reduce Th1 autoimmunity, re-duce infarct size, and improve outcomes [3].

Additionally, eliciting a Th2/Th3 response, character-ized by the secretion of immunomodulatory cytokines (IL-4, IL-10, transforming growth factor $\beta1$ (TGF-$\beta1$), promotes the immunological tolerance of CNS antigens and may augment neuroregeneration [13, 17]. These findings have led to the experimental application of drugs known to elicit Th2 immune responses for the treatment of stroke and other CNS diseases [13, 17]. Most of this work has been pioneered in *in vitro* studies and ischemic stroke models; however, the application of these theories to SAH has only begun [39]. Interestingly, statins have been described as being able to elicit a Th2 immune response [1, 15], and this may help explain their reported efficacy in treating SAH patients [56, 57]. The concept of immunomodulation may prove to be benefi-cial while avoiding the pitfalls blanket immunosuppres-sion [10].

Cell death and brain infarction

As mentioned above, apoptosis in the cells comprising the neurovascular unit is one of the key factors to BBB disruption and the development of edema. However, the apoptotic cell death of neurons in the acute phase of SAH has been demonstrated as well. Prunell *et al.* [44] demonstrated the progression of apoptosis at 2 and 7 days after SAH. The degree of neuronal apoptosis was linked to events following the initial bleed by correlating it with the severity of acute cerebral blood flow reduc-tion. In light of the results of the CONSCIOUS-1 trial, this evidence lends itself to the hypothesis that the cell death signaling initiated during acute injury may at least partially be responsible for the neurological decline traditionally attributed to vasospasm and manifesting as delayed ischemic neurological deficits. This would also mean that these acute events play a significant role in long-term outcome. Evidence from several studies demonstrates significant long-term neurological disability following SAH without the occurrence of cerebral vasospasm [8, 21, 26]. Many potential opportunities for intervention exist as more about the apoptotic cascades initiated in SAH are revealed. Yatsushige *et al.* [60] demonstrated the programmed cell death of neurons mediated through the activation of a JNK/cJun pathway, while Cahill *et al.* [6] demonstrated that activation of the 3 classical apoptotic pathways following SAH results in the loss of cortical and hippocampal neurons 72 h after SAH. Each of these studies demonstrated that the inhibition of apoptotic pathways not only reduced cellular death, but also resulted in a significant improvement in functional outcome.

The most obvious indication of cell death, albeit from apoptosis or necrosis, is the development of an infarction, and its appearance following SAH has been well documented [26, 43, 50]. Infarction is widely recognized to occur following severe vasospasm [45], but its occurrence as a result of the initial bleed is also recognized [50], and it presence under these circumstances is a clear indicator for poor outcome [26]. Some skeptics may believe that addressing this sequel of SAH is not an effective approach to improving outcome, but studies have shown that the acute administration of neuroprotectants, such as nimodipine, reduces the incidence of infarction whether it is from early brain injury or cerebral vasospasm [43]. Additionally, the cascade of events leading to infarction probably results in a continuum of cellular damage, of which infarction is the most extreme outcome. Addressing the processes leading up to infarction will not only reduce its incidence, but also reduce the more subtle sequel.

Perspectives

Aneurysmal SAH continues to be a devastating neurological event, but recent studies are continuing to shed light on the importance of early brain injury and its determination on patient survival and long-term functional outcome. Cerebral vasospasm after SAH and its clinical consequences should no longer be recognized as the only treatable cause of poor outcome following SAH. Early brain injury should perhaps now be considered to have an equal or more significant impact on outcome. The development of therapies targeting patho-

logical signal transduction, oxidative stress, and immune reaction are certain to be challenging, owing to the complexity of the disease. However, addressing early brain injury in conjunction with continued treatment for vasospasm bodes well for continued improvement in the treatment of aneurysmal SAH.

Acknowledgments

This study was partially supported by grants from the National Institutes of Health (NS45694, NS43338, and NS53407) to JHZ.

References

1. Arora M, Chen L, Paglia M, Gallagher I, Allen JE, Vyas YM, Ray A, Ray P (2006) Simvastatin promotes Th2-type responses through the induction of the chitinase family member Ym1 in dendritic cells. Proc Natl Acad Sci USA 103: 7777–7782
2. Becker KJ, Kindrick DL, Lester MP, Shea C, Ye ZC (2005) Sensitization to brain antigens after stroke is augmented by lipopolysaccharide. J Cereb Blood Flow Metab 25: 1634–1644
3. Becker KJ, McCarron RM, Ruetzler C, Laban O, Sternberg E, Flanders KC, Hallenbeck JM (1997) Immunologic tolerance to myelin basic protein decreases stroke size after transient focal cerebral ischemia. Proc Natl Acad Sci USA 94: 10873–10878
4. Broderick JP, Brott TG, Duldner JE, Tomsick T, Leach A (1994) Initial and recurrent bleeding are the major causes of death following subarachnoid hemorrhage. Stroke 25: 1342–1347
5. Busch E, Beaulieu C, de Crespigny A, Moseley ME (1998) Diffusion MR imaging during acute subarachnoid hemorrhage in rats. Stroke 29: 2155–2161
6. Cahill J, Calvert JW, Zhang JH (2006) Mechanisms of early brain injury after subarachnoid hemorrhage. J Cereb Blood Flow Metab 26: 1341–1353
7. Claassen J, Carhuapoma JR, Kreiter KT, Du EY, Connolly ES, Mayer SA (2002) Global cerebral edema after subarachnoid hemorrhage: frequency, predictors, and impact on outcome. Stroke 33: 1225–1232
8. Claassen J, Vu A, Kreiter KT, Kowalski RG, Du EY, Ostapkovich N, Fitzsimmons BF, Connolly ES, Mayer SA (2004) Effect of acute physiologic derangements on outcome after subarachnoid hemorrhage. Crit Care Med 32: 832–838
9. Endo H, Nito C, Kamada H, Yu F, Chan PH (2007) Reduction in oxidative stress by superoxide dismutase overexpression attenuates acute brain injury after subarachnoid hemorrhage via activation of Akt/glycogen synthase kinase-3beta survival signaling. J Cereb Blood Flow Metab 27: 975–982
10. Feigin VL, Anderson N, Rinkel GJ, Algra A, van Gijn J, Bennett DA (2005) Corticosteroids for aneurysmal subarachnoid haemorrhage and primary intracerebral haemorrhage. Cochrane Database Syst Rev (3): CD004583
11. Feigin VL, Lawes CM, Bennett DA, Anderson CS (2003) Stroke epidemiology: a review of population-based studies of incidence, prevalence, and case-fatality in the late 20th century. Lancet Neurol 2: 43–53
12. Figueroa S, Oset-Gasque MJ, Arce C, Martinez-Honduvilla CJ, González MP (2006) Mitochondrial involvement in nitric oxide-induced cellular death in cortical neurons in culture. J Neurosci Res 83: 441–449
13. Gee JM, Kalil A, Shea C, Becker KJ (2007) Lymphocytes: potential mediators of postischemic injury and neuroprotection. Stroke 38: 783–788

14. Germanò A, Imperatore C, d'Avella D, Costa G, Tomasello F (1998) Antivasospastic and brain-protective effects of a hydroxyl radical scavenger (AVS) after experimental subarachnoid hemorrhage. J Neurosurg 88: 1075–1081

15. Hakamada-Taguchi R, Uehara Y, Kuribayashi K, Numabe A, Saito K, Negoro H, Fujita T, Toyo-oka T, Kato T (2003) Inhibition of hydroxymethylglutaryl-coenzyme a reductase reduces Th1 development and promotes Th2 development. Circ Res 93: 948–956

16. Haley EC Jr, Kassell NF, Apperson-Hansen C, Maile MH, Alves WM (1997) A randomized, double-blind, vehicle-controlled trial of tirilazad mesylate in patients with aneurysmal subarachnoid hemorrhage: a cooperative study in North America. J Neurosurg 86: 467–474

17. Hendrix S, Nitsch R (2007) The role of T helper cells in neuroprotection and regeneration. J Neuroimmunol 184: 100–112

18. Heuer GG, Smith MJ, Elliott JP, Winn HR, LeRoux PD (2004) Relationship between intracranial pressure and other clinical variables in patients with aneurysmal subarachnoid hemorrhage. J Neurosurg 101: 408–416

19. Hop JW, Rinkel GJ, Algra A, van Gijn J (1997) Case-fatality rates and functional outcome after subarachnoid hemorrhage: a systematic review. Stroke 28: 660–664

20. Horstmann S, Su Y, Koziol J, Meyding-Lamadé U, Nagel S, Wagner S (2006) MMP-2 and MMP-9 levels in peripheral blood after subarachnoid hemorrhage. J Neurol Sci 251: 82–86

21. Hütter BO, Kreitschmann-Andermahr I, Mayfrank L, Rohde V, Spetzger U, Gilsbach JM (1999) Functional outcome after aneurysmal subarachnoid hemorrhage. Acta Neurochir Suppl 72: 157–174

22. Imperatore C, Germanò A, d'Avella D, Tomasello F, Costa G (2000) Effects of the radical scavenger AVS on behavioral and BBB changes after experimental subarachnoid hemorrhage. Life Sci 66: 779–790

23. Kamiya K, Kuyama H, Symon L (1983) An experimental study of the acute stage of subarachnoid hemorrhage. J Neurosurg 59: 917–924

24. Kassell NF, Haley EC Jr, Apperson-Hansen C, Alves WM (1996) Randomized, double-blind, vehicle-controlled trial of tirilazad mesylate in patients with aneurysmal subarachnoid hemorrhage: a cooperative study in Europe, Australia, and New Zealand. J Neurosurg 84: 221–228

25. Kassell NF, Torner JC, Haley EC Jr, Jane JA, Adams HP, Kongable GL (1990) The international cooperative study on the timing of aneurysm surgery. Part 1: Overall management results. J Neurosurg 73: 18–36

26. Kreiter KT, Copeland D, Bernardini GL, Bates JE, Peery S, Claassen J, Du YE, Stern Y, Connolly ES, Mayer SA (2002) Predictors of cognitive dysfunction after subarachnoid hemorrhage. Stroke 33: 200–208

27. Kubota T, Handa Y, Tsuchida A, Kaneko M, Kobayashi H, Kubota T (1993) The kinetics of lymphocyte subsets and macrophages in subarachnoid space after subarachnoid hemorrhage in rats. Stroke 24: 1993–2001

28. Kusaka G, Ishikawa M, Nanda A, Granger DN, Zhang JH (2004) Signaling pathways for early brain injury after subarachnoid hemorrhage. J Cereb Blood Flow Metab 24: 916–925

29. Lagares A, Gómez PA, Lobato RD, Alén JF, Alday R, Campollo J (2001) Prognostic factors on hospital admission after spontaneous subarachnoid haemorrhage. Acta Neurochir (Wien) 143: 665–672

30. Lanzino G, Kassell NF (1999) Double-blind, randomized, vehicle-controlled study of high-dose tirilazad mesylate in women with aneurysmal subarachnoid hemorrhage. Part II: A cooperative study in North America. J Neurosurg 90: 1018–1024

31. Lanzino G, Kassell NF, Dorsch NW, Pasqualin A, Brandt L, Schmiedek P, Truskowski LL, Alves WM (1999) Double-blind,

randomized, vehicle-controlled study of high-dose tirilazad mesylate in women with aneurysmal subarachnoid hemorrhage. Part I: A cooperative study in Europe, Australia, New Zealand, and South Africa. J Neurosurg 90: 1011–1017

32. Macdonald RL (2007) Prevention of cerebral vasospasm after aneurysmal subarachnoid hemorrhage with clazosentan, and ednothelin receptor antagonist (abstract #800). Neurosurgery 59: a453

33. Macdonald RL (2007) Randomized trial of clazosentan for prevention vasospasm after aneurysmal subarachnoid hemorrhage (abstract #462). Stroke 38: a453–a607

34. Mandal M, Mandal A, Das S, Chakraborti T, Sajal C (2003) Clinical implications of matrix metalloproteinases. Mol Cell Biochem 252: 305–329

35. Mathiesen T, Lefvert AK (1996) Cerebrospinal fluid and blood lymphocyte subpopulations following subarachnoid haemorrhage. Br J Neurosurg 10: 89–92

36. Mayhan WG (1999) VEGF increases permeability of the blood–brain barrier via a nitric oxide synthase/cGMP-dependent pathway. Am J Physiol 276: C1148–C1153

37. McGirt MJ, Lynch JR, Blessing R, Warner DS, Friedman AH, Laskowitz DT (2002) Serum von Willebrand factor, matrix metalloproteinase-9, and vascular endothelial growth factor levels predict the onset of cerebral vasospasm after aneurysmal subarachnoid hemorrhage. Neurosurgery 51: 1128–1135

38. Mocco J, Prickett CS, Komotar RJ, Connolly ES, Mayer SA (2007) Potential mechanisms and clinical significance of global cerebral edema following aneurysmal subarachnoid hemorrhage. Neurosurg Focus 22: E7

39. Nakayama T, Illoh K, Ruetzler C, Auh S, Sokoloff L, Hallenbeck J (2007) Intranasal administration of E-selectin to induce immunological tolerization can suppress subarachnoid hemorrhage-induced vasospasm implicating immune and inflammatory mechanisms in its genesis. Brain Res 1132: 177–184

40. Oruckaptan HH, Caner HH, Kilinc K, Ozgen T (2000) No apparent role for neutrophils and neutrophil-derived myeloperoxidase in experimental subarachnoid haemorrhage and vasospasm: a preliminary study. Acta Neurochir (Wien) 142: 83–90

41. Ostrowski RP, Colohan AR, Zhang JH (2006) Molecular mechanisms of early brain injury after subarachnoid hemorrhage. Neurol Res 28: 399–414

42. Park S, Yamaguchi M, Zhou C, Calvert JW, Tang J, Zhang JH (2004) Neurovascular protection reduces early brain injury after subarachnoid hemorrhage. Stroke 35: 2412–2417

43. Pickard JD, Murray GD, Illingworth R, Shaw MD, Teasdale GM, Foy PM, Humphrey PR, Lang DA, Nelson R, Richards P (1989) Effect of oral nimodipine on cerebral infarction and outcome after subarachnoid haemorrhage: British aneurysm nimodipine trial. BMJ 298: 636–642

44. Prunell GF, Svendgaard NA, Alkass K, Mathiesen T (2005) Delayed cell death related to acute cerebral blood flow changes following subarachnoid hemorrhage in the rat brain. J Neurosurg 102: 1046–1054

45. Rabinstein AA, Weigand S, Atkinson JL, Wijdicks EF (2005) Patterns of cerebral infarction in aneurysmal subarachnoid hemorrhage. Stroke 36: 992–997

46. Rosenberg GA (1995) Matrix metalloproteinases in brain injury. J Neurotrauma 12: 833–842

47. Rosenberg GA, Yang Y (2007) Vasogenic edema due to tight junction disruption by matrix metalloproteinases in cerebral ischemia. Neurosurg Focus 22: E4

48. Satoh M, Date I, Ohmoto T, Perkins E, Parent AD (2005) The expression and activation of matrix metalloproteinase-1 after subarachnoid haemorrhage in rats. Acta Neurochir (Wien) 147: 187–193

49. Schievink WI (1997) Intracranial aneurysms. N Engl J Med 336: 28–40

50. Schmidt JM, Rincon F, Fernandez A, Resor C, Kowalski RG, Claassen J, Connolly ES, Fitzsimmons BF, Mayer SA (2007) Cerebral infarction associated with acute subarachnoid hemorrhage. Neurocrit Care 7: 10–17

51. Scozzafava J, Brindley PG, Mehta V, Findlay JM (2007) Decompressive bifrontal craniectomy for malignant intracranial pressure following anterior communicating artery aneurysm rupture: two case reports. Neurocrit Care 6: 49–53

52. Sehba FA, Mostafa G, Knopman J, Friedrich V Jr, Bederson JB (2004) Acute alterations in microvascular basal lamina after subarachnoid hemorrhage. J Neurosurg 101: 633–640

53. Shigeno T, Fritschka E, Brock M, Schramm J, Shigeno S, Cervos-Navarro J (1982) Cerebral edema following experimental subarachnoid hemorrhage. Stroke 13: 368–379

54. Sudlow CL, Warlow CP (1997) Comparable studies of the incidence of stroke and its pathological types: results from an international collaboration. International Stroke Incidence Collaboration. Stroke 28: 491–499

55. Trabold B, Rothoerl R, Wittmann S, Woertgen C, Fröhlich D (2005) Cerebrospinal fluid and neutrophil respiratory burst after subarachnoid hemorrhage. Neuroimmunomodulation 12: 152–156

56. Tseng MY, Czosnyka M, Richards H, Pickard JD, Kirkpatrick PJ (2005) Effects of acute treatment with pravastatin on cerebral vasospasm, autoregulation, and delayed ischemic deficits after aneurysmal subarachnoid hemorrhage: a phase II randomized placebo-controlled trial. Stroke 36: 1627–1632

57. Tseng MY, Hutchinson PJ, Czosnyka M, Richards H, Pickard JD, Kirkpatrick PJ (2007) Effects of acute pravastatin treatment on intensity of rescue therapy, length of inpatient stay, and 6-month outcome in patients after aneurysmal subarachnoid hemorrhage. Stroke 38: 1545–1550

58. Turner CP, Panter SS, Sharp FR (1999) Anti-oxidants prevent focal rat brain injury as assessed by induction of heat shock proteins (HSP70, HO-1/HSP32, HSP47) following subarachnoid injections of lysed blood. Brain Res Mol Brain Res 65: 87–102

59. Voldby B, Enevoldsen EM (1982) Intracranial pressure changes following aneurysm rupture. Part 1: Clinical and angiographic correlations. J Neurosurg 56: 186–196

60. Yatsushige H, Ostrowski RP, Tsubokawa T, Colohan A, Zhang JH (2007) Role of c-Jun N-terminal kinase in early brain injury after subarachnoid hemorrhage. J Neurosci Res 85: 1436–1448

61. Zhang Z, Chopp M (2002) Vascular endothelial growth factor and angiopoietins in focal cerebral ischemia. Trends Cardiovasc Med 12: 62–66

62. Zhang ZG, Zhang L, Jiang Q, Zhang R, Davies K, Powers C, Bruggen N, Chopp M (2000) VEGF enhances angiogenesis and promotes blood–brain barrier leakage in the ischemic brain. J Clin Invest 106: 829–838

Acta Neurochir Suppl (2008) 105: 185–189
© Springer-Verlag 2008
Printed in Austria

Development of a cerebral microvascular dysplasia model in rodents

H. Su[1], Q. Hao[1], F. Shen[1], Y. Zhu[1], C. Z. Lee[1], W. L. Young[1,2,3], G. Y. Yang[1,2]

[1] Center for Cerebrovascular Research, Department of Anesthesia and Perioperative Care, University of California, San Francisco, CA, USA
[2] Department of Neurological Surgery, University of California, San Francisco, CA, USA
[3] Department of Neurology, University of California, San Francisco, CA, USA

Summary

Normal vasculature development of the central nervous system is extremely important because patients with vascular malformations are at life-threatening risk for intracranial hemorrhage or cerebral ischemia. The etiology and pathogenesis of abnormal vasculature development in the central nervous system are unknown, and progress is hampered by the lack of animal models for human cerebrovascular diseases. Here, we report our current study on cerebral microvascular dysplasia (CMVD) development. Using vascular endothelial growth factor hyper-stimulation, we demonstrated that aberrant microvessels could be developed in the rodent brain under certain conditions (such as genetic deficient background, local cytokine and chemokine release, or exogenous vessel dilating stimulation) that may speed up focal angiogenesis and lead to cerebral vascular dysplasia.

Keywords: Cerebral; dysplasia; microvascular; mice; vascular endothelial growth factor.

Introduction

Brain microvascular dysplasia is one of the most critical situations because the aberrant angiogenesis can cause epilepsy, focal ischemia, and even intracranial hemorrhage. During the disease process in cases such as brain trauma, ischemia, or inflammation, local angiogenic factors, e.g., growth factors such as vascular endothelial growth factor [VEGF], platelet derived growth factor [PDGF]; cytokines such as interleukin-1 beta [IL-1β], interleukin-6 [IL-6], transforming growth factor-beta [TGF-β], tumor necrosis factor-alpha [TNFα]; chemokines such as monocyte chemotactic protein-1 [MCP-1], macrophage inflammatory protein-1 [MIP-1]; and others such as netrin-1; matrix metalloproteinases [MMPs], and integrin, etc., are greatly increased [7]. These angiogenic mediators initially activate focal angiogenesis in the body, including brain tissue. Under certain conditions, such as genetic deficiency (endoglin [ENG] and activin-like kinase [ALK] mutation), vessel dilation stimulation (endothelial nitric oxide synthase [eNOS], hydralazine, or nicardipine), or micro-environmental changes (increased VEGF, MMP, integrin, homeobox gene expression), normal angiogenesis then turns to abnormal growth and develops to form cerebral microvascular dysplasia (CMVD). When this process takes place, increased blood–brain barrier (BBB) permeability and focal hemodynamic changes exacerbate existing dysplasia, enhance region of the dysplasia lesion, or even cause focal hemorrhage. Currently, several angiogenic mediators are being used to stimulate CMVD formation in the experimental animal brain. This strategy has provided a unique model for mechanistic studies.

Development of CMVD animal models that phenocopy human disease

Experimental animal models for arteriovenous malformations (AVMs) were first developed by surgeons seeking to understand the complex hemodynamics of arteriovenous shunting and its relationship to "normal perfusion pressure breakthrough," an infrequent but morbid complication of AVM resection [29, 30]. Further model development included attempts to model aspects of the disease related to potential therapy development, such as a target for radiosurgery or embolic agents. A wide variety of models, generally extracranial

Correspondence: Guo-Yuan Yang MD, PhD, UCSF Department of Anesthesia and Perioperative Care, 1001 Potrero Avenue, Rm. 3C-38, San Francisco, CA 94110, USA. e-mail: ccr@anesthesia.ucsf.edu

arteriovenous fistulas between the common or internal carotid artery and the external jugular vein [1, 3, 6, 13, 16, 22] and/or dural fistulas [32, 33], has been described in a number of species, including rats, swine, cats, sheep, chickens, rabbits, pigs, and goats [15, 19–21, 23, 24]. With few exceptions, they are extradural in nature [26]. Of particular note is that they do not display the clinical syndrome of recurrent hemorrhage into the brain parenchyma or cerebrospinal fluid (CSF) spaces. Therefore, a parenchymal nidus is not formed; nidus growth and hemorrhage mimicking the human disease do not occur.

To optimally study pathogenesis and disease progression, a model system is needed to test mechanistic questions. An ideal model system would have the following attributes by phenocopying the clinical cerebrovascular disease: 1) possess a nidus of abnormal vessels of varying sizes, encompassing both micro- and macro-circulatory levels; 2) display spontaneous hemorrhage into the brain parenchyma or CSF spaces (but not preferentially subarachnoid and in basal cisterns); 3) display arteriovenous shunting, including early visualization of efferent veins relative to normal venous circulation; 4) possess flow rates that are sufficient to reproduce lower proximal feeding artery pressure [9, 27]; 5) display high angiogenic and inflammatory signal expression consistent with human surgical specimens [11, 12].

TGF-β signaling is of particular interest (see companion article by Kim *et al.*). Hereditary hemorrhagic telangiectasia (HHT; Osler-weber-Rendu disease) is an autosomal dominant syndrome of mucocutaneous fragility that is strongly associated with both pulmonary and brain AVMs. The 2 common subtypes of HHT (HHT-1 and -2) are caused by well-characterized loss-of-function mutations in 2 genes [18]: ENG, which codes for an accessory protein of TGF-β receptor complexes; and ALK1 or ACVLR1, a transmembrane kinase that participates with TGF-β receptor II in TGF-β signaling. Recently, 2 reports indicate that ALK1 can signal through bone morphogenetic protein 9 (BMP9), and that ENG can potentiate the signal. These newer data suggest that BMP9 may represent the most physiologically relevant *endothelial* signaling pathway for HHT pathogenesis [5, 28]. The downstream target effector for both TGF-β and BMP signaling for AVM pathogenesis is the mothers against decapentaplegic homolog 4 (SMAD4) gene, which is associated with juvenile polyposis and has recently been described for SMAD. This gene is mutated in a combined syndrome of juvenile polyposis and HHT [8].

Approaches to CMVD model development

Based on the above attributes of human lesion tissue, we aimed our model development toward establishing the means by which we simulated relevant aspects of the human disease, either by phenocopying aspects of the vascular phenotype or by genetic manipulation to provide an intermediate phenotype.

Conceptually, dysplasia represents enlarged, dysmorphic vascular structures that have structural instability. Our model was initially based on growth factor hyperstimulation of murine brain by viral transfection. Although many exciting studies have been conducted on the initiation, formation, and growth of angiogenesis, the nature of vascular signaling pathways in abnormal cerebral vascular phenotypes in both human disease and experimental animals is still unclear [17]. The main causes of pathologic angiogenesis in the central nervous system include vascular malformations, tissue ischemia, traumatic damage, and neoplasm. Angiogenesis is a rapidly growing field with some 4477 publications listed in PubMed for the year 2007, 6 times the number from the previous 10 years [2]. Development of a non-tumor brain angiogenesis model is therefore timely.

Hyper-stimulation of angiogenesis can induce abnormal vessel formation in a variety of tissues including the brain [25, 34]. We began our modeling efforts by introducing VEGF into a normal adult circulatory bed by an adenoviral (Ad) or adeno-associated viral (AAV) vector to hyper-stimulate naive tissue, thus deregulating paracrine homeostasis. Although viral vector-delivered hyper-stimulation of VEGF can cause some degree of morphological changes [31], and other kinds of VEGF delivery cause dysmorphic vessels, a combination of the VEGF delivery system with altered genetic background may more reliably produce vascular dysplasia.

To develop a feasible and reproducible focal brain microvessel dysplasia model, we performed the following experiment based on the understanding of multi-systemic focal vascular lesions in HHT disease [10, 17]. Following induction of anesthesia, AAVVEGF was stereotactically injected into the right hemisphere of ENG$^{+/-}$ or ALK1$^{+/-}$ or ENG/ALK1$^{+/-}$ mice. Animals were sacrificed following 3–6 weeks of AAVVEGF gene transfer. Lectin staining was performed for microvessel counting. We found much more abnormal microvessel patterns in the ENG$^{+/-}$, ALK1$^{+/-}$ or ENG/ALK1$^{+/-}$ mice brain following VEGF hyper-stimulation. Our result thus indicated that VEGF hyper-stimulation could induce microvessel dysplasia in the genetic deficient situation.

To develop a CMVD model, we tested the effect of flow-augmentation in VEGF-transduced mice. Using a micro-osmotic pump infusion technique, we observed the effect of hydralazine on microvessel dysplasia formation. We counted microvessel numbers in AAVVEGF-transduced ALK1$^{+/-}$ mice with hydralazine or nicardipine or saline treatment. We found that microvessel counts were greatly increased in the AAVVEGF-transduced mice compared to the AAVlacZ plus saline infusion group; hydralazine or nicardipine did not further increase microvessel counts in hydralazine-treated AAVVEGF or AAVlacZ-transduced ALK1$^{+/-}$ mice. We then counted the number of dilated microvessels (>8 μm in diameter), which increased after treatment with hydralazine or nicardipine in both AAVlacZ and AAVVEGF-transduced mice compared to the saline infusion group mice ($p < 0.05$). BrdU staining showed CD31-positive cells were well-merged with the BrdU-positive staining, indicating active proliferation of endothelial cells in hydralazine or nicardipine infusion in AAVVEGF-transduced ALK1$^{+/-}$ mice.

We further examined the microvascular morphologic changes. Interestingly, we detected much more abnormal microvasculature, such as a massive or single enlarged node, or clustered, twisted, or spiral microvessels, following hydralazine or nicardipine micro-pump infusion in the AAVVEGF-transduced ALK$^{+/-}$ mice than in the saline-infused mice. These abnormal microvessels usually developed in the ipsilateral cortex and caudate putamen adjacent to the needle track. Confocal microscope demonstrated that these abnormal microvessels were not overlapped, confirming the abnormal microvessel morphology.

eNOS is critical for vascular remodeling, mural cell recruitment, and blood flow reserve [36]. eNOS-derived NO can serve as a vasodilator to reduce vascular resistance, improve blood flow, and maintain proportional remodeling of blood vessels during changes in blood flow. In addition, eNOS exerts a second messenger role in VEGF signaling and is necessary for many of the actions of VEGF in cultured endothelial cells or in postnatal mice. PI3K mediates a critical pathway in NO- and VEGF-mediated angiogenesis. *In vivo* results demonstrate that elevated eNOS expression or activity is sufficient to activate the PI3K/Akt signaling pathway via protein kinase G, leading to neovascularization in ischemic tissues [14].

Using adenoviral vector delivering eNOS gene (AdeNOS) transfer, AdeNOS was injected into basal ganglia region in the mouse brain. The result demonstrated that dilated microvessels are increased in the AdeNOS-transduced mouse brain compared to the control (AdlacZ), and eNOS-positive staining is mainly located in the vessel wall. In addition, less eNOS-positive staining was found in the lowest dose group, suggesting that eNOS expression is dose-dependent. We also examined microvessel morphology by lectin staining. Dilated and abnormal microvessels were identified under the hyper-stimulation of eNOS.

Functional consequences of vascular dysplasia

Morphological characterizations are the most visible and widely accepted evidence for vascular dysplasia. However, the functional consequence of vascular dysplasia is important evidence supporting dysplasia vas-

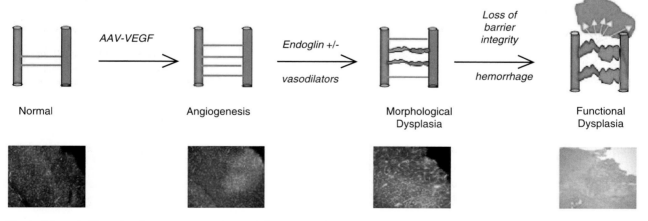

Fig. 1. Schematic illustrating the current approach to modeling vascular dysplasia in the adult brain. Main steps include initiation of angiogenesis with VEGF hyper-stimulation, and induction of morphological dysplastic changes (deficit endoglin in genetic background or local flow increases), which leads to loss of barrier integrity and micro-hemorrhage

culature as being detrimental. Within this functional determination, we decided to examine BBB permeability and micro-hemorrhage because these are often detected in vascular dysplasia.

The main dilemma of pathologic angiogenesis is consistent BBB leakage, which exacerbates brain edema and tissue damage. We demonstrated that BBB disruption occurred during active angiogenesis. BBB permeability was determined using albumin staining, as previously described [35]. BBB permeability also can be determined quantitatively using a measurement of Evans blue with similar results.

Micro-hemorrhage is another complication during active angiogenesis. We also found that micro-hemorrhage occurred in the AdVEGF-transduced mouse brain. The extent of cerebral hemorrhage can be quantified using a spectrophotometric assay with Drabkin's reagent [4]. We demonstrated that hemorrhage was in the mouse brain after injection of AdVEGF, but not in the viral vector control group after AdFc injection. The pattern of intracranial hemorrhage induced by focal VEGF hyper-stimulation in the brain is illustrated using hematoxylin-eosin staining

Conclusions and further considerations for model development

Our primary approach to creating our intermediate brain AVM phenotype has been to combine viral hyper-stimulation with manipulation of genetic background (e.g., ENG-deficient mice), or by manipulation of local hemodynamics (e.g., increased tissue perfusion by local vasodilator infusion), as illustrated in Fig. 1. We hypothesize that with further development of these experimental conditions to achieve a focal vascular lesion, we will detect direct arteriovenous shunting and spontaneous ruptures, which mimic human disease. Continually integrating hemodynamic influences on vascular remodeling is also important.

Furthermore, dysplastic abnormalities are now present in the microcirculation and need to be brought to the level of macrocirculation, as seen in human disease. These *in vivo* animal models will provide us with an opportunity to discern causal relationships in the formation of an abnormal vascular phenotype and to comprehensively investigate the pathways involved. The relationship of vascular dysplasia to the disease remains to be clarified, but this is a first step toward generating a morphological correlate of the human phenotype.

References

1. Bederson JB, Wiestler OD, Brüstle O, Roth P, Frick R, Yasargil MG (1991) Intracranial venous hypertension and the effects of venous outflow obstruction in a rat model of arteriovenous fistula. Neurosurgery 29: 341–350
2. Carmeliet P (2005) Angiogenesis in life, disease and medicine. Nature 438: 932–936
3. Chaloupka JC, Viñuela F, Robert J, Duckwiler GR (1994) An in vivo arteriovenous malformation model in swine: preliminary feasibility and natural history study. Am J Neuroradiol 15: 945–950
4. Choudhri TF, Baker KZ, Winfree CJ, Hoh BL, Simon A, Solomon RA, Berman M, Connolly ES (1997) Intraoperative mild hypothermia is not associated with increased craniotomy wound infection rate or length of hospitalization. Surg Forum 48: 548–551
5. David L, Mallet C, Mazerbourg S, Feige JJ, Bailly S (2007) Identification of BMP9 and BMP10 as functional activators of the orphan activin receptor-like kinase 1 (ALK1) in endothelial cells. Blood 109: 1953–1961
6. De Mey JG, Schiffers PM, Hilgers RH, Sanders MM (2005) Toward functional genomics of flow-induced outward remodeling of resistance arteries. Am J Physiol Heart Circ Physiol 288: H1022–H1027
7. Fan Y, Yang GY (2007) Therapeutic angiogenesis for brain ischemia: a brief review. J Neuroimmune Pharmacol 2: 284–289
8. Gallione CJ, Richards JA, Letteboer TG, Rushlow D, Prigoda NL, Leedom TP, Ganguly A, Castells A, Ploos van Amstel JK, Westermann CJ, Pyeritz RE, Marchuk DA (2006) SMAD4 mutations found in unselected HHT patients. J Med Genet 43: 793–797
9. Gao E, Young WL, Ornstein E, Pile-Spellman J, Ma Q (1997) A theoretical model of cerebral hemodynamics: application to the study of arteriovenous malformations. J Cereb Blood Flow Metab 17: 905–918
10. Guttmacher AE, Marchuk DA, White RI Jr (1995) Hereditary hemorrhagic telangiectasia. N Engl J Med 333: 918–924
11. Hashimoto T, Young WL (2004) Roles of angiogenesis and vascular remodeling in brain vascular malformations. Semin Cerebrovasc Dis Stroke 4: 217–225
12. Hashimoto T, Wu Y, Lawton MT, Yang GY, Barbaro NM, Young WL (2005) Co-expression of angiogenic factors in brain arteriovenous malformations. Neurosurgery 56: 1058–1065
13. Herman JM, Spetzler RF, Bederson JB, Kurbat JM, Zabramski JM (1995) Genesis of a dural arteriovenous malformation in a rat model. J Neurosurg 83: 539–545
14. Kawasaki K, Smith RS Jr, Hsieh CM, Sun J, Chao J, Liao JK (2003) Activation of the phosphatidylinositol 3-kinase/protein kinase Akt pathway mediates nitric oxide-induced endothelial cell migration and angiogenesis. Mol Cell Biol 23: 5726–5737
15. Kutluk K, Schumacher M, Mironov A (1991) The role of sinus thrombosis in occipital dural arteriovenous malformations – development and spontaneous closure. Neurochirurgia (Stuttg) 34: 144–147
16. Lawton MT, Jacobowitz R, Spetzler RF (1997) Redefined role of angiogenesis in the pathogenesis of dural arteriovenous malformations. J Neurosurg 87: 267–274
17. Lim M, Cheshier S, Steinberg GK (2006) New vessel formation in the central nervous system during tumor growth, vascular malformations, and Moyamoya. Curr Neurovasc Res 3: 237–245
18. Marchuk DA, Srinivasan S, Squire TL, Zawistowski JS (2003) Vascular morphogenesis: tales of two syndromes. Hum Mol Genet 12: R97–R112
19. Massoud TF, Ji C, Viñuela F, Guglielmi G, Robert J, Duckwiler GR, Gobin YP (1994) An experimental arteriovenous malformation model in swine: anatomic basis and construction technique. Am J Neuroradiol 15: 1537–1545
20. Massoud TF, Ji C, Vinuela F, Turjman F, Guglielmi G, Duckwiler GR, Gobin YP (1996) Laboratory simulations and training in

endovascular embolotherapy with a swine arteriovenous malformation model. Am J Neuroradiol 17: 271–279

21. Morgan MK, Anderson RE, Sundt TM Jr (1989) The effects of
    hyperventilation on cerebral blood flow in the rat with an open and
    closed carotid-jugular fistula. Neurosurgery 25: 606–612
22. Morgan MK, Anderson RE, Sundt TM Jr (1989) A model of the
    pathophysiology of cerebral arteriovenous malformations by a
    carotid-jugular fistula in the rat. Brain Res 496: 241–250
23. Murayama Y, Massoud TF, Viñuela F (1998) Hemodynamic
    changes in arterial feeders and draining veins during embolotherapy
    of arteriovenous malformations: an experimental study in a swine
    model. Neurosurgery 43: 96–106
24. Nagasawa S, Kawanishi M, Kondoh S, Kajimoto S, Yamaguchi K,
    Ohta T (1996) Hemodynamic simulation study of cerebral arterio-
    venous malformations. Part 2. Effects of impaired autoregulation
    and induced hypotension. J Cereb Blood Flow Metab 16: 162–169
25. Ozawa CR, Banfi A, Glazer NL, Thurston G, Springer ML, Kraft
    PE, McDonald DM, Blau HM (2004) Microenvironmental VEGF
    concentration, not total dose, determines a threshold between
    normal and aberrant angiogenesis. J Clin Invest 113: 516–527
26. Pietilä TA, Zabramski JM, Thèllier-Janko A, Duveneck K,
    Bichard WD, Brock M, Spetzler RF (2000) Animal model for
    cerebral arteriovenous malformation. Acta Neurochir (Wien) 142:
    1231–1240
27. Quick CM, Leonard EF, Young WL (2002) Adaptation of cerebral
    circulation to brain arteriovenous malformations increases feeding
    artery pressure and decreases regional hypotension. Neurosurgery
    50: 167–175
28. Scharpfenecker M, van Dinther M, Liu Z, van Bezooijen RL, Zhao
    Q, Pukac L, Löwik CW, ten Dijke P (2007) BMP-9 signals via
    ALK1 and inhibits bFGF-induced endothelial cell proliferation and
    VEGF-stimulated angiogenesis. J Cell Sci 120: 964–972
29. Scott BB, McGillicuddy JE, Seeger JF, Kindt GW, Giannotta SL
    (1978) Vascular dynamics of an experimental cerebral arteriove-
    nous shunt in the primate. Surg Neurol 10: 34–38
30. Spetzler RF, Wilson CB, Weinstein P, Mehdorn M, Townsend J,
    Telles D (1978) Normal perfusion pressure breakthrough theory.
    Clin Neurosurg 25: 651–672
31. Stiver SI, Tan X, Brown LF, Hedley-Whyte ET, Dvorak HF (2004)
    VEGF-A angiogenesis induces a stable neovasculature in adult
    murine brain. J Neuropathol Exp Neurol 63: 841–855
32. Terada T, Higashida RT, Halbach VV, Dowd CF, Tsuura M, Komai
    N, Wilson CB, Hieshima GB (1994) Development of acquired
    arteriovenous fistulas in rats due to venous hypertension. J Neuro-
    surg 80: 884–889
33. TerBrugge KG, Lasjaunias P, Hallacq P (1991) Experimental
    models in interventional neuroradiology. Am J Neuroradiol 12:
    1029–1033
34. Xu B, Wu YQ, Huey M, Arthur HM, Marchuk DA, Hashimoto T,
    Young WL, Yang GY (2004) Vascular endothelial growth factor
    induces abnormal microvasculature in the endoglin heterozygous
    mouse brain. J Cereb Blood Flow Metab 24: 237–244
35. Yang GY, Betz AL (1994) Reperfusion-induced injury to the blood–
    brain barrier after middle cerebral artery occlusion in rats. Stroke
    25: 1658–1665
36. Yu J, deMuinck ED, Zhuang Z, Drinane M, Kauser K, Rubanyi GM,
    Qian HS, Murata T, Escalante B, Sessa WC (2005) Endothelial
    nitric oxide synthase is critical for ischemic remodeling, mural cell
    recruitment, and blood flow reserve. Proc Natl Acad Sci USA 102:
    10999–11004

Acta Neurochir Suppl (2008) 105: 191–196
© Springer-Verlag 2008
Printed in Austria

Hyperbaric oxygen preconditioning protects against traumatic brain injury at high altitude

S. L. Hu, R. Hu, F. Li, Z. Liu, Y. Z. Xia, G. Y. Cui, H. Feng

Department of Neurosurgery, Southwest Hospital of the Third Military Medical University, Chongqing, P.R. China

Summary

Background. Recent studies have shown that preconditioning with hyperbaric oxygen (HBO) can reduce ischemic and hemorrhagic brain injury. We investigated effects of HBO preconditioning on traumatic brain injury (TBI) at high altitude and examined the role of matrix metalloproteinase-9 (MMP-9) in such protection.

Methods. Rats were randomly divided into 3 groups: HBO preconditioning group (HBOP; $n = 13$), high-altitude group (HA; $n = 13$), and high-altitude sham operation group (HASO; $n = 13$). All groups were subjected to head trauma by weight-drop device, except for HASO group. HBOP rats received 5 sessions of HBO preconditioning (2.5 ATA, 100% oxygen, 1 h daily) and then were kept in hypobaric chamber at 0.6 ATA (to simulate pressure at 4000 m altitude) for 3 days before operation. HA rats received control pretreatment (1 ATA, room air, 1 h daily), then followed the same procedures as HBOP group. HASO rats were subjected to skull opening only without brain injury. Twenty-four hours after TBI, 7 rats from each group were examined for neurological function and brain water content; 6 rats from each group were killed for analysis by H&E staining and immunohistochemistry.

Results. Neurological outcome in HBOP group (0.71 ± 0.49) was better than HA group (1.57 ± 0.53; $p < 0.05$). Preconditioning with HBO significantly reduced percentage of brain water content (86.24 ± 0.52 vs. 84.60 ± 0.37; $p < 0.01$). Brain morphology and structure seen by light microscopy was diminished in HA group, while fewer pathological injuries occurred in HBOP group. Compared to HA group, pretreatment with HBO significantly reduced the number of MMP-9-positive cells (92.25 ± 8.85 vs. 74.42 ± 6.27; $p < 0.01$).

Conclusions. HBO preconditioning attenuates TBI in rats at high altitude. Decline in MMP-9 expression may contribute to HBO preconditioning-induced protection of brain tissue against TBI.

Keywords: Traumatic brain injury; hyperbaric oxygen; matrix metalloproteinase-9; preconditioning.

Introduction

It is widely accepted that a number of preconditioning stimuli, including ischemia [21], hypoxia [4, 15], and drugs (such as cytokines [11], potassium chloride [25], and morphine [9]), can induce ischemic tolerance. While the previously described preconditioning methods are good for protection of the central nervous system, the application of ischemia and hypoxia preconditioning is ethically problematic in a clinical setting, and pharmacological preconditioning is questionable because of drug toxicity and side effects [2].

Accumulated evidence from recent studies shows that preconditioning with hyperbaric oxygen (HBO) can reduce ischemic brain injury [21, 24]. In addition, Qin and colleagues [13] found that preconditioning with HBO can induce tolerance to brain edema formation after experimental intracerebral hemorrhage. It is well-known that the critical factors influencing the prognosis of traumatic brain injury (TBI) are ischemia, hypoxia, hemorrhage, and edema [6, 18]. What is more, there is evidence to prove that the reduced supply of oxygen at high altitudes may lead to brain damage [3]. Therefore, we hypothesized that preconditioning with HBO can induce protective effects against TBI in rats at high altitudes.

Matrix metalloproteinase-9 (MMP-9) is one kind of zinc-dependent endopeptidases and is associated with blood–brain barrier opening and brain edema formation after TBI. Hyperbaric oxygenation can reduce expression of MMP-9 following TBI [20], suggesting a role for MMP-9 in the effects of pretreatment with repeated hyperbaric oxygenation.

This study was conducted to determine whether HBO preconditioning can induce brain protection against TBI in rats at simulated high altitude, and the role of MMP-9 in HBO preconditioning-induced protection of brain tissue against TBI.

Correspondence: H. Feng, Department of Neurosurgery, Southwest Hospital, Chongqing 400038, P.R. China. e-mail: fenghua8888@sohu.com

Materials and methods

The animal study protocol used in this research was approved by the Ethics Committee for Animal Experimentation and was conducted according to the Guidelines for Animal Experimentation of our institution. The animals were studied at Southwest Hospital of the Third Military Medical University, Chongqing, China.

Animal preparation

Thirty-nine males Sprague-Dawley rats (Experimental Animal Center of the Third Military Medical University) weighing between 200 and 240 g were used in this study. Rats were allowed free access to food and water before and after the surgical procedure. Animals were anesthetized with an intraperitoneal injection of pentobarbital (40 mg/kg). Rectal temperature was maintained at 37–37.5 °C using overhead lamps during the experiment. Arterial blood was sampled from the right femoral artery for analysis of arterial oxygen tension (PaO_2), arterial carbon dioxide tension ($PaCO_2$), pH, hematocrit, and plasma glucose levels 24 h after surgical operation.

Surgical procedures

The rats were subjected to head trauma using a weight-drop device based on the technique described by Queen and colleagues [14]. After removal from the hypobaric chamber, rats were anesthetized with an intraperitoneal injection of pentobarbital (40 mg/kg) and then placed in a stereotactic apparatus. A 4-cm long skin incision was made in the midline, and a 1-mm burr hole was drilled in the skull (2 mm anterior to lambdoid suture and 2 mm lateral to midline). The hole was then enlarged to 5 mm in diameter using a hemostatic forceps, leaving the dura intact. An area in the parietal and temporal lobe was contused by delivery of a 600 g × cm force, produced by dropping a 30-g weight a distance of 20 cm through a stainless steel guide tube onto a 4-mm diameter steel cylinder. The sham-operated rats were treated identically except for the contusion. After impact, the skull hole was filled with bone wax, and the skin incision was closed using sutures.

Experimental protocol

Thirty-nine males Sprague-Dawley rats were randomly assigned to 1 of 3 groups: HBO preconditioning group (HBOP; $n = 13$), high-altitude group (HA; $n = 13$) and high-altitude sham operation group (HASO; $n = 13$). The rats in the HBOP group received 1 h of HBO at 2.5 atmosphere absolute (ATA) in 100% oxygen each day for 5 days using an animal hyperbaric chamber, and then were kept in a hypobaric chamber at a pressure of 0.6 ATA for 3 days before operation. The rats were subjected to head trauma using a weight-drop device. The animals in the HA group were placed in a chamber (21% O_2), which was not pressurized for sham treatments, using the same 5-day schedule and the same procedures as the HBOP group. In the HASO group, rats received skull opening without brain injury. Twenty-four hours after TBI, 7 rats from each group were examined for neurological function and brain water content, and 6 rats from each group were killed for analysis by hematoxylin and eosin (H&E) staining and immunohistochemistry.

Hyperbaric and hypobaric oxygen procedure

Animals in HBOP group were placed in a small rodent HBO chamber (Binglun Corp., China). The chamber was pressurized for 20 min to a pressure of 2.5 ATA with 100% oxygen supplied continuously and maintained for 60 min. Decompression was then performed for 30 min. Animals in the other 2 groups were also transferred into the HBO chamber but received normobaric room air. Decompression

and pressurization of the hypobaric chamber (Binglun Corp.) were performed for 30 and 20 min, respectively.

Neurological evaluation and brain water content measurement

Twenty-four hours after TBI, 7 rats from each group were neurologically assessed by an observer who was unaware of the grouping, using the modified Longa criteria [28]: 0 = no deficit; 1 = failure to extend left forepaw fully; 2 = circling to the left; 3 = falling to the left; 4 = no spontaneous walking with a depressed level of consciousness; 5 = dead. dead. After completion of the neurological evaluation, animals were re-anesthetized using an intraperitoneal injection of 50 mg/kg of pentobarbital, then decapitated to measure brain water, as described previously [23]. The rat brains were removed and cortical tissue (about 150 mg) 4.5 mm from the center of the wound was cut with a blade. Brain samples were immediately weighed on an electronic analytical balance (analytical fidelity 0.1 mg; Jingtian Instruments Corp., China) to obtain wet weight (WW). Dried weight (DW) of the samples was determined after the tissues were heated for 48 h at 80 °C in an electronic homeothermic oven. The percentage of tissue water content was then calculated according to the following formula: $100 \times (WW - DW)/WW$.

Histopathologic examination

Twenty-four hours after TBI, 6 rats from each group were re-anesthetized and perfused intracardially with 4% paraformaldehyde in 0.1 M phosphate-buffered saline (PBS; pH 7.4). Brains were removed and immersed in 10% formaldehyde for 3 to 6 days at 4 °C. After dehydration in graded concentrations of ethanol and butanol, each brain was embedded in paraffin. Coronal sections of brain tissue (with the wound as center) were cut at a thickness of 5 μm and H by a blinded observer.

Immunohistochemical analyses

Twenty-four hours after TBI, 6 rats from each group were re-anesthetized and perfused intracardially with 4% paraformaldehyde in 0.1 M PBS (pH 7.4). Brains were removed and immersed in 10% formaldehyde for 3 to 6 days at 4 °C. After dehydration in graded concentrations of ethanol and butanol, each brain was embedded in paraffin. Coronal sections of the brain tissue (with the wound as center) were cut at a thickness of 5 μm. Sections were incubated according to the SP technique. The primary antibody was polyclonal rabbit anti-MMP-9 (1:100 dilution; Santa Cruz Biotechnology, Santa Cruz, CA). The second antibody was goat anti-rabbit immunoglobulin-G (Reactant kit; Zhongshan Corp., China). PBS (0.1 M, pH 7.4) was used as a negative control. The staining of cells was evaluated at a magnification of 250× by a blinded investigator. Positive cells were identified by the brown color of staining. In each slice, positive cells were counted in 2 sections for each animal and then averaged.

Statistical analyses

Data are expressed as mean ± standard deviation. Changes in arterial pH, PaO_2, $PaCO_2$, hematocrit, blood glucose concentration, neurological deficit scores, brain water content, and number of MMP-9 positive cells were compared using independent samples t test or one-way ANOVA and a Tukey multiple comparison test.

Results

Physiological variables

Physiological parameters in all groups were recorded 24 h after TBI. Variables included blood pH, PaO_2,

Table 1. *Physiological variables recorded 24 h after traumatic brain injury in rats*

Treatment group	pH	PaO_2 (mmHg)	$PaCO_2$ (mmHg)	Hematocrit (%)	Glucose (mmol/L)
High-altitude sham operation	7.41 ± 0.05	82 ± 7.8	39.9 ± 5.5	45.5 ± 3.5	7.54 ± 1.57
High altitude	7.35 ± 0.03	73 ± 9.4	46.0 ± 7.0	42.1 ± 2.4	8.35 ± 2.70
Hyperbaric oxygen preconditioning	7.32 ± 0.07	85 ± 5.0	42.2 ± 4.9	43.0 ± 3.9	7.72 ± 2.21

Data are expressed as mean ± SD.

$PaCO_2$, hematocrit, and plasma glucose level, and values were similar in all groups (Table 1).

HBO preconditioning improved neurological outcome

All animals survived until neurological assessment at 24 h after TBI. Neurological outcome in HBOP group (0.71 ± 0.49) was better than that of HA group (1.57 ± 0.53; $p < 0.05$; 7 rats per group; Fig. 1). Two animals in HBOP group showed completely normal neurological function 24 h after TBI. No animals in HA group showed normal neurological function. All animals in HASO group had normal function.

HBO preconditioning reduced brain water content

Preconditioning with HBO significantly reduced the percentage of brain water content in cortex 24 h after TBI (84.60 ± 0.37 in HBOP group compared with 86.24 ± 0.52 in HA group; $p < 0.01$; 7 rats per group; Fig. 2).

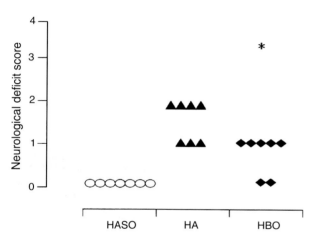

Fig. 1. Neurological outcome 24 h after TBI. *HA* group exposed to 21% O_2 at 1 ATA for 1 h each day for 5 days; *HBO* group exposed to HBO in 100% O_2 at 2.5 ATA for 1 h each day for 5 days. *$p < 0.05$ compared with HA group

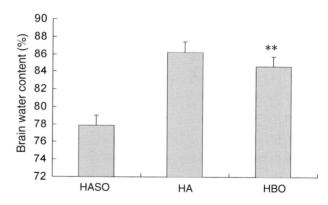

Fig. 2. Percentage of brain water content in brain cortex 24 h after TBI in rats. *HA* group exposed to 21% O^2 at 1 ATA for 1 h each day for 5 days; *HBO* group exposed to HBO in 100% O_2 at 2.5 ATA for 1 h each day for 5 days. **$p < 0.01$ compared with HASO group, compared with HA group ($p < 0.01$)

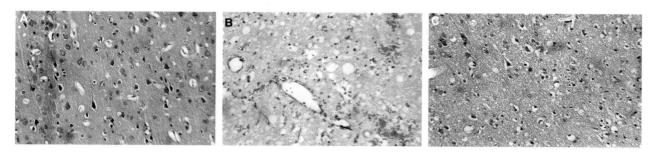

Fig. 3. Photomicrographs showing brain morphology and structure, stained with hematoxylin and eosin 24 h after TBI in rats. (A) HASO group; minimal change. (B) HA group exposed to 21% O_2 at 1 ATA for 1 h each day for 5 days; dramatic decrease in number of cells, conspicuous edema of interstitium, and hemorrhage. (C) HBO group exposed to HBO in 100% O_2 at 2.5 ATA for 1 h each day for 5 days; fewer pathological injuries occurred

HBO preconditioning improved histopathologic outcome

Brain morphology and structure as shown by light microscopy was greatly diminished in HA group, with massive cells necrosis, dramatic decrease in neurons, and conspicuous edema of interstitium, while fewer pathological injuries occurred in HBOP group. There was little change in HASO group (Fig. 3).

HBO preconditioning decreased number of MMP-9 positive cells

To examine the role of MMP-9 in HBO preconditioning-induced brain protection, expression of MMP-9 was observed using immunohistochemical techniques. We found that, compared to HA group, pretreatment with HBO significantly reduced the number of MMP-9-positive cells (92.25 ± 8.85 vs. 74.42 ± 6.27; $p < 0.01$; 6 rats per group; Fig. 4). There was minimal expression of MMP-9 in the HASO group (Fig. 5).

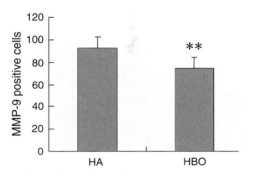

Fig. 4. Number of MMP-9 positive cells by immunohistochemical analysis in brain cortex 24 h after TBI in rats. *HA* Group exposed to 21% O_2 at 1 ATA for 1 h each day for 5 days. *HBO* group exposed to HBO in 100% O_2 at 2.5 ATA for 1 h each day for 5 days. $**p < 0.01$ compared with HA group

Discussion

The major findings of this study are that repeated exposure to HBO before TBI in rats at simulated high altitude can induce tolerance to TBI, and that the mechanism of HBO preconditioning-induced neuroprotection may be related to its inhibiting effect on the expression of MMP-9.

In 1996, Wada *et al.* [21] first reported ischemic tolerance could be obtained in the brain by HBO preconditioning. Further research found that the same phenomenon occurs in spinal cord [2], heart [26], liver [27], and kidney [5]. Recently, Qin and coworkers [13] reported that repeated administration of HBO can produce protective effects against brain edema formation after experimental intracerebral hemorrhage. However, it is important to choose the optimal stimulus intensity and interval between preconditioning treatment and subsequent insult. To determine the preferential conditions for induction of ischemic tolerance by HBO, Wada *et al.* [22] compared the effects of preconditioning with 5 sessions of HBO (100% oxygen, 2 ATA), 10 sessions of HBO (100% oxygen, 3 ATA), and 1 session of HBO (100% oxygen, 2 ATA), and found that preconditioning with 5 sessions of HBO (100% oxygen, 2 ATA) induced ischemic tolerance and the other session numbers did not. Qin *et al.* [13] also found that 5 sessions rather than 2 or 3 sessions of preconditioning with HBO can induce brain protection against hemorrhagic edema formation. However, to date, it is unclear whether or not repeated hyperbaric oxygenation can reduce brain damage after TBI at high altitude. In this study, we demonstrated that HBO preconditioning can induce tolerance to TBI.

Past studies have suggested that the mechanisms by which preconditioning with HBO results in neuroprotection involved increased expression of heme oxygenase-1 [8], upregulation of antioxidant enzymes such as cata-

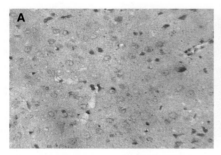
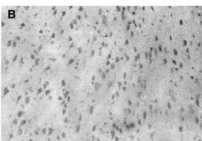
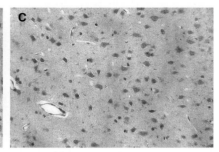

Fig. 5. Photomicrographs showing immunohistochemical analysis of MMP-9 positive cells in brain cortex 24 h after TBI in rats. (A) HASO group. (B) HA group exposed to 21% O_2 at 1 ATA for 1 h each day for 5 days. (C) HBO group exposed to HBO in 100% O_2 at 2.5 ATA 1 h each day for 5 days

lase and superoxide dismutase [12], activation of p44/p42 mitogen-activated protein kinases (p44/p42 MAPK) [13], or inhibition of infiltration of polymorphonuclear neutrophils [10]. However, relatively little is known regarding the exact mechanism. Our current study suggests the role of MMP-9 in HBO preconditioning-induced brain protection. MMP-9 is a member of the MMP family, which are zinc-dependent endopeptidases that cleave protein components of extracellular matrix such as collagens, laminin, fibronectin, and proteoglycans. Recent evidence suggests that MMPs contribute to acute edema and lesion formation following TBI, and MMP-9 levels increase significantly in brain 24 h after trauma [17, 19]. Hyperbaric oxygenation can reduce expression of MMP-9 in the rat [20], which implies that HBO preconditioning-induced tolerance to TBI might be associated with its inhibiting effects on expression of MMP-9. Previous studies have demonstrated preconditioning with HBO can activate p44/p42 MAPK [13] in the brain and decrease infiltration of neutrophils [10]. Shin *et al.* [16] found that activation of p38 MAPK resulted in down-regulation of MMP-9. P38 MAPK is closely related in structure and function to p44/p42 MAPK. Therefore, although the precise mechanisms by which HBO preconditioning leads to decreased expression of MMP-9 are unknown, the effects may be caused partially through activation of MAPK or attenuation of neutrophil inflammatory response, which provide the main source of MMP-9 [20].

There are many high-altitude districts in the world, such as the Qinghai-Tibet Plateau in western China. With the economic development of the Qinghai-Tibet Plateau and the building up of Qinghai-Tibet railway, more and more people travel to Tibet for pleasure or business, which may lead to a rise in morbidity for TBI at high altitudes. Our results indicate that repeated HBO as pretreatment may be beneficial to people traveling to Qinghai-Tibet Plateau.

Surgical operations, like traumatic injuries, may result in hemorrhage, edema, ischemia, and/or hypoxia. HBO, as a new preconditioning stimulus, has many advantages compared with ischemic preconditioning and pharmacological preconditioning and may be a potential method for preconditioning before surgery if proven safe and helpful. Kurir *et al.* [7] found that repeated hyperbaric oxygenation before partial hepatectomy promotes liver regeneration and improves liver function postoperatively. To evaluate the effects of HBO preconditioning on brain ischemia in patients undergoing cardiopulmonary bypass, Alex *et al.* [1] compared the effects of precon-

ditioning with HBO (oxygen, 2.4 ATA) and control air (atmospheric air, 1.5 ATA), and found that preconditioning with HBO rather than control air can reduce neuropsychometric dysfunction and also modulate the inflammatory response after cardiopulmonary bypass.

In conclusion, serial exposure to HBO as preconditioning can attenuate TBI in rats at simulated high altitude. The decline in MMP-9 expression may contribute to HBO preconditioning-induced protection of brain tissue against TBI. Pretreatment with HBO might be beneficial for people traveling to high altitude districts.

Acknowledgments

This work was supported by the key technologies R&D program of China (2006BAI01A13) and the medical research program of PLA of China (06MB241, 01L049). The authors thank Jiasi Bai, M.D. (Technician, Department of Central Laboratory, Southwest Hospital, Chongqing, China), Rong Zhang (Technician, Department of Pathology, Southwest Hospital, Chongqing, China), and Shibing Zhang and Jiexiang Pan, B.S. (Technicians, Hyperbaric Oxygen Center, Southwest Hospital, Chongqing, China) for their technical assistance.

References

1. Alex J, Laden G, Cale AR, Bennett S, Flowers K, Madden L, Gardiner E, McCollum PT, Griffin SC (2005) Pretreatment with hyperbaric oxygen and its effect on neuropsychometric dysfunction and systemic inflammatory response after cardiopulmonary bypass: a prospective randomized double-blind trial. J Thorac Cardiovasc Surg 130: 1623–1630

2. Dong H, Xiong L, Zhu Z, Chen S, Hou L, Sakabe T (2002) Preconditioning with hyperbaric oxygen and hyperoxia induces tolerance against spinal cord ischemia in rabbits. Anesthesiology 96: 907–912

3. Fayed N, Modrego PJ, Morales H (2006) Evidence of brain damage after high-altitude climbing by means of magnetic resonance imaging. Am J Med 119: 168.e1–6

4. Freiberger JJ, Suliman HB, Sheng H, McAdoo J, Piantadosi CA, Warner DS (2006) A comparison of hyperbaric oxygen versus hypoxic cerebral preconditioning in neonatal rats. Brain Res 1075: 213–222

5. Gurer A, Ozdogan M, Gomceli I, Demirag A, Gulbahar O, Arikok T, Kulacoglu H, Dundar K, Ozlem N (2006) Hyperbaric oxygenation attenuates renal ischemia-reperfusion injury in rats. Transplant Proc 38: 3337–3340

6. Krishnappa IK, Contant CF, Robertson CS (1999) Regional changes in cerebral extracellular glucose and lactate concentrations following severe cortical impact injury and secondary ischemia in rats. J Neurotraum 16: 213–224

7. Kurir TT, Markotić A, Katalinić V, Bozanić D, Cikes V, Zemunik T, Modun D, Rincić J, Boraska V, Bota B, Salamunić I, Radić S (2004) Effect of hyperbaric oxygenation on the regeneration of the liver after partial hepatectomy in rats. Braz J Med Biol Res 37: 1231–1237

8. Li Q, Li J, Zhang L, Wang B, Xiong L (2007) Preconditioning with hyperbaric oxygen induces tolerance against oxidative injury via increased expression of heme oxygenase-1 in primary cultured spinal cord neurons. Life Sci 80: 1087–1093

9. Lim YJ, Zheng S, Zuo Z (2004) Morphine preconditions Purkinje cells against cell death under in vitro simulated ischemia-reperfusion conditions. Anesthesiology 100: 562–568

10. Miljkovic-Lolic M, Silbergleit R, Fiskum G, Rosenthal RE (2003) Neuroprotective effects of hyperbaric oxygen treatment in experimental focal cerebral ischemia are associated with reduced brain leukocyte myeloperoxidase activity. Brain Res 971: 90–94

11. Nawashiro H, Tasaki K, Ruetzler CA, Hallenbeck JM (1997) TNF-alpha pretreatment induces protective effects against focal cerebral ischemia in mice. J Cereb Blood Flow Metab 17: 483–490

12. Nie H, Xiong L, Lao N, Chen S, Xu N, Zhu Z (2006) Hyperbaric oxygen preconditioning induces tolerance against spinal cord ischemia by upregulation of antioxidant enzymes in rabbits. J Cereb Blood Flow Metab 26: 666–674

13. Qin Z, Song S, Xi G, Silbergleit R, Keep RF, Hoff JT, Hua Y (2007) Preconditioning with hyperbaric oxygen attenuates brain edema after experimental intracerebral hemorrhage. Neurosurg Focus 22: E13

14. Queen SA, Chen MJ, Feeney DM (1997) d-Amphetamine attenuates decreased cerebral glucose utilization after unilateral sensorimotor cortex contusion in rats. Brain Res 777: 42–50

15. Rauca C, Zerbe R, Jantze H, Krug M (2000) The importance of free hydroxyl radicals to hypoxia preconditioning. Brain Res 868: 147–149

16. Shin CY, Lee WJ, Choi JW, Choi MS, Park GH, Yoo BK, Han SY, Ryu JR, Choi EY, Ko KH (2007) Role of p38 MAPK on the downregulation of matrix metalloproteinase-9 expression in rat astrocytes. Arch Pharm Res 30: 624–633

17. Sifringer M, Stefovska V, Zentner I, Hansen B, Stepulak A, Knaute C, Marzahn J, Ikonomidou C (2007) The role of matrix metalloproteinases in infant traumatic brain injury. Neurobiol Dis 25: 526–535

18. Tan S, Zhou F, Nielsen VG, Wang Z, Gladson CL, Parks DA (1999) Increased injury following intermittent fetal hypoxia-reoxygenation is associated with increased free radical production in fetal rabbit brain. J Neuropathol Exp Neurol 58: 972–981

19. Truettner JS, Alonso OF, Dalton Dietrich W (2005) Influence of therapeutic hypothermia on matrix metalloproteinase activity after traumatic brain injury in rats. J Cereb Blood Flow Metab 25: 1505–1516

20. Vlodavsky E, Palzur E, Soustiel JF (2006) Hyperbaric oxygen therapy reduces neuroinflammation and expression of matrix metalloproteinase-9 in the rat model of traumatic brain injury. Neuropathol Appl Neurobiol 32: 40–50

21. Wada K, Ito M, Miyazawa T, Katoh H, Nawashiro H, Shima K, Chigasaki H (1996) Repeated hyperbaric oxygen induces ischemic tolerance in gerbil hippocampus. Brain Res 740: 15–20

22. Wada K, Miyazawa T, Nomura N, Tsuzuki N, Nawashiro H, Shima K (2001) Preferential conditions for and possible mechanisms of induction of ischemic tolerance by repeated hyperbaric oxygenation in gerbil hippocampus. Neurosurgery 49:160–167

23. Xi G, Keep RF, Hoff JT (1998) Erythrocytes and delayed brain edema formation following intracerebral hemorrhage in rats. J Neurosurg 89: 991–996

24. Xiong L, Zhu Z, Dong H, Hu W, Hou L, Chen S (2000) Hyperbaric oxygen preconditioning induces neuroprotection against ischemia in transient not permanent middle cerebral artery occlusion rat model. Chin Med J (Engl) 113: 836–839

25. Yanamoto H, Hashimoto N, Nagata I, Kikuchi H (1998) Infarct tolerance against temporary focal ischemia following spreading depression in rat brain. Brain Res 784: 239–249

26. Yogaratnam JZ, Laden G, Madden LA, Seymour AM, Guvendik L, Cowen M, Greenman J, Cale A, Griffin S (2006) Hyperbaric oxygen: a new drug in myocardial revascularization and protection? Cardiovasc Revasc Med 7: 146–154

27. Yu SY, Chiu JH, Yang SD, Yu HY, Hsieh CC, Chen PJ, Lui WY, Wu CW (2005) Preconditioned hyperbaric oxygenation protects the liver against ischemia-reperfusion injury in rats. J Surg Res 128: 28–36

28. Longa EZ, Weinstein PR, Carlson S, Cummins R (1989) Reversible middle cerebral artery occlusion without craniectomy in rats. Stroke 20: 84–91

Human intracranial hemorrhage (non-intracerebral hemorrhage)

Acta Neurochir Suppl (2008) 105: 199–206
© Springer-Verlag 2008
Printed in Austria

Genetic considerations relevant to intracranial hemorrhage and brain arteriovenous malformations

H. Kim[1,2], **D. A. Marchuk**[3], **L. Pawlikowska**[1], **Y. Chen**[1], **H. Su**[1], **G. Y. Yang**[1,4], **W. L. Young**[1,2,5]

[1] Center for Cerebrovascular Research, Department of Anesthesia and Perioperative Care, University of California, San Francisco, CA, USA
[2] Institute for Human Genetics, University of California, San Francisco, CA, USA
[3] Department of Molecular Genetics and Microbiology, Duke University School of Medicine, Durham, NC, USA
[4] Department of Neurological Surgery, University of California, San Francisco, CA, USA
[5] Department of Neurology, University of California, San Francisco, CA, USA

Summary

Brain arteriovenous malformations (AVMs) cause intracranial hemorrhage (ICH), especially in young adults. Molecular characterization of lesional tissue provides evidence for involvement of both angiogenic and inflammatory pathways, but the pathogenesis remains obscure and medical therapy is lacking. Abnormal expression patterns have been observed for proteins related to angiogenesis (e.g., vascular endothelial growth factor, angiopoietin-2, matrix metalloproteinase-9), and inflammation (e.g., interleukin-6 [IL-6] and myeloperoxidase). Macrophage and neutrophil invasion have also been observed in the absence of prior ICH. Candidate gene association studies have identified a number of germline variants associated with clinical ICH course and AVM susceptibility. A single nucleotide polymorphism (SNP) in activin receptor-like kinase-1 (ALK-1) is associated with AVM susceptibility, and SNPs in IL-6, tumor necrosis factor-α (TNF-α), and apolipoprotein-E (APOE) are associated with AVM rupture. These observations suggest that even without a complete understanding of the determinants of AVM development, the recent discoveries of downstream derangements in vascular function and integrity may offer potential targets for therapy development. Further, biomarkers can now be established for assessing ICH risk. These data will generate hypotheses that can be tested mechanistically in model systems, including surrogate phenotypes, such as vascular dysplasia and/or models recapitulating the clinical syndrome of recurrent spontaneous ICH.

Keywords: Angiogenesis; inflammation; vascular malformations.

Introduction

Brain arteriovenous malformations (AVMs) represent a relatively infrequent but important source of neurological morbidity in relatively young adults [4]. Brain AVMs

have a population prevalence of 10 to 18 per 100,000 adults [3, 7], and a new detection rate of approximately 1.3 per 100,000 person-years [58]. The basic morphology is that of a vascular mass, called the nidus, that directly shunts blood between the arterial and venous circulations without a true capillary bed. There is usually high flow through the feeding arteries, nidus, and draining veins. The nidus is a complex tangle of abnormal, dilated channels, not clearly artery or vein, with intervening gliosis.

Seizures, mass effect, and headache are causes of associated morbidity, but prevention of new or recurrent intracranial hemorrhage (ICH) is the primary rationale to treat AVMs, usually with some combination of surgical resection, embolization, and stereotactic radiotherapy. The risk of spontaneous ICH has been estimated in retrospective and prospective observational studies to range approximately from 2 to 4% per year [31]. Other than non-specific control of symptomatology, such as headache and seizures, primary medical therapy is lacking.

Etiology and pathogenesis

The genesis of AVMs has been enigmatic. Unlike the association of antecedent head trauma or other injuries with the pathogenesis of dural arteriovenous fistulae (DAVF), environmental risk factors for AVMs are lacking. There is remarkably little evidence for the common assertion that AVMs are congenital lesions arising during the fourth to eighth week of embryonic development,

Correspondence: William L. Young, MD, UCSF Department of Anesthesia and Perioperative Care, 1001 Potrero Avenue, Room 3C-38, San Francisco, CA 94110, USA. e-mail: ccr@anesthesia.ucsf.edu

considering the widespread use of prenatal ultrasound (Vein of Galen lesions are not true AVMs). Further, there have been multiple reports of AVMs that grow or regress, including de novo AVM formation [19]. Inciting event(s) might include the sequelae of even relatively modest injury from an otherwise unremarkable episode of trauma, infection, inflammation, irradiation, or compression. In susceptible individuals, one might posit some degree of localized venous hypertension [34, 68] from microvascular thrombosis, perhaps associated with a state of relative thrombophilia [56]. The scarce data available on longitudinal assessment of AVM growth suggests that approximately 50% of cases display interval growth [25]. Consistent with growth is the many-fold greater endothelial proliferation rate (Ki-67) in AVM surgical specimens, compared to control brain [25].

Characterization of lesional tissue

Available evidence points toward an active angiogenic and inflammatory lesion rather than a static congenital

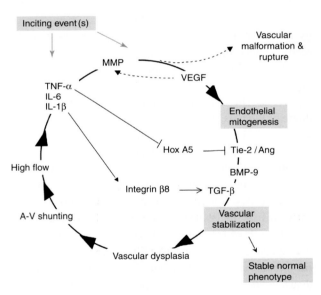

Fig. 1. Speculative synthesis of experimental observations relevant to AVM pathogenesis is presented in a simplified, conceptual fashion. After an inciting event or events, inflammatory or angiogenic activity (MMP, VEGF) initiates microvascular growth and remodeling, which are stabilized through interplay of pathways that include TIE-2/ANG and ALK-1/ENG. TGF-β signaling occurs primarily through ALK-5 in smooth muscle and BMP-9 signaling through ALK-1 in the endothelium (see Fig. 2). Normal vessels stabilize, but a region that represents an incipient AVM undergoes a dysplastic response. Arteriovenous (A–V) shunting and high flow rates synergize with the dysplastic response and involve classical inflammatory signals, causing a vicious cycle in a localized area destined to become the AVM nidus. Eventually, the human disease phenotype results. Genetic variation can influence any and all of the pathways

anomaly. A conceptual, speculative synthesis of these observations is shown in Fig. 1. Our group and others [27] have shown that a prominent feature of the AVM phenotype is relative overexpression of vascular endothelial growth factor-A (VEGF-A), at both the mRNA and protein level. VEGF may contribute to the hemorrhagic tendency of AVMs, extrapolating from animal models [35]. Other upstream factors that may contribute to AVM formation might include Homeobox genes, such as excess pro-angiogenic Hox D3 or deficient anti-angiogenic Hox A5 [12]. The vascular phenotype of AVM tissue may be explained, in part, by inadequate recruitment of peri-endothelial support structure, which is mediated by angiopoietins and TIE-2 signaling. For example, angiopoietin-2 (Ang-2), which allows loosening of cell-to-cell contacts, is over-expressed in the perivascular region in AVM vascular channels [24].

A key downstream consequence of VEGF and Ang-2 activity, contributing to the angiogenic phenotype, is matrix metalloproteinase (MMP) expression. MMP-9 expression in particular appears to be orders of magnitude higher in AVM than control tissue [13, 26], with levels of naturally-occurring MMP inhibitors, TIMP-1 and TIMP-3, also higher, but to a lesser degree. Additional inflammatory markers that are over-expressed include myeloperoxidase (MPO) and interleukin (IL)-6, both of which are highly correlated with MMP-9 [13, 14]. MMP-9 expression is correlated with the lipocalin-MMP-9 complex, suggesting neutrophils as a major source. In a subset of unruptured, non-embolized AVMs, neutrophils (MPO), macrophages/microglia (CD68), T-lymphocytes (CD3), and B-lymphocytes (CD20) were clearly evident in the vascular wall and intervening stroma of AVM tissue, whereas T- and B-lymphocytes were rarely observed [15].

Genetic considerations relevant to AVMs

The majority of brain AVMs are sporadic; however, there is some evidence supporting a familial component to the AVM phenotype and there is evidence that genetic variation is relevant to the study of the disease. A simplified summary of relevant pathways is shown in Fig. 2.

Mendelian disease

To date, the most significant candidate genes/pathways for brain AVM pathogenesis have come from Mendelian disorders that exhibit AVMs as part of their clinical phenotype. AVMs are highly prevalent in patients with

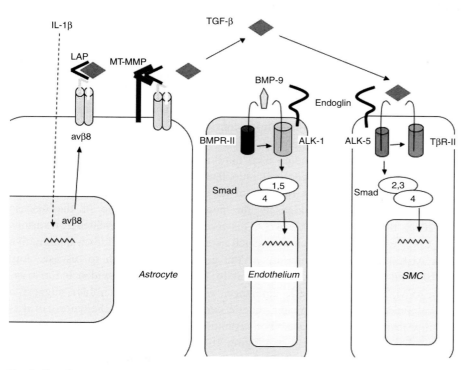

Fig. 2. Signaling pathways and speculative synthesis of signaling pathways. The $\alpha v \beta 8$ gene, which has an IL-1β responsive region in human and mouse $\beta 8$ promoters, is critical for liberation of TGF-β from LAP. MMP-9 activity and inflammation are associated with IL-1β, TNF-α, and IL-6. TGF-β signaling proceeds through the ALK-5 receptor expressed primarily on vascular smooth muscle. Endothelial cells express primarily ALK-1, which signals via the BMP-9 ligand. The ALK-1 signal is required for EC maturation, which when abrogated, leads to inappropriate EC migration and proliferation. ENG is an accessory receptor that can modulate both TGF-β and ALK-1 signaling. ALK-1 and ALK-5 signal via distinct SMAD effector pathways converge on the common co-effector, SMAD4, in order to effect gene expression

hereditary hemorrhagic telangiectasia (HHT), an autosomal dominant disorder of mucocutaneous fragility and AVMs in various organs, including the brain. The 2 main subtypes of HHT (HHT-1 and -2) are caused by loss-of-function mutations in 2 genes [38] originally implicated in tumor growth factor (TGF)-β signaling pathways (Fig. 1). The first is endoglin (ENG), which codes for an accessory protein of TGF-β receptor complexes. The second is activin-like kinase-1 (ALK-1 or ACVLR1), which codes for a transmembrane kinase also thought to participate in TGF-β signaling.

Two recent reports show that ALK-1 may instead signal through bone morphogenetic protein (BMP)-9 and that ENG can potentiate the signal, suggesting that BMP-9 may represent a physiologically relevant *endothelial* signaling pathway for HHT pathogenesis [17, 52]. Endothelial cell (EC)-specific ablation of the murine ALK-1 gene causes AVM formation during development, whereas mice harboring an EC-specific knockout of ALK-5 (the type I TGF-β receptor) or TbRII (the type II TGF-β receptor) show neither AVM formation nor any other perturbation in vascular morphogenesis [42].

A third candidate for AVM pathogenesis is the SMAD4 gene, encoding the downstream effector for both TGF-β and BMP signaling. This gene is mutated in a combined syndrome of juvenile polyposis and HHT [21]. Two additional independent loci, termed HHT-3 and HHT-4, have recently been described [5, 16], but the genes underlying these less-common forms of HHT have yet to be identified.

In HHT, defects in either ENG or ALK-1 may affect a common pathway. By inference, this common pathway, which includes BMP-9, is also implicated in sporadic brain AVM development. A potential *mechanism* for the role of this pathway in AVM pathogenesis would include the requirement of ALK-1 for EC maturation [18, 32]. Disruption of this signaling pathway by mutation or possibly through physiological perturbation would result in a block in the maturation process, leading to inappropriate EC migration and proliferation. This suggests that aberrant EC migration and proliferation may be one of the earliest events in the development of an AVM.

The pathways involved in TGF-β signaling are complex and interconnected [59]. In addition to direct effects of abnormal ENG and ALK-1 signaling that result in abnormal angiogenic function [60], insufficient ENG may affect local hemodynamics through its interaction with nitric oxide signaling [61]. A loss of local microvascular flow regulation may in and of itself lead to the development of arteriovenous shunts, as predicted by computational modeling studies [46].

As a class, the inherited AVMs in HHT have some distinguishing morphological features, but are generally similar to the sporadic lesions and cannot be distinguished individually on the basis of their angioarchitecture [37, 40]. Brain AVMs are approximately 10 times more common in HHT-1/ENG ($\sim$20%) than HHT-2/ALK-1 ($\sim$2%) patients [6, 36, 50]. Compared to sporadic lesions, presence of an ENG or ALK-1 mutation results in an approximate 1000- or 100-fold increased risk, respectively, of developing a brain AVM. The greatly elevated risk of brain AVM development in the Mendelian disorders raises the possibility that germline *sequence variants* of these and other genes may likewise pose a significant risk for *sporadic* brain AVM development.

Because the population prevalence of HHT is roughly 1/10,000, and approximately 10% of all HHT cases harbor brain AVMs [36], this would yield a population prevalence of HHT-related AVMs of 1/100,000. Therefore, given the total AVM population prevalence of 10 to 18 per 100,000 adults [3, 7], the fraction of HHT-AVMs in large referral series should be approximately 5% to 10%. Interestingly, HHT accounts for less than 1% of the University of California San Francisco (UCSF) [31] and Columbia [39] AVM databases (unpublished data), suggesting that systematic underestimation of undiagnosed HHT may occur in the large referral cohorts.

Familial aggregation

Although rare, familial cases of AVM outside the context of HHT have been reported in the literature [30, 63]. A recent review article examined all case reports and identified 53 patients without HHT in 25 families with AVMs, mostly of first-degree relationships (79%) [63]. While no clear pattern of inheritance emerged from the pedigrees, the clinical characteristics of familial AVM patients did not differ significantly from sporadic AVM, except for a younger age at diagnosis. In addition, linkage and association analysis of 6 Japanese families, each with 2 affected relatives, was recently reported [30]. Linkage analysis revealed 7 candidate

regions, with the strongest signal at chromosome 6q25 (LOD = 1.88; $p = 0.002$) under a dominant genetic model. However, no association was observed with markers in the candidate linkage regions likely due to the small sample size.

Further evidence for a genetic component to AVMs comes from considering the excess risk of disease in relatives compared to the general population. A commonly used familial aggregation measure is the recurrence risk ratio, lambda (λ), defined as the risk of disease in relatives of an individual with disease ($K_{relative}$), divided by the population prevalence of the disease (K) [47]. This measure can be calculated for various relatives, such as siblings, and provides a quantitative measure of the genetic contribution to disease. Any λ value equal to 1.0 indicates no evidence for a genetic influence, whereas higher λ values suggest a greater genetic component to the pathogenesis of disease. For example, complex diseases have $\lambda_{sibling}$ values ranging from 2.0 to 5.0 for ischemic stroke [41], 58 for ankylosing spondylitis [11], and 215 for autism [48].

The lack of published population-based studies of AVM with family history information makes it difficult to assess familial aggregation. However, we estimated $\lambda_{sibling}$ for the recently reported linkage and association study of AVM by Inoue *et al.* [30], which included cases from a region of Japan thought to have a high prevalence of AVM. Five of 31 cases (assuming 26 cases included in the association analysis had no family history) had affected siblings, yielding a sibling recurrence risk (K_s) of 16%. Given a population risk of AVM (K) of 18 per 100,000 (0.018%) [3], the excess sibling risk ($\lambda_{sibling} = K_{sibling}/K$) is estimated to be 889 (16%/0.018%). As a sensitivity analysis, we calculated $\lambda_{sibling}$ varying the recurrence risk to siblings from 0.01% to 50% and assuming a population prevalence of AVM of 0.018%. A sibling recurrence risk even as low as 0.05% would yield a $\lambda_{sibling}$ of 2.78, which would still support a genetic contribution to the disease.

Taken together, there is modest evidence supporting familial aggregation for the AVM phenotype, although definitive proof is lacking. The high relative risk to siblings suggests a significant genetic influence, although this could also be the result of random chance, shared environmental factors, shared genetic factors, or any combination of these. The challenge is identifying enough families with imaging-confirmed AVM cases and genetic data to perform classical genetic studies.

An alternative genetic mechanism for sporadic AVMs

An alternative hypothesis for sporadic AVM pathogenesis would posit that the relevant genes/pathways are disrupted by *somatic*, rather than germline mutations. This genetic mechanism would parallel that found for venous malformations, where germline TIE-2 mutations are found in autosomal dominant families with venous malformations [9, 64], but somatic mutations are found in *tissue* isolated from sporadic venous malformations [8, 65]. The somatic mutation mechanism might also explain the rarity of families with AVMs outside the context of HHT. The occasional but rare familial occurrence of the usually sporadic AVM is similar to that found with other vascular traits such as Klippel-Trenaunay syndrome. This pattern has been termed paradominant inheritance and invokes a crucial role for somatic mutation as its underlying mechanism [22, 23]. In the paradominant model, heterozygous individuals for a germline mutation are phenotypically normal, but zygotes that are homozygous for the mutation die during early embryogenesis. Thus, the mutation rarely manifests as familial inheritance of a trait, but instead is usually "silently" transmitted through many generations. However, the trait becomes manifest in an individual when a somatic mutation occurs at a later stage during embryogenesis, giving rise to a mutant cell population being either homozygous or hemizygous for the mutation. This clone of mutant cells has bypassed the developmental block, and these cells can now seed the development of the vascular anomaly. This intriguing hypothesis has yet to be explored for sporadic AVMs.

Another consideration is the way one construes the nature of an "inherited disease". Even if the mechanism of AVM initiation – as yet unknown – is a structural or mechanical insult, which is not in itself a heritable trait, the subsequent growth and behavior of the lesion can still be influenced by genetic variation in mechanistic pathways important in vascular biology. For example, there are multiple genetic loci that control VEGF-induced angiogenesis [49, 53]. Genetic influences on AVM pathobiology may therefore be evaluated in a case-control study design comparing affected patients to normal controls, or in cross-sectional or longitudinal cohort designs to investigate genetic influences on clinical course, such as propensity to rupture.

Candidate gene studies in AVM patients

We have pursued 2 general classes of candidates for examination: (a) genes in pathways found to be upregulated in lesional tissue, i.e., inflammatory or angiogenic genes; and (b) genes mutated in Mendelian disorders affecting the cerebral circulation, e.g., HHT. Such genes provide a starting point for hypothesis generation for both clinical studies and laboratory experiments. Common polymorphisms may subtly alter protein function or expression, resulting in phenotypes relevant to the human disease. For example, abnormal vascular development has been observed in murine models with insufficient ALK-1 [57, 62] and ENG [51]. Importantly, adenoviral-mediated VEGF gene transfer in ENG-deficient mice causes enhancement of vascular abnormalities, suggesting a synergism between TGF-β and VEGF signaling pathways in development of abnormal or "dysplastic" vessels [66]. Structural integrity may also be influenced by upstream influences on TGF-β signaling. For example, of interest is the interaction of astrocytic integrin $\alpha V\beta 8$ and its role in TGF-β transport; its abrogation results in vascular instability leading to developmental ICH [10]. Preliminary data suggest decreased $\alpha V\beta 8$ expression in resected AVM tissue (unpublished data).

We recently provided the first description of a common genetic variant associated with the sporadic disease: an intronic variant of ALK-1 (IVS3 -35 A>G) was present at a higher frequency in AVM cases compared to healthy controls [44]. This association was independently replicated [54, 55]. Preliminary data suggest that this single nucleotide polymorphism (SNP) is associated with alternative splicing (unpublished data). Other SNPs we have found to be associated with AVM susceptibility include common promoter polymorphisms in IL-1β (IL-1β -31 T>C and -511 C>T) [29].

There are also genetic influences on clinical course of AVM rupture resulting in ICH in 3 settings: presentation with ICH [28, 43], new ICH after diagnosis [1, 45], and ICH after treatment [2]. We found that the GG genotype of the IL-6 (IL-6 -174 G>C) promoter polymorphism was associated with clinical presentation of ICH [43]. The high-risk IL-6 -174 GG genotype was also associated with the highest IL-6 mRNA and protein levels in AVM tissue [14]. We have not yet identified any associations of sporadic AVM with polymorphisms in genes coding for important angiogenesis-related proteins, such as VEGF, TIE-2, or the angiopoietins.

We have further explored use of genotype to predict new ICH in the natural course after presentation, but before any treatment had been initiated [1, 45]. We found that the A allele of the TNF-α -238 G>A promoter SNP was associated with new hemorrhage in the natural course of a sample of 280 AVM cases. Adjusting for initial presentation with hemorrhage, age, and race/ethnicity, resulted in an adjusted hazards ratio (HR) of 4.0 (95% CI = 1.3–12.3; $p = 0.015$) [1].

Additionally, the apolipoprotein (APOE) $\varepsilon 2$, but not APOE $\varepsilon 4$ allele, was associated with new hemorrhage ($n = 284$) in the natural course, with an adjusted HR of 5.1 (95% CI = 1.5–17.7; $p = 0.01$) [45]. When examined together in a multivariate model, both the APOE $\varepsilon 2$ and TNF-α -238 A alleles were independent predictors of ICH risk [45]. The TNF-α and APOE results are exciting, because they represent the first description of a genotype associated with increased natural history hemorrhagic risk in AVM patients. Newer evidence also associates IL-1β with increased risk of new ICH [28]. In addition to their association with spontaneous ICH in the natural, untreated course, both APOE $\varepsilon 2$ and TNF-α -238 A alleles appear to confer greater risk for post-radiosurgery and post-surgical hemorrhage [2].

All of these genetic association results require replication and larger sample sizes, considerable challenges for a rare disease such as AVM. The largest cohorts to date have been assembled from clinical series. Although the large clinical series have not directly studied genetics, there may be indirect evidence of a genetic influence, in that race/ethnic background appears to affect spontaneous bleeding rate [31]. This association could be explained by genetic, socio-economic, and environmental factors, or a complex combination of all three. However, no specific factors have been identified in case series, with the possible exception of essential hypertension [33].

Conclusions

Considering the tissue expression data together with the genetic studies, the available data are consistent with the hypothesis that angiogenic and inflammatory processes – including ENG and ALK-1 signaling pathways – contribute to AVM pathogenesis and clinical course. Although the data do not prove that such activity is causative, involvement of these pathways appears highly plausible. Replication studies are needed for the genetic association findings and animal models are needed for mechanistic studies.

A prevailing view is that AVM pathophysiology is governed to a large extent by chronic hemodynamic derangements [20, 67] imposed on a relatively fixed congenital lesion. Our findings raise the possibility that angiogenic and inflammatory pathways can either synergize with underlying defects or hemodynamic injury to

result in the clinical phenotype and behavior. Further, it may be the case that the angiogenic and inflammatory components are actually the driving causal force in disease initiation and progression, perhaps in conjunction with as yet undetermined environmental influences. Progress in elucidating these pathways and mechanisms not only offer promise for developing innovative, safer treatments for the disease, but also may provide insights into the vascular failure seen in other hemorrhagic brain disorders.

References

1. Achrol AS, Pawlikowska L, McCulloch CE, Poon KY, Ha C, Zaroff JG, Johnston SC, Lee C, Lawton MT, Sidney S, Marchuk DA, Kwok PY, Young WL (2006) Tumor necrosis factor-alpha-238G > A promoter polymorphism is associated with increased risk of new hemorrhage in the natural course of patients with brain arteriovenous malformations. Stroke 37: 231–234
2. Achrol AS, Kim H, Pawlikowska L, Trudy Poon KY, McCulloch CE, Ko NU, Johnston SC, McDermott MW, Zaroff JG, Lawton MT, Kwok PY, Young WL (2007) Association of tumor necrosis factor-alpha-238G > A and apolipoprotein E2 polymorphisms with intracranial hemorrhage after brain arteriovenous malformation treatment. Neurosurgery 61: 731–740
3. Al-Shahi R, Fang JS, Lewis SC, Warlow CP (2002) Prevalence of adults with brain arteriovenous malformations: a community based study in Scotland using capture-recapture analysis. J Neurol Neurosurg Psychiatry 73: 547–551
4. Arteriovenous Malformation Study Group (1999) Arteriovenous malformations of the brain in adults. N Engl J Med 340: 1812–1818
5. Bayrak-Toydemir P, McDonald J, Akarsu N, Toydemir RM, Calderon F, Tuncali T, Tang W, Miller F, Mao R (2006) A fourth locus for hereditary hemorrhagic telangiectasia maps to chromosome 7. Am J Med Genet A 140: 2155–2162
6. Bayrak-Toydemir P, McDonald J, Markewitz B, Lewin S, Miller F, Chou LS, Gedge F, Tang W, Coon H, Mao R (2006) Genotype-phenotype correlation in hereditary hemorrhagic telangiectasia: mutations and manifestations. Am J Med Genet A 140: 463–470
7. Berman MF, Sciacca RR, Pile-Spellman J, Stapf C, Connolly ES Jr, Mohr JP, Young WL (2000) The epidemiology of brain arteriovenous malformations. Neurosurgery 47: 389–397
8. Brouillard P, Vikkula M (2007) Genetic causes of vascular malformations. Hum Mol Genet 16(2): R140–R149
9. Calvert JT, Riney TJ, Kontos CD, Cha EH, Prieto VG, Shea CR, Berg JN, Nevin NC, Simpson SA, Pasyk KA, Speer MC, Peters KG, Marchuk DA (1999) Allelic and locus heterogeneity in inherited venous malformations. Hum Mol Genet 8: 1279–1289
10. Cambier S, Gline S, Mu D, Collins R, Araya J, Dolganov G, Einheber S, Boudreau N, Nishimura SL (2005) Integrin alpha(v)-beta8-mediated activation of transforming growth factor-beta by perivascular astrocytes: an angiogenic control switch. Am J Pathol 166: 1883–1894
11. Carter N, Williamson L, Kennedy LG, Brown MA, Wordsworth BP (2000) Susceptibility to ankylosing spondylitis. Rheumatology (Oxford) 39: 445
12. Chen Y, Xu B, Arderiu G, Hashimoto T, Young WL, Boudreau N, Yang GY (2004) Retroviral delivery of homeobox D3 gene induces cerebral angiogenesis in mice. J Cereb Blood Flow Metab 24: 1280–1287

13. Chen Y, Fan Y, Poon KY, Achrol AS, Lawton MT, Zhu Y, McCulloch CE, Hashimoto T, Lee C, Barbaro NM, Bollen AW, Yang GY, Young WL (2006) MMP-9 expression is associated with leukocytic but not endothelial markers in brain arteriovenous malformations. Front Biosci 11: 3121–3128

14. Chen Y, Pawlikowska L, Yao JS, Shen F, Zhai W, Achrol AS, Lawton MT, Kwok PY, Yang GY, Young WL (2006) Interleukin-6 involvement in brain arteriovenous malformations. Ann Neurol 59: 72–80

15. Chen Y, Zhu W, Bollen AW, Lawton MT, Barbaro NM, Dowd CF, Hashimoto T, Yang GY, Young WL (2008) Evidence for inflammatory cell involvement in brain arteriovenous malformations. Neurosurgery (in press)

16. Cole SG, Begbie ME, Wallace GM, Shovlin CL (2005) A new locus for hereditary haemorrhagic telangiectasia (HHT3) maps to chromosome 5. J Med Genet 42: 577–582

17. David L, Mallet C, Mazerbourg S, Feige JJ, Bailly S (2007) Identification of BMP9 and BMP10 as functional activators of the orphan activin receptor-like kinase 1 (ALK1) endothelial cells. Blood 109: 1953–1961

18. David L, Mallet C, Vailhé B, Lamouille S, Feige JJ, Bailly S (2007) Activin receptor-like kinase 1 inhibits human microvascular endothelial cell migration: potential roles for JNK and ERK. J Cell Physiol 213: 484–489

19. Du R, Hashimoto T, Tihan T, Young WL, Perry V, Lawton MT (2007) Growth and regression of arteriovenous malformations in a patient with hereditary hemorrhagic telangiectasia. Case report. J Neurosurg 106: 470–477

20. Duong DH, Young WL, Vang MC, Sciacca RR, Mast H, Koennecke HC, Hartmann A, Joshi S, Mohr JP, Pile-Spellman J (1998) Feeding artery pressure and venous drainage pattern are primary determinants of hemorrhage from cerebral arteriovenous malformations. Stroke 29: 1167–1176

21. Gallione CJ, Richards JA, Letteboer TG, Rushlow D, Prigoda NL, Leedom TP, Ganguly A, Castells A, Ploos van Amstel JK, Westermann CJ, Pyeritz RE, Marchuk DA (2006) SMAD4 mutations found in unselected HHT patients. J Med Genet 43: 793–797

22. Happle R (1992) Paradominant inheritance: a possible explanation for Becker's pigmented hairy nevus. Eur J Dermatol 2: 39–40

23. Happle R (1993) Klippel-Trenaunay syndrome: is it a paradominant trait? Br J Dermatol 128: 465–466

24. Hashimoto T, Lam T, Boudreau NJ, Bollen AW, Lawton MT, Young WL (2001) Abnormal balance in the angiopoietin-tie2 system in human brain arteriovenous malformations. Circ Res 89: 111–113

25. Hashimoto T, Mesa-Tejada R, Quick CM, Bollen AW, Joshi S, Pile-Spellman J, Lawton MT, Young WL (2001) Evidence of increased endothelial cell turnover in brain arteriovenous malformations. Neurosurgery 49: 124–132

26. Hashimoto T, Wen G, Lawton MT, Boudreau NJ, Bollen AW, Yang GY, Barbaro NM, Higashida RT, Dowd CF, Halbach VV, Young WL (2003) Abnormal expression of matrix metalloproteinases and tissue inhibitors of metalloproteinases in brain arteriovenous malformations. Stroke 34: 925–931

27. Hashimoto T, Lawton MT, Wen G, Yang GY, Chaly T Jr, Stewart CL, Dressman HK, Barbaro NM, Marchuk DA, Young WL (2004) Gene microarray analysis of human brain arteriovenous malformations. Neurosurgery 54: 410–425

28. Hysi PG, Kim H, Pawlikowska L, McCulloch CE, Zaroff JG, Marchuk DA, Lawton MT, Kwok PY, Young WL (2007) Association of interleukin-1 beta (IL1β) gene and risk of intracranial hemorrhage in brain arteriovenous malformation patients (Abstract #2538). 57th Annual Meeting of the American Society of Human Genetics, San Diego, CA

29. Hysi PG, Kim H, Pawlikowska L, McCulloch CE, Zaroff JG, Sidney S, Burchard EG, Marchuk DA, Lawton MT, Kwok PY, Young WL (2007) Association of interleukin-1 beta (IL1B) gene and brain arteriovenous malformation in Caucasians (abstract). Stroke 38: 456

30. Inoue S, Liu W, Inoue K, Mineharu Y, Takenaka K, Yamakawa H, Abe M, Jafar JJ, Herzig R, Koizumi A (2007) Combination of linkage and association studies for brain arteriovenous malformation. Stroke 38: 1368–1370

31. Kim H, Sidney S, McCulloch CE, Poon KY, Singh V, Johnston SC, Ko NU, Achrol AS, Lawton MT, Higashida RT, Young WL (2007) Racial/ethnic differences in longitudinal risk of intracranial hemorrhage in brain arteriovenous malformation patients. Stroke 38: 2430–2437

32. Lamouille S, Mallet C, Feige JJ, Bailly S (2002) Activin receptor-like kinase 1 is implicated in the maturation phase of angiogenesis. Blood 100: 4495–4501

33. Langer DJ, Lasner TM, Hurst RW, Flamm ES, Zager EL, King JT Jr (1998) Hypertension, small size, and deep venous drainage are associated with risk of hemorrhagic presentation of cerebral arteriovenous malformations. Neurosurgery 42: 481–489

34. Lawton MT, Jacobowitz R, Spetzler RF (1997) Redefined role of angiogenesis in the pathogenesis of dural arteriovenous malformations. J Neurosurg 87: 267–274

35. Lee CZ, Xue Z, Zhu Y, Yang GY, Young WL (2007) Matrix metalloproteinase-9 inhibition attenuates vascular endothelial growth factor-induced intracerebral hemorrhage. Stroke 38: 2563–2568

36. Letteboer TG, Mager JJ, Snijder RJ, Koeleman BP, Lindhout D, Ploos van Amstel JK, Westermann CJ (2006) Genotype–phenotype relationship in hereditary haemorrhagic telangiectasia. J Med Genet 43: 371–377

37. Maher CO, Piepgras DG, Brown RD Jr, Friedman JA, Pollock BE (2001) Cerebrovascular manifestations in 321 cases of hereditary hemorrhagic telangiectasia. Stroke 32: 877–882

38. Marchuk DA, Srinivasan S, Squire TL, Zawistowski JS (2003) Vascular morphogenesis: tales of two syndromes. Hum Mol Genet 12: R97–R112

39. Mast H, Young WL, Koennecke HC, Sciacca RR, Osipov A, Pile-Spellman J, Hacein-Bey L, Duong H, Stein BM, Mohr JP (1997) Risk of spontaneous haemorrhage after diagnosis of cerebral arteriovenous malformation. Lancet 350: 1065–1068

40. Matsubara S, Manzia JL, ter Brugge K, Willinsky RA, Montanera W, Faughnan ME (2000) Angiographic and clinical characteristics of patients with cerebral arteriovenous malformations associated with hereditary hemorrhagic telangiectasia. Am J Neuroradiol 21: 1016–1020

41. Meschia JF, Brown RD Jr, Brott TG, Chukwudelunzu FE, Hardy J, Rich SS (2002) The Siblings With Ischemic Stroke Study (SWISS) protocol. BMC Med Genet 3: 1

42. Park SO, Lee YJ, Seki T, Hong KH, Fliess N, Jiang Z, Park A, Wu X, Kaartinen V, Roman BL, Oh SP (2008) ALK5- and TGFBR2-independent role of ALK1 in the pathogenesis of hereditary hemorrhagic telangiectasia type 2. Blood 111: 633–642

43. Pawlikowska L, Tran MN, Achrol AS, McCulloch CE, Ha C, Lind DL, Hashimoto T, Zaroff J, Lawton MT, Marchuk DA, Kwok PY, Young WL (2004) Polymorphisms in genes involved in inflammatory and angiogenic pathways and the risk of hemorrhagic presentation of brain arteriovenous malformations. Stroke 35: 2294–2300

44. Pawlikowska L, Tran MN, Achrol AS, Ha C, Burchard E, Choudhry S, Zaroff J, Lawton MT, Castro R, McCulloch CE, Marchuk D, Kwok PY, Young WL (2005) Polymorphisms in transforming growth factor-beta-related genes ALK1 and ENG are associated with sporadic brain arteriovenous malformations. Stroke 36: 2278–2280

45. Pawlikowska L, Poon KY, Achrol AS, McCulloch CE, Ha C, Lum K, Zaroff JG, Ko NU, Johnston SC, Sidney S, Marchuk DA, Lawton MT, Kwok PY, Young WL (2006) Apoliprotein E epsilon 2 is

associated with new hemorrhage risk in brain arteriovenous malformations. Neurosurgery 58: 838–843

46. Quick CM, Hashimoto T, Young WL (2001) Lack of flow regulation may explain the development of arteriovenous malformations. Neurol Res 23: 641–644

47. Risch N (1990) Linkage strategies for genetically complex traits. I. Multilocus models. Am J Hum Genet 46: 222–228

48. Ritvo ER, Jorde LB, Mason-Brothers A, Freeman BJ, Pingree C, Jones MB, McMahon WM, Petersen PB, Jenson WR, Mo A (1989) The UCLA-University of Utah epidemiologic survey of autism: recurrence risk estimates and genetic counseling. Am J Psychiatry 146: 1032–1036

49. Rogers MS, D'Amato RJ (2006) The effect of genetic diversity on angiogenesis. Exp Cell Res 312: 561–574

50. Sabbà C, Pasculli G, Lenato GM, Suppressa P, Lastella P, Memeo M, Dicuonzo F, Guant G (2007) Hereditary hemorragic telangiectasia: clinical features in ENG and ALK1 mutation carriers. J Thromb Haemost 5: 1149–1157

51. Satomi J, Mount RJ, Toporsian M, Paterson AD, Wallace MC, Harrison RV, Letarte M (2003) Cerebral vascular abnormalities in a murine model of hereditary hemorrhagic telangiectasia. Stroke 34: 783–789

52. Scharpfenecker M, van Dinther M, Liu Z, van Bezooijen RL, Zhao Q, Pukac L, Löwik CW, ten Dijke P (2007) BMP-9 signals via ALK1 and inhibits bFGF-induced endothelial cell proliferation and VEGF-stimulated angiogenesis. J Cell Sci 120: 964–972

53. Shaked Y, Bertolini F, Man S, Rogers MS, Cervi D, Foutz T, Rawn K, Voskas D, Dumont DJ, Ben-David Y, Lawler J, Henkin J, Huber J, Hicklin DJ, D'Amato RJ, Kerbel RS (2005) Genetic heterogeneity of the vasculogenic phenotype parallels angiogenesis: implications for cellular surrogate marker analysis of antiangiogenesis. Cancer Cell 7: 101–111

54. Simon M, Franke D, Ludwig M, Aliashkevich AF, Köster G, Oldenburg J, Boström A, Ziegler A, Schramm J (2006) Association of a polymorphism of the ACVRL1 gene with sporadic arteriovenous malformations of the central nervous system. J Neurosurg 104: 945–949

55. Simon M, Schramm J, Ludwig M, Ziegler A (2007) Response to neurosurgical forum letter to the Editor "Arteriovenous Malformation" by Young *et al.* J Neurosurg 106: 731–733

56. Singh V, Smith WS, Lawton MT, Halbach VV, Young WL (2006) Thrombophilic mutation as a new high-risk feature in DAVF patients (abstract S-99). Ann Neurol 60(Suppl 3): S30

57. Srinivasan S, Hanes MA, Dickens T, Porteous ME, Oh SP, Hale LP, Marchuk DA (2003) A mouse model for hereditary hemorrhagic telangiectasia (HHT) type 2. Hum Mol Genet 12: 473–482

58. Stapf C, Mast H, Sciacca RR, Berenstein A, Nelson PK, Gobin YP, Pile-Spellman J, Mohr JP (2003) The New York Islands AVM Study: design, study progress, and initial results. Stroke 34: e29–e33

59. ten Dijke P, Arthur HM (2007) Extracellular control of TGFbeta signalling in vascular development and disease. Nat Rev Mol Cell Biol 8: 857–869

60. Thomas B, Eyries M, Montagne K, Martin S, Agrapart M, Simerman-Francois R, Letarte M, Soubrier F (2007) Altered endothelial gene expression associated with hereditary haemorrhagic telangiectasia. Eur J Clin Invest 37: 580–588

61. Toporsian M, Gros R, Kabir MG, Vera S, Govindaraju K, Eidelman DH, Husain M, Letarte M (2005) A role for endoglin in coupling eNOS activity and regulating vascular tone revealed in hereditary hemorrhagic telangiectasia. Circ Res 96: 684–692

62. Urness LD, Sorensen LK, Li DY (2000) Arteriovenous malformations in mice lacking activin receptor-like kinase-1. Nat Genet 26: 328–331

63. van Beijnum J, van der Worp HB, Schippers HM, van Nieuwenhuizen O, Kappelle LJ, Rinkel GJ, Berkelbach van der Sprenkel JW, Klijn CJ (2007) Familial occurrence of brain arteriovenous malformations: a systematic review. J Neurol Neurosurg Psychiatry 78: 1213–1217

64. Vikkula M, Boon LM, Carraway KL 3rd, Calvert JT, Diamonti AJ, Goumnerov B, Pasyk KA, Marchuk DA, Warman ML, Cantley LC, Mulliken JB, Olsen BR (1996) Vascular dysmorphogenesis caused by an activating mutation in the receptor tyrosine kinase TIE2. Cell 87: 1181–1190

65. Wouters V, Limaye N, Uebelhoer M, Mulliken JB, Boon LM, Vikkula M (2007) Sporadic venous malformation is caused by somatic mutations in TIE2 (Abstract). American Society of Human Genetics 57th Annual Meeting, San Diego, CA

66. Xu B, Wu YQ, Huey M, Arthur HM, Marchuk DA, Hashimoto T, Young WL, Yang GY (2004) Vascular endothelial growth factor induces abnormal microvasculature in the endoglin heterozygous mouse brain. J Cereb Blood Flow Metab 24: 237–244

67. Young WL, Kader A, Ornstein E, Baker KZ, Ostapkovich N, Pile-Spellman J, Fogarty-Mack P, Stein BM (1996) Cerebral hyperemia after arteriovenous malformation resection is related to "breakthrough" complications but not to feeding artery pressure. The Columbia University Arteriovenous Malformation Study Project. Neurosurgery 38: 1085–1095

68. Zhu Y, Lawton MT, Du R, Shwe Y, Chen Y, Shen F, Young WL, Yang GY (2006) Expression of hypoxia-inducible factor-1 and vascular endothelial growth factor in response to venous hypertension. Neurosurgery 59: 687–696

Acta Neurochir Suppl (2008) 105: 207–210
© Springer-Verlag 2008
Printed in Austria

Vasospasm after aneurysmal subarachnoid hemorrhage: need for further study

J. D. Pearl, R. L. Macdonald

Division of Neurosurgery and Keenan Research Centre, St. Michael's Hospital, and Department of Surgery, University of Toronto, Toronto, Ontario, Canada

Summary

Cerebral vasospasm is the classic cause of delayed neurological deterioration leading to cerebral ischemia and infarction, and thus, poor outcome and occasionally death, after aneurysmal subarachnoid hemorrhage (SAH). Advances in diagnosis and treatment, principally nimodipine, intensive care management, hemodynamic manipulations, and endovascular neuroradiology procedures, have improved the prospects for these patients, but outcomes remain disappointing. A phase 2b clinical trial (CONSCIOUS-1) demonstrated marked prevention of vasospasm with the endothelin antagonist, clazosentan, yet patient outcome was not improved. The most likely explanation is that the study was underpowered to detect the relatively small improvements in outcome that would be seen with prevention of vasospasm, especially when assessed using relatively insensitive measures such as the modified Rankin and Glasgow outcome scales. Other possible explanations for this result are that adverse effects of treatment affected the beneficial effects of the drug. It also is possible that alternative causes of neurological deterioration and poor outcome after SAH, including delayed effects of acute global cerebral ischemia, thromboembolism, microcirculatory dysfunction, and cortical spreading depression, play a role. Clazosentan reduced angiographic vasospasm in a dose-dependent manner in patients with aneurysmal SAH following coiling or clipping of the aneurysm. Reducing the incidence of vasospasm should have an important effect on clinical outcome. A phase 3 clinical trial (CONSCIOUS-2) will focus on quantifying this outcome in patients undergoing aneurysm clipping receiving placebo or 5 mg/h of clazosentan.

Keywords: Cerebral aneurysm; clazosentan; endothelin antagonist; subarachnoid hemorrhage; vasospasm.

Introduction

Cerebral vasospasm remains an important contributor to patient morbidity and mortality after aneurysmal subarachnoid hemorrhage (SAH), despite sizeable efforts

Correspondence: R. Loch Macdonald, Division of Neurosurgery, Department of Surgery, St. Michael's Hospital of the University of Toronto, 30 Bond Street, Toronto, Ontario, Canada M5B 1W8. e-mail: macdonaldlo@smh.toronto.on.ca

to control its occurrence. In fact, vasospasm following aneurysmal SAH is a significant independent risk factor for poor prognosis in survivors of aneurysm rupture [9]. Vasospasm can occur as early as 3 days and as late as 14 days after SAH secondary to aneurysm rupture. It is often defined radiologically or clinically. Radiologic vasospasm is diagnosed by arterial narrowing on angiography. Contrast fills vessels at a slower rate, and comparison with previous angiograms demonstrates progressively narrowing arteries that then return to normal weeks later in most cases. Clinical vasospasm, delayed ischemic neurological deficit, or delayed cerebral ischemia (DCI) is a clinical diagnosis of exclusion assigned to patients post-SAH, who show confusion, decreased level of consciousness, or present with a focal neurological deficit. It is believed, but not well documented, that clinical vasospasm can occur without radiological vasospasm. The reverse, where patients have radiological vasospasm and no symptoms, occurs in about half of cases.

The pathophysiology and pathogenesis of vasospasm and DCI continues to be widely researched and debated. Though widely accepted that vessel contraction and arterial narrowing are primarily responsible for the ischemia and consequent neurologic decline seen after SAH, we know that the process is far more complicated. Immediate global cerebral ischemia occurring when the aneurysm ruptures, loss of blood-brain barrier integrity, activation of apoptosis and inflammatory pathways, microcirculatory constriction, thromboembolism, and cortical spreading depression have all been hypothesized as elements of the process [7].

Prognosis

Patient outcome after SAH is dependent upon a wide array of factors [9]. The relative contributions of various factors to outcome have been estimated and divided into those present on admission and thus perhaps less-modifiable, and those developing after admission and traditionally being considered more treatable. The most important factor present on admission is the neurological grade of the patient. All other factors such as age, amount of SAH on computed tomography, presence of intraventricular and intracerebral hemorrhage, size and location of the aneurysm, and preexisting systemic hypertension, were less important. Of the factors developing after admission, the most important was cerebral infarction (although strictly speaking, not a risk factor for poor outcome). Others, such as vasospasm and fever 8 days after SAH, contributed a similar amount, whereas use of anticonvulsants and various hemodynamic treatments were less influential. The multiple factors and relatively small overall effect of vasospasm leads to very large sample sizes when traditional clinical trials are designed for agents to prevent vasospasm with endpoints such as the Glasgow Outcome Scale [6]. Further complicating the picture are additional, as yet unidentified factors that are not directly modifiable by treating physicians, such as genetic predispositions to brain injury [5]. Another issue is that the above retrospective multivariable analysis does not give any information about the causative nature of any of the features to outcome but simply measures association. Fever after SAH is a good example. The uncertainty lies in whether we consider the febrile patient in such condition as a cause or a consequence of the underlying aneurysmal pathology. Certainly, SAH and the resulting neurological deficits will have an effect on physiological homeostasis. In fact, the extent of neurological insult will determine the magnitude of dysfunction systemically [11]. A vicious cycle thus develops, where the increasing systemic disorder results in further neurological injury. This may be a consequence of one known manifestation of systemic disease: fever. Other work has identified poor clinical neurological grade and the presence of intraventricular hemorrhage as key risk factors in the development of fever after SAH [3]. Importantly, these febrile patients are often refractory to the usual treatments for fever, such as acetaminophen. Further study on patient management and the development of medical complications such as fever is certainly warranted.

Pathogenesis of vasospasm

Given the correlation between vasospasm of cerebral arteries and poor outcome, much interest has focused on the etiologic factors that propagate vasospasm and the possibility of selectively targeting and interrupting their mechanism of action. Endothelin-1 is an important mediator of vasospasm and is known to be a potent and long-lasting vasoconstrictor. Clazosentan, a selective endothelin-A receptor antagonist, has proven to be an interesting candidate in the treatment of vasospasm owing to its ability to reverse vasoconstriction in experimental [10] and phase 2a clinical trials [12]. Much focus has turned to the possibility of using clazosentan in the prevention angiographic cerebral vasospasm following aneurysmal SAH.

Vajkoczy et al. [12] randomized 76 patients with aneurysmal SAH to clazosentan, 0.2 mg/kg/h, or placebo. In blinded analysis, moderate and severe angiographic vasospasm was reduced significantly from 88% in the placebo to 40% in the clazosentan-treated patients. Regional cerebral blood flow was also measured [1]. It was the same in placebo (23 ± 4 mL/100 g/min) and clazosentan (24 ± 1) patients acutely after the SAH, but by day 8 was significantly lower in the placebo group (11 ± 7 versus 24 ± 13). In an open-label component of the study, clazosentan was infused intravenously in some of the placebo patients after vasospasm had developed and it was found to reverse established vasospasm in 50% of cases. Furthermore, new infarctions were observed in 15% of patients in the clazosentan group compared to 44% in the placebo group (not statistically significant). Toxicity seemed to be minimal.

CONSCIOUS-1

The effects of clazosentan on the occurrence of vasospasm were tested further in the CONSCIOUS-1 study (clazosentan to overcome neurological ischemia and infarction occurring after subarachnoid hemorrhage). Here, a double-blind, randomized placebo-controlled approach was employed for patients with ruptured aneurysms treated with either coiling or clipping. Clazosentan, 1, 5, or 15 mg/h was tested in patients for up to 14 days. The primary efficacy endpoint was moderate or severe cerebral vasospasm, as measured by digital subtraction catheter angiography (DSCA) at day 9 ± 2 post-aneurysm rupture. Of note, this is one of few [4, 12], and possibly the largest trial to evaluate an experimental treatment for cerebral vasospasm using DSCA. Recruitment involved 413 patients from 52 centers worldwide. All 3 doses significantly reduced moderate or severe cerebral vasospasm. The effect was proportional to the dose of the drug administered, with a relative risk reduction of 65% (as compared to placebo) in the group of patients receiving 15 mg/h of clazosentan ($p < 0.0001$).

While the reduction in vasospasm occurred in a dose-dependent manner, clinical outcome was not favorably changed. One somewhat implausible explanation for this is that moderate and severe vasospasm defined angiographically does not necessarily cause poor outcome. A review of the literature as well as clinical experience shows that patients with severe vasospasm that is not treated develop large cerebral infarctions. Cerebral infarction is strongly associated with poor outcome, and angioplasty to reverse vasospasm almost certainly saves lives, suggesting that this is not true [2, 8]. Another possibility is that clinical benefit may be balanced by side effects of the drug. This seems unlikely, because there was a trend for reduction in cerebral infarct number and volume among the clazosentan-treated patients compared to placebo. There may be other causes for DCI as aforementioned. Reducing the degree of vasospasm can only reduce its contribution to the clinical outcome that is dependent upon a number of modifiable and unmodifiable factors. Finally, and perhaps most likely, is the fact that the study was not powered to detect an effect on the Glasgow Outcome Scale, which would require many more patients [6].

CONSCIOUS-2

The benefit of clazosentan in reducing vasospasm is strongly supported now in 2 blinded clinical trials. Since vasospasm is a well-documented adverse prognostic factor for outcome after aneurysmal SAH, it remains important to further study preventive treatments. CONSCIOUS-2 is the next study of clazosentan and is a phase 3 randomized, blinded, placebo-controlled trial. It aims to measure clinical outcome using the primary endpoint of vasospasm morbidity and all-cause mortality. Vasospasm morbidity is defined as delayed neurological deterioration, new cerebral infarction, and/or commencement of valid rescue therapy for vasospasm. Patients suffering from aneurysmal SAH who have had their aneurysm clipped and do not suffer any severe intraoperative complications that would compromise neurological evaluation will be randomized 2:1 to receive clazosentan (5 mg/h) or placebo. One design advantage of this study is that the patients entered will represent a homogenous group, with a unique treatment for their ruptured aneurysm (neurosurgical clipping). Additionally, multiple secondary endpoints of this study include the extended Glasgow Outcome Scale assessed at 3 months, as well as total volume of new cerebral infarcts and each of the primary endpoint components as determined by a central critical events committee. This way, we will be able to measure the longer term effects of clazosentan, as well as the clinical outcome of patients with reduced vasospasm months after the initial hemorrhage.

Conclusions

Two of every 3 patients with aneurysmal SAH will experience vasospasm, and 1 of these will suffer morbidity and mortality that decreases their chance for meaningful recovery [7]. This is in spite of nimodipine and complicated, expensive hemodynamic therapy and intensive care monitoring. Currently, treatment for SAH remains supportive and the treatment options for vasospasm are limited. Vasospasm is a well-established complication of SAH and clazosentan has statistically shown to be effective in reducing its incidence. Hopefully, the CONSCIOUS-2 study will elucidate whether and how this translates into clinical benefit for our patients.

References

1. Barth M, Capelle HH, Munch E, Thome C, Fiedler F, Schmiedek P, Vajkoczy P (2007) Effects of the selective endothelin A (ET(A)) receptor antagonist Clazosentan on cerebral perfusion and cerebral oxygenation following severe subarachnoid hemorrhage – preliminary results from a randomized clinical series. Acta Neurochir (Wien) 149: 911–918
2. Fergusen S, Macdonald RL (2007) Predictors of cerebral infarction in patients with aneurysmal subarachnoid hemorrhage. Neurosurgery 60: 658–667
3. Fernandez A, Schmidt JM, Claassen J, Pavlicova M, Huddleston D, Kreiter KT, Ostapkovich ND, Kowalski RG, Parra A, Connolly ES, Mayer SA (2007) Fever after subarachnoid hemorrhage: risk factors and impact on outcome. Neurology 68: 1013–1019
4. Findlay JM, Kassell NF, Weir BK, Haley EC Jr, Kongable G, Germanson T, Truskowski L, Alves WM, Holness RO, Knuckey NW (1995) A randomized trial of intraoperative, intracisternal tissue plasminogen activator for the prevention of vasospasm. Neurosurgery 37: 168–178
5. Leung CH, Poon WS, Yu LM, Wong GK, Ng HK (2002) Apolipoprotein E genotype and outcome in aneurysmal subarachnoid hemorrhage. Stroke 33: 548–552
6. Macdonald RL, Kreiter KT, Mayer SA, Knappertz V (2005) Methodology for phase 3 clinical trial planning: powering treatment studies of vasospasm in SAH. J Neurosurg 102: A416
7. Macdonald RL, Pluta RM, Zhang JH (2007) Cerebral vasospasm after subarachnoid hemorrhage: the emerging revolution. Nat Clin Pract Neurol 3: 256–263

8. Nolan CP, Macdonald RL (2006) Can angiographic vasospasm be used as a surrogate marker in evaluating therapeutic interventions for cerebral vasospasm? Neurosurg Focus 21: E1

9. Rosengart AJ, Schultheiss KE, Tolentino J, Macdonald RL (2007) Prognostic factors for outcome in patients with aneurysmal subarachnoid hemorrhage. Stroke 38: 2315–2321

10. Roux S, Breu V, Giller T, Neidhart W, Ramuz H, Coassolo P, Clozel JP, Clozel M (1997) Ro 61-1790, a new hydrosoluble endothelin antagonist: general pharmacology and effects on experimental cerebral vasospasm. J Pharmacol Exp Ther 283: 1110–1118

11. Stevens RD, Nyquist PA (2007) The systemic implications of aneurysmal subarachnoid hemorrhage. J Neurol Sci 261: 143–156

12. Vajkoczy P, Meyer B, Weidauer S, Raabe A, Thome C, Ringel F, Breu V, Schmiedek P (2005) Clazosentan (AXV-034343), a selective endothelin A receptor antagonist, in the prevention of cerebral vasospasm following severe aneurysmal subarachnoid hemorrhage: results of a randomized, double-blind, placebo-controlled, multicenter phase IIa study. J Neurosurg 103: 9–17

Acta Neurochir Suppl (2008) 105: 211–215
© Springer-Verlag 2008
Printed in Austria

Regional cerebral blood flow and oxygen metabolism in aneurysmal subarachnoid hemorrhage: positron emission tomography evaluation of clipping versus coiling

N. Kawai, T. Nakamura, T. Tamiya, S. Nagao

Department of Neurological Surgery, Kagawa University School of Medicine, Kagawa, Japan

Summary

Objective. We investigated early postoperative hemodynamic and metabolic values using positron emission tomography (PET) scanning in subarachnoid hemorrhage (SAH) patients treated with clipping or coiling, and evaluated usefulness of PET studies in predicting late ischemic events and neurological outcome in SAH patients.

Methods. We examined 14 SAH patients treated with neurosurgical clipping (CLIP group) and 16 patients treated with endovascular coiling (COIL group). Cerebral blood flow (CBF), cerebral metabolic rate for oxygen (CMRO$_2$), and oxygen extraction fraction (OEF) were determined using ^{15}O-PET scanning about 8.5 days after SAH.

Results. 1) Mean regional CBF (rCBF) in the middle cerebral artery (MCA) territory was significantly higher in CLIP group compared with COIL group; regional CMRO$_2$ (rCMRO$_2$) and regional OEF (rOEF) were also higher. Four clipped patients showed true hyperemia in the MCA territory; none of the coiled patients showed hyperemia. 2) Surgical intervention significantly decreased mean rCMRO$_2$ and rOEF in the operated frontal lobe compared with the unoperated side. 3) Nine of 30 patients (40%) developed subsequent clinical vasospasm after SAH. Significant differences between the spasm group and non-spasm group were not observed in the MCA territory before vasospasm.

Conclusion. A wide range of cerebral perfusion patterns including hyperemia were found in the CLIP group. Surgical manipulation of the brain significantly reduced oxygen metabolism in the operated frontal lobe. PET data alone may not have independent prognostic value for detecting delayed cerebral ischemia or in predicting neurological outcome.

Keywords: Cerebral blood flow; cerebral oxygen metabolism; endovascular coiling; subarachnoid hemorrhage; surgical clipping.

Introduction

Clipping has been considered the most reliable and common treatment for subarachnoid hemorrhage (SAH) resulting from ruptured aneurysm. In the past decade, however, endovascular coiling has grown in popularity as an alternative to clipping. Outcome studies are necessary to ascertain the relative benefits of endovascular coiling over neurosurgical clipping.

The International Subarachnoid Aneurysm Trial (ISAT), a randomized trial comparing neurosurgical clipping with endovascular coiling in patients with ruptured intracranial aneurysm, has shown the benefit of endovascular treatment on the primary outcome: death or dependency at 1 year [11]. Many studies of reportedly good neurological outcome have demonstrated that a significant number of SAH patients show impairments in neuropsychological functioning [7, 9]. To fully understand the clinical outcome and relative efficacy of these treatments, evaluation of neuropsychological status, including cognitive outcome, is necessary. A recent study showed that coiled patients may have slightly better cognitive outcome than clipped patients in the acute phase after treatment [3]. However, there are minimal differences in long-term cognitive outcome between the 2 groups because of the post-acute stage of recovery in the both groups [3]. This finding indicates that there might be differences in cerebral blood flow (CBF) and metabolism that occur shortly after clipping or coiling of a ruptured aneurysm.

The primary aim of our study was to investigate early hemodynamic and metabolic values using positron emission tomography (PET) scanning in patients with SAH. Regional cortical values of CBF, cerebral metabolic rate of oxygen (CMRO$_2$), and oxygen extraction fraction (OEF) were evaluated within 14 days after SAH and compared between the surgical clipping (CLIP) group and the endovascular coiling (COIL) group. The second-

Correspondence: Nobuyuki Kawai, M.D., Department of Neurological Surgery, Kagawa University School of Medicine, 1750-1 Miki-cho, Kita-gun, Kagawa 761-0793, Japan. e-mail: nobu@med.kagawa-u.ac.jp

ary aim of this study was to evaluate the correlation be-tween the PET findings and delayed cerebral ischemia due to cerebral vasospasm and to determine the useful-ness of PET studies in predicting late ischemic events and neurological outcome.

Materials and methods

Patients, study design, and treatment

Thirty consecutive patients with SAH attributable to aneurysm rupture (20 women, 10 men) with a mean age of 61.6 ± 13.4 years (range, 32–79 years) were enrolled in this study. The protocol excluded patients who had large intracerebral hematoma or were World Federation of Neurological Surgeons (WFNS) grade V.

Decisions on how to treat an aneurysm were made on a case-by-case fashion, depending on angiographic and clinical data. Fourteen patients were treated by neurosurgical clipping using the standard pterional approach (10 women, 4 men; mean age 54.0 ± 12.4 years) (CLIP group) and 16 patients were treated by endovascular coiling with Guglielmi detachable coil (GDC) (10 women, 6 men; mean age 68.1 ± 10.5 years) (COIL group). As the treatment strategy was decided on a case-by-case fashion, the COIL group was found to be significantly older than the CLIP group ($p < 0.01$). The 2 groups were compared with 13 disease control patients (CONTROL group) without SAH, where a cerebral pan-angiography did not show any vascular lesions (6 women, 7 men; mean age 60.8 ± 11.7 years). The clinical status of the patients was assessed using the WFNS grading scale, and mean WFNS grade on admission was similar in the CLIP group (2.6 ± 0.7) and in the COIL group (2.4 ± 0.7). Four patients bearing posterior circulation aneurysm were all treated by endovascular coiling.

Postoperatively, all patients were monitored in neurological intensive care units, usually until day 14 post-SAH. Regardless of the method of securing the ruptured aneurysm, every patient was treated in the same way with hypervolemia/hypertension and intermittent fasudil hydro-chloride (Rho-kinase inhibitor) administration. Continuous cerebrospinal fluid drainage from the lumbar subarachnoid space was placed when necessary. Neurological examinations were performed daily to detect delayed ischemic neurological deterioration (DIND). DIND was defined as a new or aggravating neurological deficit or a reduced level of consciousness and confirmed with digital angiography. Once cerebral

vasospasm was revealed on angiography, fasudil hydrochloride or pa-paverine hydrochloride was selectively administered to relax constricted arteries and intensive hypervolemia/hypertension therapy was per-formed to maintain adequate CBF. Regional CBF (rCBF) and metabo-lism was determined using positron emission tomography (PET), usually within 10 days after SAH. Patients who already exhibited DIND and had cerebral infarction on CT scan at the time of PET examination were excluded from this study. Outcome was graded according to the Glasgow Outcome Scale at time of discharge from the hospital.

Results

One patient in the CLIP group (7%) had severe DIND resulting in cerebral infarction and 4 patients (29%) had mild to moderate symptoms from DIND without radio-logical consequences. On the other hand, 3 patients in the COIL group (19%) had moderate to severe DIND with subsequent cerebral infarction, and 1 patient (6%) had minor symptoms from DIND without permanent radiological findings. Therefore, the incidence of clinical vasospasm was not significantly different between the 2 groups. The outcome of the patients at discharge was similar in the CLIP group (GR:9, MD:3, SD:1, VS:1) and in the COIL group (GR:10, MD:4, SD:2).

PET studies were performed usually within 10 days after SAH in both groups (8.4 ± 3.4 days in the CLIP group and 8.6 ± 2.4 days in the COIL group). Physio-logical parameters including blood pressure, arterial pH, PaO_2, $PaCO_2$, hemoglobin concentration, and he-matocrit level were within normal values and did not differ significantly between the 2 groups. Mean rCBF in the middle cerebral artery (MCA) territory was sig-nificantly higher in the CLIP group (49.9 ± 4.5 ml/100 g/min) compared with the COIL group (44.1 ± 4.1 ml/100 g/min, $p < 0.01$) (Fig. 1A). The mean rCBF

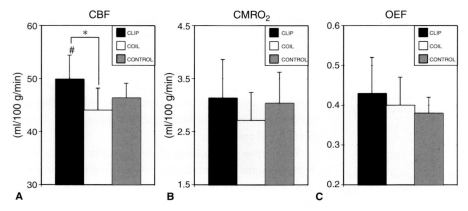

Fig. 1. Comparison of rCBF (A), rCMRO$_2$ (B), and rOEF (C) in the MCA territory examined using ^{15}O-PET in SAH patients treated with surgical clipping (CLIP) or endovascular coiling (COIL) and controls (CONTROL). PET scanning was performed about 8.5 days after SAH in the CLIP and COIL patient groups. Mean rCBF was significantly higher in the CLIP group compared with the COIL group ($^*p < 0.01$). The rCBF value observed in the CLIP group was also significantly higher than that in the CONTROL group ($^\#p < 0.05$). Mean rCMRO$_2$ and rOEF were higher in the CLIP group compared with the COIL group, but the differences between the 2 groups were not statistically significant

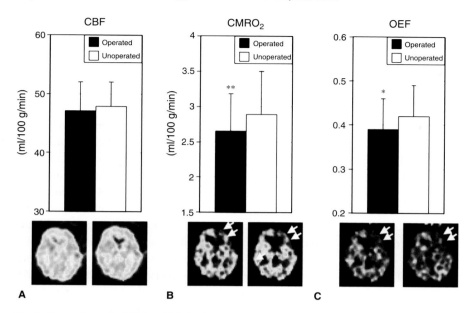

Fig. 2. Comparison of rCBF (A), rCMRO$_2$ (B) and rOEF (C) in operated and unoperated frontal lobes of SAH patients treated with surgical clipping ($n = 14$). Mean rCBF in the operated frontal lobe did not significantly differ from the value in the unoperated frontal lobe. Mean rCMRO$_2$ and rOEF in the operated frontal lobe were significantly lower compared with values in the unoperated frontal lobe ($^{**}p < 0.01$ and $^{*}p < 0.05$). Comparison was made by paired t-test. The bottom row of images is from a representative case showing decreased rCMRO$_2$ and rOEF in the operated frontal lobe (*double arrow*)

value observed in the CLIP group was also significantly higher than that in the CONTROL group (46.4 ± 2.7 ml/100 g/min, $p < 0.05$). Four patients in the CLIP group showed hyperemia (rCBF >51.6 ml/100 g/min, mean rCBF $+ 2$ SD in the CONTROL group) in the MCA territory; however, no patients in the COIL group showed hyperemia. Mean regional CMRO$_2$ (rCMRO$_2$) in the MCA territory was higher in the CLIP group (3.14 ± 0.72 ml/100 g/min) compared with that in the COIL group (2.72 ± 0.52 ml/100 g/min), but this was not statistically significant (Fig. 1B). Again, mean regional OEF (rOEF) in the MCA territory was slightly higher in the CLIP group (0.43 ± 0.09), but was not

significantly different compared with that in the COIL group (0.40 ± 0.07) (Fig. 1C). Since only a small number of patients ($n = 4$) had poor neurological outcome (SD + VS) in both groups, we did not perform a statistical comparison of PET values between good-outcome and poor-outcome patients. Four poor-outcome patients (2 in each group) showed slightly lowered mean rCBF (44.4 ± 5.1 ml/100 g/min) in the MCA territory; their mean rCMRO$_2$ was, however, apparently low (2.40 ± 0.34 ml/100 g/min). To evaluate the effect of surgical manipulation and retraction of the brain on CBF and metabolism, we compared PET values in the bilateral frontal lobe in the CLIP group ($n = 14$). Al-

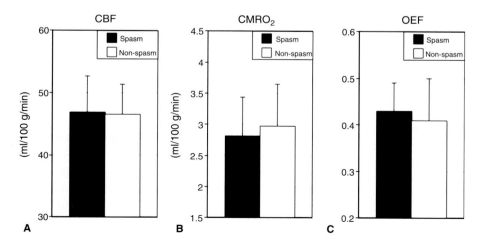

Fig. 3. Comparison of rCBF (A), rCMRO$_2$ (B) and rOEF (C) before clinical vasospasm in the MCA territory in the spasm group ($n = 12$) and non-spasm group ($n = 18$). There were no significant differences in these PET values between the 2 groups

though there was no significant difference in mean rCBF in the frontal lobe between the approach side (47.1 ± 4.9 ml/100 g/min) and non-approach side (47.9 ± 4.1 ml/100 g/min) (Fig. 2A), the values of mean rCMRO$_2$ and rOEF in the frontal lobe were significantly lower in the approach side (2.65 ± 0.53 ml/100 g/min and 0.39 ± 0.07 ml/100 g/min, respectively) compared with those in the non-approach side (2.89 ± 0.61 ml/100 g/min; $p < 0.01$, and 0.42 ± 0.07; $p < 0.05$, respectively) (Fig. 2B and C). To clarify the second aim of our study, evaluation of the usefulness of PET studies in predicting cerebral vasospasm, we compared PET values obtained before clinical vasospasm in the MCA territory between the spasm group ($n = 12$) and the non-spasm group ($n = 18$). There was no significant difference in rCBF between the spasm group (46.9 ± 5.8 ml/100 g/min) and the non-spasm group (46.6 ± 4.8 ml/100 g/min) (Fig. 3A). Again, there were no significant differences in oxygen metabolism between the spasm group (rCMRO$_2$ = 2.82 ± 0.62; rOEF = 0.43 ± 0.06) and the non-spasm group (rCMRO$_2$ = 2.98 ± 0.67; rOEF = 0.41 ± 0.09) (Fig. 3B and C).

Discussion

Our study was conducted to examine 2 questions. The first was to determine whether there are any differences in postoperative CBF and metabolism between surgically clipped and endovascularly coiled patients after aneurysmal SAH. The clinical and demographic data are identical between the 2 groups, and PET scans were obtained at similar time points in the acute stage after SAH. Regional CBF in the MCA territory was significantly higher in the CLIP group compared with the COIL group. The effect of aging on CBF might be small and could not account for the significant reduction observed in the COIL group. We found a wide variation in CBF patterns, ranging from reduced blood flow to normal CBF values to hyperemia among SAH patients treated by surgical clipping. Four of the clipped patients (29%) exhibited true hyperemia in the MCA territory; however, none of the coiled patients showed hyperemia. Hyperemia observed in the CLIP group influenced the result of significantly higher values of mean rCBF in the MCA territory compared with the COIL group. Several pervious studies have demonstrated globally and gradually reduced CBF and CMRO$_2$ in the acute stage of aneurysmal SAH [5, 8]. There was, however, one report showing hyperemic CBF values in the normal cortices in surgically operated SAH patients [6]. A recent xenon-

CT study also demonstrated that global hyperemia was detected postoperatively in 14% of the aneurysmal SAH patients treated with surgical clipping [13]. To the best of our knowledge, no report has demonstrated cerebral hyperemia in SAH patients treated with coil embolization.

Although hyperemia is not a rare phenomenon following aneurysmal SAH, the precise mechanism of hyperemia has not been elucidated. A large amount of SAH causes elevated intracranial pressure and results in a severe drop in perfusion pressure [5]. Craniotomy for surgical clipping dramatically reduces intracranial pressure and this may cause reperfusion hyperemia. This does not occur in aneurysmal SAH patients treated with endovascular coiling. Our patients who showed global hyperemia after surgery also exhibited globally increased cerebral blood volume (CBV) in the brain. Hyperemia with increased CBV supports the reperfusion theory, which consists of recruitment of blood flow into the impaired cerebral vasculature with vasodilatation. In a scenario of cerebral ischemia, postischemic hyperemia is a beneficial phenomenon associated with good tissue outcome by restoring the blood flow into the impaired cerebral vasculatures when it occurs early in the acute ischemic phase. A previous study has shown that hyperemic CBF value following SAH correlates to a favorable outcome [13]. In our study, 4 clipped patients exhibited true hyperemia in the PET scan obtained 7 to 11 days after SAH, and they all showed good neurological outcome (GR) at discharge.

Animal studies have shown that marked reduction in CBF underlying a brain retractor and prolonged brain retraction can lead to tissue damage [12]. Yundt *et al.* used PET to measure rCBF, rCMRO$_2$, and rOEF in 4 patients 1 day before and 6–17 days after surgical clipping for ruptured aneurysm [14]. They compared pre- and postoperative changes and differences between operated and unoperated hemispheres. Measurements revealed that CMRO$_2$ fell 45% and OEF fell 32% after surgery in the retraction zone, while CBF remained unchanged. We observed similar results in our surgically-treated SAH patients, but the relative reductions in CMRO$_2$ and OEF in the operated frontal lobe were very mild (<10%).

The second question examined in our study is whether PET examinations have predictable values of late ischemic events and final neurological outcome. Measurement of CBF has been shown to provide useful prognostic information about patients with SAH and to help guide timing of surgery. Transcranial Doppler

(TCD) ultrasonography is a commonly used technique to measure blood flow velocities in large intracranial arteries [1]. Although TDC is the simplest and least invasive method to detect changes in CBF in patients with SAH, this technique is associated with poor sensitivity and specificity and is best used in combination with other modalities [10, 13]. We observed apparently low rCMRO$_2$ and rOEF in the MCA territory in patients with poor neurological outcome; rCBF in the MCA territory, however, did not differ between the poor- and good-outcome groups. In a primate study of cerebral ischemia, CMRO$_2$ measurement provided the best predictor of reversible or irreversible tissue damage [4]. Also, OEF and CMRO$_2$ measurements could provide a true definition of ischemia in patients with aneurysmal SAH [2]. We observed that 36 and 27% of the clipped and coiled patients, respectively, exhibited delayed clinical and/or angiographic vasospasm. However, no significant difference in CBF and metabolism in the MCA territory was observed between spasm and non-spasm patients before the vasospasm. Of course, it is important to recognize that PET studies provide a "snapshot" of cerebral perfusion and metabolism at the time of scanning, but provide no information regarding preceding or subsequent events. The number of patients in this series is insufficient for detailed quantification of this prognostic value, but our results suggest that PET data may not have independent prognostic value in the assessment of crude outcome, in terms of poor and good neurological outcome. No study has attempted to compare the PET findings and cognitive outcome in aneurysmal SAH patients treated by surgical clipping or endovascular coiling. We would like to examine the relationship between the temporal and spatial PET findings and neuropsychological consequences including cognitive function in our next study.

Conclusions

First, among patients with aneurysmal SAH, we observed that mean rCBF in the MCA territory was significantly higher in the CLIP group compared with the COIL group. A wide range of cerebral perfusion patterns including hyperemia was found in the CLIP group, while no patients in the COIL group showed hyperemia. Surgical manipulation of the brain significantly reduced rCMRO$_2$ and rOEF, but not rCBF in the operated frontal lobe compared with those in the unoperated frontal lobe.

Secondly, PET data alone may not have independent prognostic value in detecting delayed cerebral ischemia or for predicting crude neurological outcome. It is necessary to examine the relationship between PET findings and neuropsychological consequences, including cognitive function, in the future.

References

1. Aaslid R, Huber P, Nornes H (1984) Evaluation of cerebrovascular spasm with transcranial Doppler ultrasound. J Neurosurg 60: 37–41
2. Carpenter DA, Grubb RL Jr, Tempel LW, Powers WJ (1991) Cerebral oxygen metabolism after aneurysmal subarachnoid hemorrhage. J Cereb Blood Flow Metab 11: 837–844
3. Frazer D, Ahuja A, Watkins L, Cipolotti L (2007) Coiling versus clipping for the treatment of aneurysmal subarachnoid hemorrhage: a longitudinal investigation into cognitive outcome. Neurosurgery 60: 434–442
4. Frykholm P, Andersson JL, Valtysson J, Silander HC, Hillered L, Persson L, Olsson Y, Yu WR, Westerberg G, Watanabe Y, Långström B, Enblad P (2000) A metabolic threshold of irreversible ischemia demonstrated by PET in a middle cerebral artery occlusion-reperfusion primate model. Acta Neurol Scand 102: 18–26
5. Hayashi T, Suzuki A, Hatazawa J, Kanno I, Shirane R, Yoshimoto T, Yasui N (2000) Cerebral circulation and metabolism in the acute stage of subarachnoid hemorrhage. J Neurosurg 93: 1014–1018
6. Hino A, Mizukawa N, Tenjin H, Imahori Y, Taketomo S, Yano I, Nakahashi H, Hirakawa K (1989) Postoperative hemodynamic and metabolic changes in patients with subarachnoid hemorrhage. Stroke 20: 1504–1510
7. Hütter BO, Kreitschmann-Andermahr I, Gilsbach JM (1998) Cognitive deficits in the acute stage after subarachnoid hemorrhage. Neurosurgery 43: 1054–1065
8. Kawamura S, Sayama I, Yasui N, Uemura K (1992) Sequential changes in cerebral blood flow and metabolism in patients with subarachnoid haemorrhage. Acta Neurochir (Wien) 114: 12–15
9. Mavaddat N, Sahakian BJ, Hutchinson PJ, Kirkpatrick PJ (1999) Cognition following subarachnoid hemorrhage from anterior communicating artery aneurysm: relation to timing of surgery. J Neurosurg 91: 402–407
10. Minhas PS, Mennon DK, Smielewski P, Czosnyka M, Kirkpatrick PJ, Clark JC, Pickard JD (2003) Positron emission tomographic cerebral perfusion disturbances and transcranial Doppler findings among patients with neurological deterioration after subarachnoid hemorrhage. Neurosurgery 52: 1017–1024
11. Molyneux AJ, Kerr RSC, Stratton I, Sandercock P, Clarke M, Shrimpton J, Holman R; International Subarachnoid Aneurysm Trial (ISAT) Collaborative Group (2002) International Subarachnoid Aneurysm Trial (ISAT) of neurosurgical clipping versus endovascular coiling in 2143 patients with ruptured intracranial aneurysms: a randomised trial. Lancet 360: 1267–1274
12. Rosenørn J, Diemer N (1985) The risk of cerebral damage during graded brain retractor pressure in the rat. J Neurosurg 63: 608–611
13. Rothoerl RD, Woertgen C, Brawanski A (2004) Hyperemia following aneurysmal subarachnoid hemorrhage: incidence, diagnosis, clinical features, and outcome. Intens Care Med 30: 1298–1302
14. Yundt KD, Grubb RL Jr, Diringer MN, Powers WJ (1997) Cerebral hemodynamic and metabolic changes caused by brain retraction after aneurysmal subarachnoid hemorrhage. Neurosurgery 40: 442–451

Acta Neurochir Suppl (2008) 105: 217–220
© Springer-Verlag 2008
Printed in Austria

Preliminary report of the clot lysis evaluating accelerated resolution of intraventricular hemorrhage (CLEAR-IVH) clinical trial

T. Morgan[1], I. Awad[2], P. Keyl[3], K. Lane[1], D. Hanley[1]

[1] The Johns Hopkins University, Baltimore, MD, USA
[2] Evanston Northwestern University, Evanston, IL, USA
[3] Keyl Associates, East Sandwich, MA, USA

Summary

Introduction. Brain hemorrhage is the most frequent fatal form of stroke and has the highest level of morbidity of any stroke subtype. For patients with both intracerebral hemorrhage and intraventricular hemorrhage (IVH), expected mortality is 50–80%. No validated, efficacious treatment exists for humans, but animal models demonstrate substantial physiologic and functional benefits associated with rapid, near-complete removal of blood from either the ventricle or intracerebral location (i.e., ~80% removal over 48 h). The purpose of the CLEAR-IVH trial (Parts A and B) is to evaluate safety and efficacy of using multiple injections of low-dose rt-PA to accelerate lysis and evacuation of IVH.

Methods. Patients enrolled in the trial receive an injection of 1.0 mg rt-PA through an external ventricular drain every 8 h up to 12 doses, or until clot reduction or clinical endpoint is met. CT scans are taken daily to monitor clot resolution and check for unexpected bleeding events. In a previous dose-finding study where the safety profile (symptomatic re-bleeding) was 0%, 1 mg rt-PA every 8 h was determined the appropriate dose.

Results. Comprehensive analyses of 36 patients in the recently completed CLEAR-IVH Part B are currently being conducted. Adverse events are within safety limits, including 30-day mortality, 8%; symptomatic re-bleeding, 8%; and bacterial ventriculitis, 0%.

Conclusion. Preliminary analyses show that use of low-dose rt-PA can be safely administered to stable IVH clots and may increase lysis rates.

Keywords: Intraventricular hemorrhage; thrombolysis; tissue plasminogen activator.

Introduction

Intraventricular hemorrhage (IVH) occurs in about 40% of primary intracerebral hemorrhage (ICH) cases and 15% of aneurysmal subarachnoid hemorrhage (SAH)

Correspondence: Timothy Morgan, B.Sc., Johns Hopkins University, 1550 Orleans Street, CRB II 3M50 South, Baltimore, MD 21231, USA. e-mail: tmorga10@jhmi.edu

cases [1, 6, 8, 17]. The incidence of IVH in ICH is about twice that of SAH; respectively they account for about 10 and 5% of the 500,000 strokes occurring yearly in the United States [5, 6]. Thus, an IVH occurs in about 22,000 people every year in the United States. Most recent research supports the assertion that IVH is a significant and independent contributor to morbidity and mortality in both ICH and aneurysmal SAH [1, 7, 8, 15, 22, 23, 25]. Mortality estimates for this condition range from 50 to 80% [2, 23].

Current practice in the management of IVH involves the use of an extraventricular drain (EVD) to treat obstructive hydrocephalus; however, an EVD is often inadequate in the setting of IVH because the catheter becomes occluded with blood clots. Conventional therapy for catheter occlusion with blood is removal of the occluded catheter and insertion of a second catheter in another location, preferably one that is free of blood. This technique does little to address inflammatory reactions caused by the breakdown of blood clots in ventricles that often lead to communicating hydrocephalus [4, 9, 10, 14]. The severity of communicating hydrocephalus appears to be related to the amount of blood present and the amount of time that the cerebrospinal fluid (CSF) is exposed to the clotted blood [3, 11–13, 21, 24]. In the CLEAR-IVH trial, the aim is to use recombinant tissue plasminogen activator (rt-PA; CathFlo Activase, Genetech Inc., South San Francisco, CA) to accelerate the lysis of IVH and effectively drain lysed blood products, thereby alleviating the effects of obstructive hydrocephalus and reducing the incidence of communicating hydrocephalus.

Background

Pang *et al.* [18–20] developed a model of intraventricular thrombolysis by treating clotted blood injected into the ventricles of adult dogs. In this study, more rapid clearance of intraventricular blood occurred in lytic-treated versus control animals. Similarly, Mayfrank *et al.* [16] showed ventricular dilatation and an association of blood clot volume with mass effect in a pig model. In that study, significant decline in this mass effect was noted at 1.5 h and 7 days when rt-PA was used for intraventricular thrombolysis. Importantly, in both canine and porcine models, the greater the volume of blood clot injected into the ventricles, the greater the likelihood of animal death [16, 20]. Initial data from the CLEAR-IVH Part B study ($n = 36$), and findings from the preceding safety study ($n = 48$) and CLEAR-IVH Part A study (dose-finding, $n = 16$), shows a similar proportional effect between greater clot volume and increased mortality in human IVH patients.

Methods

Inclusion criteria for the study are as follows: patients aged 18–75 with an intraventricular catheter placed as standard of care, using less than or equal to 2 complete passes. The eligible patient's diagnostic computed tomography (CT) scan must show evidence of either third or fourth ventricle obstruction, and an ICH volume ≤ 30 cc (volume calculated using the $A \times B \times C/2$ method) and stable at least 6 h later by a second CT scan. If an aneurysm is suspected, magnetic resonance angiography or CT angiography must be obtained prior to enrollment to rule out aneurysm, arteriovenous malformation, or any other vascular anomaly. The patient must have a historical Rankin score of 0 or 1 and a negative pregnancy test. Exclusion criteria include: any infratentorial hemorrhage, coagulopathy, platelet count <100,000, international normalized ratio >1.7, abnormal prothrombin time (PT), or an elevated activated partial thromboplastin time (APTT). Reversal of warfarin is permitted. If SAH is suspected, an angiogram is obtained to rule out any possibility of a bleeding source not strongly associated with hypertension.

Patients meeting enrollment criteria have an EVD placed as standard of care for treatment of acute obstructive hydrocephalus. Before dosing, the investigator is required to view the most recent CT scan, confirming that the catheter does not deliver rt-PA into tissue or subarachnoid space. Once catheter placement is confirmed and CSF outflow is observed to follow normal pressure wave forms, the first dose of drug is administered no sooner than 12 h and no later than 48 h after the diagnostic CT scan. Pharmacokinetic samples are drawn at doses 1 and 4 to assess drug-blood interaction (Fig. 1). After injection, the system is closed for 1 h to allow for drug-clot interaction. After 1 h, the system is opened for drainage. Isovolumetric injections continue every 8 h up to 12 doses, or until a clinical endpoint is met. Clinical endpoints include: (1) clot reduction to 80% of initial clot volume, (2) clearance of all obstruction of the third and fourth ventricles, and (3) any instance of re-bleeding in which stability cannot be re-established. A CT scan is taken every 24 h to assess whether an endpoint has been met. Follow-up scans are scheduled at 30 days and 180 days after treatment to monitor any subsequent bleeding event and track continuing changes in residual clot.

Results

One hundred patients (22 placebo, 78 treatment) have been treated using the described protocol. Results from

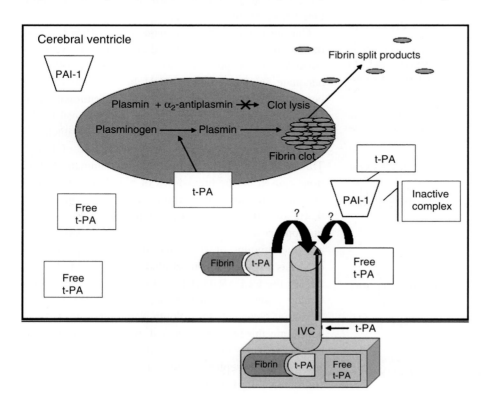

Fig. 1. rt-PA in the ventricle; the biochemistry of drug-blood interactions

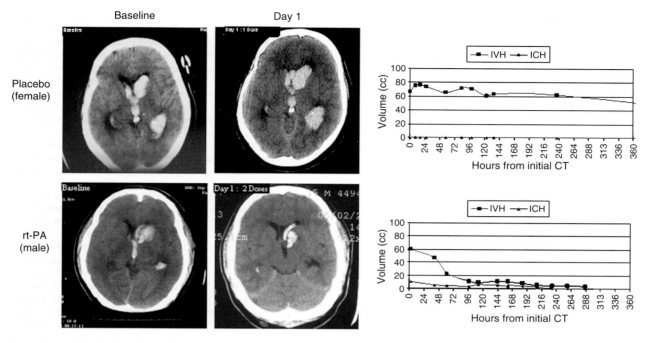

Fig. 2. Comparison of placebo patient and rt-PA patient

the recently concluded Phase II CLEAR-IVH, Part B, trial are not yet available. However, preliminary analyses indicate that low-dose treatment with rt-PA shows an expected safety profile, with the incidence of ventriculitis, cerebritis, re-bleeding, and 30-day mortality below predetermined study thresholds. One additional finding is that intraventricular blood closest to the drug-delivering EVD, as well as blood in the third and fourth ventricles, resolves more quickly than blood in areas of the ventricular system further from the EVD. Furthermore, once obstruction of the third and fourth ventricles is removed, clot lysis rates dissipate more rapidly in the treated patients (Fig. 2).

Conclusion

Enrollment in Phase II of the study concluded in March 2008. Early analyses have shown that areas closest to the catheter delivering drug and the third and fourth ventricles are the first to resolve with intraventricular rt-PA dosing. Furthermore, areas near the EVD catheter and the third and fourth ventricles show a clear dose response. This suggests that appropriate dosage and catheter placement are both important in achieving optimal clot lysis. Complete analyses are forthcoming.

Acknowledgments

This trial is funded by grant FD-R-001693-06 from the Food and Drug Administration Office of Orphan Products Development and Genentech Inc., South San Francisco, CA, through donation of the study drug.

References

1. Adams HP, Torner JC, Kassell NF (1992) Intraventricular hemorrhage among patients with recently ruptured aneurysms: a report of the Cooperative Aneurysm Study. Stroke 23: 140 (abstract)
2. Adams RE, Diringer MN (1998) Response to external ventricular drainage in spontaneous intracerebral hemorrhage with hydrocephalus. Neurology 50: 519–523
3. Ahmann PA, Lazzara A, Dykes FD, Brann AW Jr, Schwartz JF (1980) Intraventricular hemorrhage in the high-risk preterm infant: incidence and outcome. Ann Neurol 7: 118–124
4. Bagley C (1928) Blood in cerebrospinal fluid. Resultant functional and organic alterations in the central nervous system. Arch Surg 17: 39–81
5. Broderick JP, Brott T, Tomsick T, Miller R, Huster G (1993) Intracerebral hemorrhage more than twice as common as subarachnoid hemorrhage. J Neurosurg 78: 188–191
6. Brott T, Thalinger K, Hertzberg V (1986) Hypertension as a risk factor for spontaneous intracerebral hemorrhage. Stroke 17: 1078–1083
7. Conway JE, Oshiro EM, Piantadosi S (1998) Ventricular blood is an admission ct variable which predicts poor clinical outcome after aneurysmal subarachnoid hemorrhage. American Association of Neurological Surgeons Annual Meeting, Philadelphia, PA. J Neurosurg 88: 398A (abstract)
8. Daverat P, Castel JP, Dartigues JF, Orgogozo JM (1991) Death and functional outcome after spontaneous intracerebral hemorrahge. A prospective study of 166 cases using multivariate analysis. Stroke 22: 1–6
9. DeLand FH, James AE Jr, Ladd DJ, Konigsmark BW (1972) Normal pressure hydrocephalus: a histologic study. Am J Clin Pathol 58: 58–63

10. Ellington E, Margolis G (1969) Block of arachnoid villus by subarachnoid hemorrhage. J Neurosurg 30: 651–657
11. Findlay JM, Weir BK, Gordon P, Grace M, Baughman R (1989) Safety and efficacy of intrathecal thrombolytic therapy in a primate model of cerebral vasospasm. Neurosurgery 24: 491–498
12. Fisher CM, Kistler JP, Davis JM (1980) Relation of cerebral vasospasm to subarachnoid hemorrhage visualized by computerized tomographic scanning. Neurosurgery 6: 1–9
13. Kassell NF, Torner JC, Adams HP Jr (1984) Antifibrinolytic therapy in the acute period following aneurysmal subarachnoid hemorrhage. Preliminary observations from the Cooperative Aneurysm Study. J Neurosurg 61: 225–230
14. Kibler RF, Couch RS, Crompton MR (1961) Hydrocephalus in the adult following spontaneous subarachnoid hemorrhage. Brain 84: 45–61
15. Lisk DR, Pasteur W, Rhoades H, Putnam RD, Grotta JC (1994) Early presentation of hemispheric intracerebral hemorrhage: prediction of outcome and guidelines for treatment allocation. Neurology 44: 133–139
16. Mayfrank L, Kissler J, Raoofi R, Delsing P, Weis J, Küker W, Gilsbach JM (1997) Ventricular dilatation in experimental intraventricular hemorrhage in pigs. Characterization of cerebrospinal fluid dynamics and the effects of fibrinolytic treatment. Stroke 28: 141–148
17. Mohr G, Ferguson G, Khan M, Malloy D, Watts R, Benoit B, Weir B (1983) Intraventricular hemorrhage from ruptured aneurysm. J Neurosurg 58: 482–487
18. Pang D, Sclabassi RJ, Horton JA (1986) Lysis of intraventricular blood clot with urokinase in a canine model: Part 1. Canine intraventricular blood cast model. Neurosurgery 19: 540–546
19. Pang D, Sclabassi RJ, Horton JA (1986) Lysis of intraventricular blood clot with urokinase in a canine model: Part 2. In vivo safety study of intraventricular urokinase. Neurosurgery 19: 547–552
20. Pang D, Sclabassi RJ, Horton JA (1986) Lysis of intraventricular blood clot with urokinase in a canine model: Part 3. Effects of intraventricular urokinase on clot lysis and posthemorrhagic hydrocephalus. Neurosurgery 19: 553–572
21. Papile LA, Burstein J, Burstein R, Koffler H (1978) Incidence and evolution of subependymal and intraventricular hemorrhage: a study of infants with birth weights less than 1,500 g. J Pediatr 92: 529–534
22. Tuhrim S, Dambrosia JM, Price TR, Mohr JP, Wolf PA, Hier DB, Kase CS (1991) Intracerebral hemorrhage: external validation and extension of a model for prediction of 30-day survival. Ann Neurol 29: 658–663
23. Tuhrim S, Horowitz DR, Sacher M, Godbold JH (1995) Validation and comparison of models predicting survival following intracerebral hemorrhage. Crit Care Med 23: 950–954
24. Yasargil MG, Yonekawa Y, Zumstein B, Stahl HJ (1973) Hydrocephalus following spontaneous subarachnoid hemorrhage. Clinical features and treatment. J Neurosurg 39: 474–479
25. Young WB, Lee KP, Pessin MS, Kwan ES, Rand WM, Caplan LR (1990) Prognostic significance of ventricular blood in supratentorial hemorrhage: a volumetric study. Neurology 40: 616–619

Acta Neurochir Suppl (2008) 105: 221–224
© Springer-Verlag 2008
Printed in Austria

Leptin plays a role in ruptured human brain arteriovenous malformations

Q. Xie, X. C. Chen, Y. Gong, Y. X. Gu

Department of Neurosurgery, Huashan Hospital, Fudan University, Shanghai, China

Summary

Introduction. Intracerebral hemorrhage (ICH) is one of the most common clinical manifestations of human brain arteriovenous malformation (BAVM). However, the hemorrhagic mechanism of BAVM is still unclear. Leptin, first discovered in obesity research, has not been systematically studied in BAVM and ICH. We investigated expression and effect of leptin on human BAVM.

Methods. Specimens were obtained from 6 BAVM patients, who had been divided into either hemorrhagic or non-hemorrhagic groups. Leptin, leptin receptor, and signal transducers and activators of transcription-3 (STAT3) were analyzed by different methods, such as gene chips, reverse transcription-polymerase chain reaction (RT-PCR), immunohistochemistry, and Western blot. Perinidal brain tissue around each BAVM served as control.

Results. Gene chips and RT-PCR found transcriptional leptin raised at least 2 levels in hemorrhagic BAVM. Immunohistochemical slices also showed higher expression of leptin, leptin receptor, and STAT3 on nidus part of hemorrhagic BAVM than non-hemorrhagic ones. On Western blot analysis, hemorrhagic BAVMs had higher levels of leptin ($p < 0.01$).

Conclusions. The transcriptional and translational levels of leptin, leptin receptor, and STAT3 were higher in hemorrhagic BAVM, suggesting that leptin may play an important role in the hemorrhagic mechanism of BAVM.

Keywords: Brain arteriovenous malformations; leptin; intracerebral hemorrhage.

Introduction

Intracerebral hemorrhage (ICH) is one of the most common clinical manifestations of human brain arteriovenous malformation (BAVM) [1]. The primary goal of modern treatments, including surgical resection, interventional embolism and radiotherapy, or multidisciplinary therapy, is to lessen occurrences of BAVM bleeding [3]. However, the hemorrhagic mechanism of BAVM rupture is still unclear.

Correspondence: Xian-cheng Chen, Department of Neurosurgery, Huashan Hospital, Shanghai 200040, China. e-mail: xcchen58@yahoo.com.cn

Leptin was once classified as a key endocrine factor in regulating metabolism and was originally discovered in obesity research [11], but it has not been systematically studied in the field of BAVM and ICH [10]. Previously, we screened leptin as a significantly upregulated factor in the nidus part of BAVM by angiogenesis microarray. Also, Soderberg et al. [8] found there was positive relationship between leptin levels in serum and first-occurrence ICH, which is another independent risk factor of hemorrhagic stroke. These findings caused us to consider the possibility of a relationship between leptin and bleeding of BAVM. Therefore, the goal of our study was to investigate expression and effect of leptin and its related signaling pathway on human BAVM.

Methods

Samples

Specimens from 6 BAVM patients were obtained, with informed consent, for the period November, 2006 to March, 2007 at our hospital. Clinical data for these patients are listed in Table 1. According to each patient's history and imaging data, the patients were divided into 2 groups: hemorrhagic (3 patients) and non-hemorrhagic (3 patients). None of them had ever received either embolization or radiotherapy prior to their surgery.

The nidus and perinidal brain tissue of each BAVM was identified and then carefully dissected by the same experienced surgeon. Samples were collected individually and stored in liquid nitrogen, and later transferred to a $-80\,°C$ refrigerator, while the remainder of the specimen underwent routine pathological examination and immunohistochemistry to confirm BAVM, as follows.

Microarray analysis

Total ribonucleic acid (RNA) was extracted from the stored frozen tissue of nidus (N), supplying artery (A), draining vein (V), and perinidal brain tissue (B) individually using TRIzol reagent (Invitrogen, Carlsbad, CA). Yield and quality of total RNA were assessed by ultraviolet absorbance and denaturing agarose gel electrophoresis. Oligo GEArray Human Angiogenesis Microarray (OHS-024; SuperArray Biosciences Corp.,

Table 1. *Clinical data for BAVM study patients*

Pt. no.	Age/ Sex	Hemorrhage	Epilepsy	Radiotherapy	Embolization	BAVM site	BAVM diameter (cm)	Spetzler-Martin scale [9]	Gene chips	IHC	RT-PCR	Western blot
1	30/M	yes	no	no	no	L Fr	4.0	2	√	√	√	√
2	17/F	yes	no	no	no	L T&P	5.5	2	√	√	–	√
3	49/M	yes	no	no	no	L T	4.5	2	√	√	–	√
4	60/F	no	no	no	no	L Fr	7.0	3	–	√	–	–
5	35/M	no	yes	no	no	L P&O	4.0	2	–	√	–	–
6	30/F	no	yes	no	no	L T	3.5	2	–	√	–	–

BAVM Brain arteriovenous malformation; *F* female; *Fr* frontal; *IHC* immunohistochemistry; *L* left; *M* male; *O* occipital; *P* parietal; *Pt* patient; *RT-PCR* reverse transcription-polymerase chain reaction; *T* temporal.

Frederick, MD) was used to test 113 key genes involved in modulating the biological processes of angiogenesis. Particularly, the leptin gene bands were compared among the 4 tissues. After mean values of N, A, V, and B parts of 3 hemorrhagic BAVM specimens were concluded as N′, A′, V′, B′, we calculated values of N′/B′, A′/B′, V′/B′, making B′ as control and β-actin as internal control.

Semi-quantitative reverse transcription-polymerase chain reaction (RT-PCR)

A randomly selected nidus part of hemorrhagic BAVM underwent semi-quantitative RT-PCR, while the perinidal brain tissue of the same patient served as control.

After mRNA sequence of human leptin gene was copied from the National Center for Biotechnology Information (NCBI) GeneBank on-line, Primer Express version 1.0 software (Applied Biosystems, Foster City, CA) was used to design specific primers, which were manufactured by SBS Company (Beijing, China) and stored at $-20\,^\circ$C. Forward primer is 5′-GAA GGTTTGGTGTGTGGAGATG-3′, and reverse primer is 5′-GCCTGATTAGGTGGTTGTGAGG-3′.

In RT-PCR system A, RNase-free H_2O 11 μL, 10× reaction buffer 2 μL, dNTP 2 μL, oligo $(dT)_{18}$ 2 μL, RNA inhibitor 1 μL, sample RNA 1 μL, and sensicript RTase 1 μL, were added to a 20-μL final volume. The contents were mixed well at $37\,^\circ$C for an hour, so that sample RNA was reverse transcribed and amplified to cDNA. Then in PCR system B, ddH_2O 15.62 μL, 10X reaction buffer 2 μL, dNTP 0.4 μL, forward primer 0.4 μL, reverse primer 0.4 μL, sample cDNA 1 μL, and Hotstar-ase 0.18 μL, were added to a 20-μL final volume. The contents were mixed and the conditions of the PCR thermocycler were programmed at $94\,^\circ$C for 15 min, $94\,^\circ$C for 30 sec, $54\,^\circ$C for 30 sec, and $72\,^\circ$C for 40 sec; after 35 cycles, maintain $72\,^\circ$C for 10 min. mRNA levels were normalized to β-actin as outlined by the manufacturer.

To every 10-μL sample, 2 μL loading dye (Fermentas Life Sciences, Glen Burnie, MD) was added into the well and DNA marker DL2,000 (TaKaRa) 7 μL was used as control. After electrophoresis for 30 min, the gel was visualized on an ultraviolet transilluminator and pictures were saved to compare expression of leptin gene in different samples semi-quantitatively.

Immunohistochemical studies

Immunostaining was performed strictly following Strept-Avidin-Biotin-Peroxidase Complex (SABC) method using reagent kits. Sections of all specimens were incubated with primary antibodies of either leptin or leptin receptor diluted at the following concentrations: rabbit polyclonal anti-human leptin antibody, 1:20 diluted (Chemicon International, Temecula, CA); rabbit polyclonal anti-rat leptin receptor antibody, 1:20 diluted (Abcam Inc., Cambridge, MA); rabbit monoclonal anti-rat signal transducers and activators of transcription-3 (STAT3) antibody, 1:100 diluted (Cell Signaling Technology, Inc., Beverly, MA). The sec-

tions were mounted and photographed under fluorescent microscope. Negative controls were performed without adding primary antibodies.

Western blot analysis

Protein was extracted from all 3 hemorrhagic BAVM specimens and Western blot analysis was performed. Extracted protein from perinidal brain tissues served as controls. Briefly, concentration of sample protein was measured by bovine serum albumin method. The protein sample (50 μg) was run on 12% polyacrylamide gels with a 4% stacking gel after denaturing in $100\,^\circ$C water for 5 min. The protein was transferred to pure nitrocellulose membrane (Amersham Biosciences, Piscataway, NJ), and membranes were probed with a 1:5000 dilution of the primary antibody (rabbit anti-human leptin antibody; Chemicon International) and a 1:2000 dilution of the secondary antibody (peroxidase-conjugated goat anti-rabbit antibody). Finally, the antigen-antibody complexes were visualized with a chemiluminescence system and exposed to photosensitive film. The relative densities of leptin protein bands were analyzed.

Statistical analysis

Data are presented as mean ± standard deviation. We used SPSS version 10.0 software (SPSS, Inc., Chicago, IL) to analyze and F-test for comparison among groups. p-value of <0.05 was considered significant.

Results

With microarray analysis, values of N′/B′, A′/B′, V′/B′ were calculated, and N′/B′ was found to be about 4 times higher than the others, suggesting that mRNA ex-

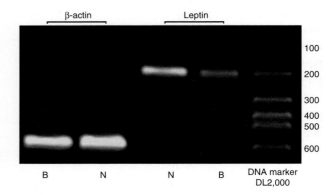

Fig. 1. RT-PCR compared to expression of leptin. Expression of leptin on nidus is higher than in perinidal brain tissue

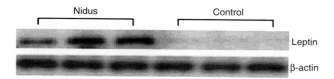

Fig. 2. Expression of leptin on nidus part of BAVM and slight expression on perinidal tissue on Western blot

pression of leptin gene in the nidus part of BAVM was about 4-fold higher than in artery, vein, or perinidal brain tissue ($p < 0.01$).

In Fig. 1, semi-quantitative RT-PCR indicates that the band of leptin gene in nidus part of BAVM was clearer than in perinidal brain tissue under the ultraviolet transilluminator, proving that the nidus part had higher expression of leptin gene than perinidal brain tissue.

The vascular walls of the nidus part in non-hemorrhagic BAVM were thicker than in hemorrhagic ones. Leptin antibody was positive on matrix of BAVM, but negative on vascular walls and sporadically positive on perinidal brain tissue. The stains of leptin antibody were much stronger in hemorrhagic BAVM than in non-hemorrhagic, suggesting that expression of leptin in hemorrhagic BAVM was higher. Leptin receptor antibody had a similar expression. STAT3 antibody was positive on both matrix and vascular walls, and sporadically positive on perinidal brain tissue. There was no significant difference in its staining on hemorrhagic and non-hemorrhagic BAVM.

Western blot analysis showed that there was expression of leptin on the nidus part of BAVM and slight expression on perinidal tissue, which concurs with the results above (Fig. 2).

Discussion

Leptin gene is coded by ob gene, which is on chromosome 7q31.3 in humans [10]. It has 146 amino acid residues and its molecular weight is about 16 kD [2]. In serum, leptin molecules mostly combine with protein for its strong hydrophilic activity, while only the free leptin has its biological effects within a 10-min half-life [10]. Leptin has to bind to its receptor to activate downstream effectors, such as the nuclear transcriptor, STAT3 [10]. Leptin receptor distributes widely in the human body, mainly in choroid plexus, hypothalamus, liver, kidney, heart, spleen, testis, fat tissue, and pancreatic cells [2]. However, there has been no report of leptin expression on BAVM. In our study, we found that the transcription and translation levels of leptin, leptin receptor, and STAT3 were higher in hemorrhagic BAVM

than in non-hemorrhagic ones, suggesting that leptin might play a role in rupture of BAVM.

The origin of leptin in BAVM may be similar to that of other general endocrine hormones, and secreted in several ways. First, after leptin is secreted by peripheral white fat cells, it is transferred to BAVM. Since the flow rate of blood in the nidus part of BAVM is faster, more leptin deposits there. Secondly, several kinds of cells are capable of secreting leptin by paracrine approach, such as vascular endothelial cells, smooth muscle cells, fibroblasts, and macrophages. Third, the nidus itself secrets leptin through an autocrine approach. The results of immunohistochemical analysis showed leptin antibody was negative on vascular walls of the nidus part but positive on matrix and perinidal brain tissue. Since the half-life of leptin is rather short, about 10 min, the secretion of leptin is probably from matrix cells of nidus. According to different methods of secretion, leptin deposits at the nidus part mostly because of fast flow, high pressure, and disruption of blood-brain barrier of BAVM.

We also found that expression of leptin, leptin receptor, and STAT3 is greater in the nidus part of BAVMs. Generally, the signal transduction pathway induced by leptin is JAK/STAT, MAPK, PI3K, and so on [2]. JAK/STAT3 is the main pathway after leptin combines with its receptor [4]. The transcriptional and translational levels of leptin, leptin receptor, and STAT3 are higher in hemorrhagic BAVM, suggesting that leptin may play an important role in the hemorrhagic mechanism of BAVM, probably acting through the JAK-STAT3 signaling pathway.

Several hypotheses are proposed to explain why leptin has a higher expression in BAVM. First, it is a specific elevation. Leptin may promote angiogenesis and remodeling of vascular walls, such as hyperplasia of vascular endothelial cells and smooth muscle cells, so that the vascular walls are unstable [5, 7]. Leptin can activate several pathways to release nitric monoxide, which dilates vascular walls and thus leads to rupture [2]. Furthermore, leptin is the result of BAVM bleeding, which may facilitate hyperplasia and calcification of vascular walls and stable matrix, in order to prevent further bleeding [2, 4, 5, 7]. Second, it is a non-specific process. The deposition of leptin is the result of high flow volume and disruption of blood-brain barrier. We are more inclined toward the first explanation.

We chose perinidal brain tissue as our controls for a reason. Sato et al. [6] proposed the term 'perinidal dilated capillary networks' (PDCN), and proved PDCN is abnormally dilated to about 10- to 25-fold greater than normal capillary vessels adjacent to nidus, and is composed of micro-vessels communicating with nidus, supplying artery, draining vein, and normal brain tissue. In our experience, we usually resect these abnormal tissues for fear of postoperative perfusion pressure breakthrough and recurrence of BAVM. Of course, these perinidal brain tissues are not normal brain tissue and may still be subject to controversy, for they may have gliosis, scar, or hemosiderosis, and are apt to change by bleeding, hemodynamics, and interference by surgery, but this is an ethically agreeable self-control.

In summary, we explored the effect of leptin and its relative factors on bleeding of BAVMs, which may help in the development of new therapeutic strategies for predicting and preventing hemorrhagic BAVM.

References

1. Choi JH, Mohr JP (2005) Brain arteriovenous malformations in adults. Lancet Neurol 4: 299–308
2. Fruhbeck G (2006) Intracellular signaling pathways activated by leptin. Biochem J 393: 7–20
3. Gault J, Sarin H, Awadallah NA, Shenkar R, Awad IA (2004) Pathobiology of human cerebrovascular malformations: basic mechanisms and clinical relevance. Neurosurgery 55: 1–17
4. Mütze J, Roth J, Gerstberger R, Matsumura K, Hübschle T (2006) Immunohistochemical evidence of functional leptin receptor expression in neuronal and endothelial cells of the rat brain. Neurosci Lett 394: 105–110
5. Park HY, Kwon HM, Lim HJ, Hong BK, Lee JY, Park BE, Jang Y, Cho SY, Kim HS (2001) Potential role of leptin in angiogenesis: leptin induces endothelial cell proliferation and expression of matrix metalloproteinases in vivo and in vitro. Exp Mol Med 33: 95–102
6. Sato S, Kodama N, Sasaki T, Matsumoto M, Ishikawa T (2004) Perinidal dilated capillary networks in cerebral arteriovenous malformations. Neurosurgery 54: 163–170
7. Schäfer K, Halle M, Goeschen C, Dellas C, Pynn M, Loskutoff DJ, Konstantinides S (2004) Leptin promotes vascular remodeling and neointimal growth in mice. Arterioscler Thromb Vasc Biol 24: 112–117
8. Söderberg S, Ahrén B, Stegmayr B, Johnson O, Wiklund PG, Weinehall L, Hallmans G, Olsson T (1999) Leptin is a risk marker for first-ever hemorrhagic stroke in a population-based cohort. Stroke 30: 328–337
9. Spetzler RF, Martin NA (1986) A proposed grading system for arteriovenous malformations. J Neurosurg 65: 476–483
10. Werner N, Nickenig G (2004) From fat fighter to risk factor: the zigzag trek of leptin. Arterioscler Thromb Vasc Biol 24: 7–9
11. Zhang Y, Proenca R, Maffei M, Barone M, Leopold L, Friedman JM (1994) Positional cloning of the mouse obese gene and its human homologue. Nature 372: 425–432

Acta Neurochir Suppl (2008) 105: 225–228
© Springer-Verlag 2008
Printed in Austria

Novel treatments for cerebral vasospasm following aneurysmal subarachnoid hemorrhage

E. Lehmann, O. Sagher

Department of Neurosurgery, University of Michigan Health System, Ann Arbor, MI, USA

Summary

Cerebral vasospasm is a major cause of cerebral ischemia and poor outcomes in the setting of aneurysmal subarachnoid hemorrhage (SAH). Despite advances in diagnosis and treatment of SAH, the pathophysiology of vasospasm is still poorly understood and outcomes remain disappointing. Recent advances in understanding the role of hemoglobin in initiating an inflammatory cascade in the subarachnoid space open new avenues for therapy. Preliminary experimental and clinical evidence indicate that targets in the inflammatory and oxidative cascades hold promise in reducing the incidence and impact of cerebral vasospasm.

Keywords: Edaravone; haptoglobin; hemoglobin; ibuprofen; leflunomide; subarachnoid hemorrhage; vasospasm.

Introduction

Despite decades of intensive research, cerebral vasospasm due to subarachnoid hemorrhage (SAH) continues to pose a formidable clinical problem. There are approximately 30,000 cases of ruptured cerebral aneurysms in the United States every year, and a significant number of these cases are complicated by ischemia due to delayed vasospasm. In fact, cerebral vasospasm likely accounts for the fact that, while responsible for only 3% of all strokes, SAH represents a significant proportion of poor outcomes related to stroke [4, 7, 17, 30]. Moreover, considering that the average age of the SAH patient is decades younger than for other types of stroke, many more years of functional life are lost as a result of aneurysm rupture and subsequent vasospasm [30, 33, 35]. As such, cerebral vasospasm is a promising target for treatments to reduce the morbidity and mortality associated with the rupture of cerebral aneurysms.

Conventional treatments for cerebral vasospasm have focused on the fluid dynamics of cerebral vasculature, affecting vascular resistance, flow viscosity, and blood pressure. Current medical management of vasospasm typically involves hypervolemia, hypertension, and hemodilution [19, 22, 29]. While it is capable of reducing adverse outcomes related to vasospasm, hemodynamic therapy is unable to prevent the vasospastic process [21, 24]. Patients must be monitored carefully through treatment to evaluate for signs of congestive heart failure related to the hemodynamic stress placed on the myocardium with this therapy. In addition to hemodynamic therapy, current medical management involves the use of calcium channel blockers that ostensibly act on smooth muscle cells to cause relaxation [5, 11, 14, 25, 27, 28, 38]. The calcium channel blocker nimodipine preferentially vasodilates cerebral blood vessels, leaving it less likely to cause systemic hypotension than other calcium channel blockers. While this medication has not been shown to alter the incidence of angiographic vasospasm, studies have shown that it decreases the incidence of cerebral ischemia [8]. Thought to act as a calcium channel blocker as well, magnesium sulfate infusion has also been shown in randomized controlled trials to reduce the incidence of symptomatic vasospasm, and preliminary evidence indicates that it may lead to improved outcomes [31, 36, 37].

Medical and hemodynamic therapies are augmented nowadays with interventional procedures, including angioplasty and intra-arterial vasodilator treatment. These have shown efficacy in treating vasospasm. Balloon angioplasty, while only available for larger vessels, is ef-

Correspondence: Oren Sagher, Department of Neurosurgery, University of Michigan Health System, 1500 E. Medical Center Drive, Room 3552 TC, Ann Arbor, MI 48109-5338, USA. e-mail: osagher@umich.edu

fective in reversing focal vasospasm [18, 20]. While these therapies have shown efficacy in treatment of vasospasm, each acts to affect hemodynamics in cerebral vasculature without addressing the pathophysiology of cerebral vasospasm.

Newer research has focused on the role of oxidative damage and inflammation in the pathophysiology of cerebral vasospasm following the release of hemoglobin from extravasated red blood cells following SAH. It is now believed that this hemoglobin participates in attracting inflammatory cells to the perivascular space [2, 6]. In addition, it is becoming increasingly clear that iron released from the hemoglobin molecules leads directly to oxidative stress in the surrounding area [23, 34]. In this study, we focus on several novel treatment strategies that involve decreasing the quantity of subarachnoid hemoglobin, interrupting the attraction of inflammatory cells, or decreasing oxidative damage to cell membranes. We do not intend for this to be an encyclopedic description of novel research on this topic. For a thorough review of the panoply of current treatment strategies in cerebral vasospasm, the reader is encouraged to read 2 recently-published, excellent reviews on the topic [18, 20].

New treatments

Thrombolytics

Since the extravasation of blood into the subarachnoid space is ultimately the cause of vasospasm, one strategy to reduce spasm involves decreasing the burden of subarachnoid blood using thrombolytics to lyse clot. In Japan, it is not uncommon to place drainage catheters in the basal cisterns of patients with SAH. These may then be used to instill thrombolytic agents, such as recombinant tissue plasminogen activator (TPA), to help dissolve and clear the blood present in the basal cisterns. More recent trials involve irrigation of the cisterns intraoperatively immediately following aneurysm clipping, followed by cisternal drainage. A meta-analysis examining 9 studies from 1990 to 2000 showed significant decrease in the incidence of delayed ischemia and showed improved functional outcomes with decreased mortality following thrombolytic therapy [1]. Conversely, the single randomized prospective trial has not shown evidence of benefit [12]. This is an area open to more study, although preliminary data indicates a reduction in symptomatic vasospasm in patients treated with thrombolytics and drainage [16]. An obvious concern with regard to the instillation of a thrombolytic agent following rupture of

cerebral aneurysm would be complications related to bleeding. This concern has in fact been borne out in recent studies, where hemorrhagic complication rates as high as 15% have been documented [1].

Haptoglobin

While the gross removal of subarachnoid blood shows promise in the prevention of cerebral vasospasm, the microscopic removal of hemoglobin may also prove helpful. The body's endogenous system for clearance of extracorpuscular hemoglobin involves the serum protein, haptoglobin [3, 6]. Unlike other mammalian species, which harbor only 1 haptoglobin subtype, humans have 2 separate alleles of haptoglobin molecules. This leads to 3 possible protein subtypes: homozygous for type 1 (Hp1-1), heterozygous (Hp1-2), or homozygous for type 2 (Hp2-2). Each of these molecules has a very different protein structure, leading to different molecular interaction and efficiency in inactivation and clearance of hemoglobin. Since extracorpuscular hemoglobin molecules are responsible for free radical production and the induction of prostaglandin synthesis in the perivascular space, haptoglobin could prove helpful by impeding its inflammatory and oxidizing capabilities.

The haptoglobin 2 allele interferes with normal polymerization of the haptoglobin molecule. In animals and in humans with the Hp1-1 phenotype, haptoglobin forms a dimer. The presence of a second allele (Hp2) induces polymerization, creating a linear polymer in Hp1-2, and a cyclical polymer in Hp2-2. Hp1-2 and Hp2-2 polymers do not readily cross membranes, decreasing their access to the extravasated blood. Moreover, when combined with hemoglobin, Hp2-2 is more potent at activating monocytes and macrophages than Hp1-1, while it is less able to stimulate production of anti-inflammatory cytokines [6]. There is a potential therefore that the Hp2 allele may actually *exacerbate* the vasospastic process.

Recent experimental evidence has been presented to support the notion that the presence of Hp2 alleles may play a role in cerebral vasospasm. The arterial lumens of knock-in mice with Hp2-2 phenotypes were more constricted following SAH than those in Hp1-1 mice. Also, the physical activity level of the Hp2-2 mice was significantly decreased, indicating symptomatic vasospasm [6]. Other, more recent studies have indicated that haptoglobin genotype may determine the severity of the inflammatory response to blood products, leading to a prediction of those who may be more susceptible to vasospasm following SAH [3, 6, 15]. A recent clinical trial studied patients with SAH and has shown correlation of haptoglobin type with presence of vasospasm on transcranial Doppler examination [3].

This understanding of haptoglobin sub-types opens a new area of prognostic and treatment modalities. Already, haptoglobin typing has been used to predict those patients with SAH who are at increased risk of vasospasm. This may allow the tailoring of other preventive measures to those patients at highest risk [3, 15]. Haptoglobin may also be used as a therapeutic approach, with possible cisternal infusion of Hp1-1 to improve clearance of hemoglobin.

Anti-inflammatory agents

Extravascular hemoglobin is a potent pro-inflammatory agent, causing the induction of adhesion molecules and inflammatory cytokines. As such, inflammation plays an important role in the pathophysiology of cerebral vasospasm. Adhesion molecules and inflammatory cytokines, induced by free hemoglobin, act as chemo-attractants, leading to aggregation of leukocytes in the walls of cerebral blood vessels and in the perivascular space and, in turn, intimal hyperplasia and luminal narrowing with subendothelial fibrosis [2, 9, 13, 26, 32].

Once the inflammatory cascade has been initiated by free hemoglobin, treatment options may focus on interrupting continued inflammatory signals. For example, by interrupting the chemo-attractive signals that bring inflammatory cells to the site of subarachnoid blood, local administration of ibuprofen has shown promise in preventing vasospasm [13, 26, 32]. Independent of its effect on cyclooxygenase, ibuprofen in high intrathecal concentrations inhibits CAM expression, blocking the key mediator of leukocyte extravasation, decreasing inflammation in blood vessel walls. This is a property shared by other non-steroidal anti-inflammatory drugs, as well; however, attaining the concentration necessary in cerebrospinal fluid would require toxic oral doses. Recently, drug-eluting polymers have been developed for cisternal administration of these agents following aneurysm clipping. Treatment with ibuprofen-eluting polymer has been shown to prevent vasospasm when initiated within 6 h of SAH in a rabbit model [13]. Subsequent primate studies have shown similar results when the polymer was placed within 12 h of the hemorrhagic event [26]. In addition, there was no evidence of immediate systemic or local toxicity at 7 days.

Another potent anti-inflammatory agent, leflunomide, acts through inhibiting pro-inflammatory cytokines and protein kinases. It may also have an anti-proliferative ef-

fect on vascular smooth muscle and anti-angiogenic properties. Early rabbit studies showed that oral leflunomide treatment is able to reverse vasospasm by decreasing wall thickness and increasing luminal cross-sectional area [2].

Finally, preliminary data from a recent small clinical trial indicates that dexamethasone, applied topically to arteries following aneurysm clipping, reduced the incidence of symptomatic vasospasm. In this particular series, 1 patient (10%) in the treated group had vasospasm without neurological deficit, compared with 4 patients (40%) in the control group, 1 of whom had hemiplegia [10]. It remains to be seen whether a beneficial effect of this treatment could be demonstrated in larger, more well-controlled studies.

Free radical scavengers: edaravone

Oxyhemoglobin is known to release reactive oxygen species, such as superoxide, and the iron from heme actively catalyzes the reaction, forming hydroxyl radicals. When hemoglobin is released into the perivascular space following SAH, these free radicals attack endothelial cell membranes, leading to lipid peroxidation and cell membrane damage [23, 34]. Brain tissue is very sensitive to lipid peroxidation, due to the high concentration of polyunsaturated fatty acids and its high rate of oxygen consumption. Lipid peroxidation leads to changes in cell membrane structure, causing edema and cell death.

Efforts to take advantage of this mechanism are still in the early phase. One novel free radical scavenger, edaravone, acts on hydroxyl radicals and on iron-dependent lipid peroxidation. While human studies have not been completed, continuous intravenous administration of edaravone for 7 days following SAH in a canine model has shown significant reduction in cerebral vasospasm, as observed on basilar artery angiography [23].

Conclusion

Subarachnoid blood following aneurysm rupture plays an important role in the pathophysiology of cerebral vasospasm. Extracellular hemoglobin leads to increased inflammation and oxidative damage to the cerebral vasculature. The future of vasospasm prevention and treatment rests in further understanding and manipulation of these processes. By physically or chemically reducing the perivascular hemoglobin burden, or by interrupting the damaging inflammatory and oxidative cascades, it may be possible to prevent the consequences of cerebral vasospasm. This is the new frontier in the treatment of this challenging and important clinical problem.

References

1. Amin-Hanjani S, Ogilvy CS, Barker FG 2nd (2004) Does intracisternal thrombolysis prevent vasospasm after aneurysmal subarachnoid hemorrhage? A meta-analysis. Neurosurgery 54: 326–335
2. Belen D, Besalti O, Yiğitkanli K, Kösemehmetoğlu K, Simşek S, Bolay H (2007) Leflunomide prevents vasospasm secondary to subarachnoid haemorrhage. Acta Neurochir (Wien) 149: 1041–1048
3. Borsody M, Burke A, Coplin W, Miller-Lotan R, Levy A (2006) Haptoglobin and the development of cerebral artery vasospasm after subarachnoid hemorrhage. Neurology 66: 634–640
4. Broessner G, Helbok R, Lackner P, Mitterberger M, Beer R, Engelhardt K, Brenneis C, Pfausler B, Schmutzhard E (2007) Survival and long-term functional outcome in 1,155 consecutive neurocritical care patients. Crit Care Med 35: 2025–2030
5. Brown G, Carley S (2004) Best evidence topic reports. Does nimodipine reduce mortality and secondary ischaemic events after subarachnoid haemorrhage? Emerg Med J 21: 333
6. Chaichana KL, Levy AP, Miller-Lotan R, Shakur S, Tamargo RJ (2007) Haptoglobin 2-2 genotype determines chronic vasospasm after experimental subarachnoid hemorrhage. Stroke 38: 3266–3271
7. de Rooij NK, Linn FH, van der Plas JA, Algra A, Rinkel GJ (2007) Incidence of subarachnoid haemorrhage: a systematic review with emphasis on region, age, gender and time trends. J Neurol Neurosurg Psychiatry 78: 1365–1372
8. Dorhout Mees SM, Rinkel GJ, Feigin VL, Algra A, van den Bergh WM, Vermeulen M, van Gijn J (2007) Calcium antagonists for aneurysmal subarachnoid haemorrhage. Cochrane Database Syst Rev (3): CD000277
9. Dumont AS, Dumont RJ, Chow MM, Lin CL, Calisaneller T, Ley KF, Kassell NF, Lee KS (2003) Cerebral vasospasm after subarachnoid hemorrhage: putative role of inflammation. Neurosurgery 53: 123–135
10. Fei L, Golwa F (2007) Topical application of dexamethasone to prevent cerebral vasospasm after aneurysmal subarachnoid haemorrhage: a pilot study. Clin Drug Invest 27: 827–832
11. Feigin VL, Rinkel GJ, Algra A, Vermeulen M, van Gijn J (1998) Calcium antagonists in patients with aneurysmal subarachnoid hemorrhage: a systematic review. Neurology 50: 876–883
12. Findlay JM, Weir BK, Steinke D, Tanabe T, Gordon P, Grace M (1988) Effect of intrathecal thrombolytic therapy on subarachnoid clot and chronic vasospasm in a primate model of SAH. J Neurosurg 69: 723–735
13. Frazier JL, Pradilla G, Wang PP, Tamargo RJ (2004) Inhibition of cerebral vasospasm by intracranial delivery of ibuprofen from a controlled-release polymer in a rabbit model of subarachnoid hemorrhage. J Neurosurg 101: 93–98
14. Inzitari D, Poggesi A (2005) Calcium channel blockers and stroke. Aging Clin Exp Res 17: 16–30
15. Khurana VG, Fox DJ, Meissner I, Meyer FB, Spetzler RF (2006) Update on evidence for a genetic predisposition to cerebral vasospasm. Neurosurg Focus 21: E3
16. Kinouchi H, Ogasawara K, Shimizu H, Mizoi K, Yoshimoto T (2004) Prevention of symptomatic vasospasm after aneurysmal subarachnoid hemorrhage by intraoperative cisternal fibrinolysis using tissue-type plasminogen activator combined with continuous cisternal drainage. Neurol Med Chir (Tokyo) 44: 569–577
17. Koffijberg H, Buskens E, Granath F, Adami J, Ekbom A, Rinkel GJ, Blomqvist P (2008) Subarachnoid haemorrhage in Sweden 1987–2002: regional incidence and case fatality rates. J Neurol Neurosurg Psychiatry 79: 294–299
18. Komotar RJ, Zacharia BE, Valhora R, Mocco J, Connolly ES Jr (2007) Advances in vasospasm treatment and prevention. J Neurol Sci 261: 134–142
19. Lee KH, Lukovits T, Friedman JA (2006) "Triple-H" therapy for cerebral vasospasm following subarachnoid hemorrhage. Neurocrit Care 4: 68–76
20. Macdonald RL, Pluta RM, Zhang JH (2007) Cerebral vasospasm after subarachnoid hemorrhage: the emerging revolution. Nat Clin Pract Neurol 3: 256–263
21. Muench E, Horn P, Bauhuf C, Roth H, Philipps M, Hermann P, Quintel M, Schmiedek P, Vajkoczy P (2007) Effects of hypervolemia and hypertension on regional cerebral blood flow, intracranial pressure, and brain tissue oxygenation after subarachnoid hemorrhage. Crit Care Med 35: 1844–1852
22. Myburgh JA (2005) "Triple h" therapy for aneurysmal subarachnoid haemorrhage: real therapy or chasing numbers? Crit Care Resusc 7: 206–212
23. Nakagomi T, Yamakawa K, Sasaki T, Saito I, Takakura K (2003) Effect of edaravone on cerebral vasospasm following experimental subarachnoid hemorrhage. J Stroke Cerebrovasc Dis 12: 17–21
24. Ogungbo B, Prakash S, Ushewokunze S, Etherson K, Sinar J (2005) Value of triple H therapy in a patient with an ischemic penumbra following subarachnoid hemorrhage: a case study. J Neurosci Nurs 37: 326–328, 333
25. Oran I, Cinar C (2007) Continuous intra-arterial infusion of nimodipine during embolization of cerebral aneurysms associated with vasospasm. Am J Neuroradiol 29: 291–295
26. Pradilla G, Thai QA, Legnani FG, Clatterbuck RE, Gailloud P, Murphy KP, Tamargo RJ (2005) Local delivery of ibuprofen via controlled-release polymers prevents angiographic vasospasm in a monkey model of subarachnoid hemorrhage. Neurosurgery 57: 184–190
27. Rinkel GJ, Feigin VL, Algra A, Vermeulen M, van Gijn J (2002) Calcium antagonists for aneurysmal subarachnoid haemorrhage. Cochrane Database Syst Rev (4): CD000277
28. Rinkel GJ, Feigin VL, Algra A, van den Bergh WM, Vermeulen M, van Gijn J (2005) Calcium antagonists for aneurysmal subarachnoid haemorrhage. Cochrane Database Syst Rev (1): CD000277
29. Sen J, Belli A, Albon H, Morgan L, Petzold A, Kitchen N (2003) Triple-H therapy in the management of aneurysmal subarachnoid haemorrhage. Lancet Neurol 2: 614–621
30. Shea AM, Reed SD, Curtis LH, Alexander MJ, Villani JJ, Schulman KA (2007) Characteristics of nontraumatic subarachnoid hemorrhage in the United States in 2003. Neurosurgery 61: 1131–1138
31. Stippler M, Crago E, Levy EI, Kerr ME, Yonas H, Horowitz MB, Kassam A (2006) Magnesium infusion for vasospasm prophylaxis after subarachnoid hemorrhage. J Neurosurg 105: 723–729
32. Thai QA, Oshiro EM, Tamargo RJ (1999) Inhibition of experimental vasospasm in rats with the periadventitial administration of ibuprofen using controlled-release polymers. Stroke 30: 140–147
33. Topcuoglu MA, Pryor JC, Ogilvy CS, Kistler JP (2002) Cerebral vasospasm following subarachnoid hemorrhage. Curr Treat Options Cardiovasc Med 4: 373–384
34. Tosaka M, Hashiba Y, Saito N, Imai H, Shimizu T, Sasaki T (2002) Contractile responses to reactive oxygen species in the canine basilar artery in vitro: selective inhibitory effect of MCI-186, a new hydroxyl radical scavenger. Acta Neurochir (Wien) 144: 1305–1310
35. Treggiari MM, Walder B, Suter PM, Romand JA (2003) Systematic review of the prevention of delayed ischemic neurological deficits with hypertension, hypervolemia, and hemodilution therapy following subarachnoid hemorrhage. J Neurosurg 98: 978–984
36. van den Bergh WM, Dijkhuizen RM, Rinkel GJ (2004) Potentials of magnesium treatment in subarachnoid haemorrhage. Magnes Res 17: 301–313
37. van den Bergh WM, Algra A, van Kooten F, Dirven CM, van Gijn J, Vermeulen M, Rinkel GJ (2005) Magnesium sulfate in aneurysmal subarachnoid hemorrhage: a randomized controlled trial. Stroke 36: 1011–1015
38. Vergouwen MD, Vermeulen M, Roos YB (2006) Effect of nimodipine on outcome in patients with traumatic subarachnoid haemorrhage: a systematic review. Lancet Neurol 5: 1029–1032

Acta Neurochir Suppl (2008) 105: 229–232
© Springer-Verlag 2008
Printed in Austria

Relationship between serum sodium level and brain ventricle size after aneurysmal subarachnoid hemorrhage

M. Li[1], W. Li[2], L. Wang[2], Y. Hu[1], G. Chen[2]

[1] Neurological Intensive Care Unit, the 2nd Affiliated Hospital of Zhejiang University, Zhejiang, P.R. China
[2] Department of Neurosurgery, the 2nd Affiliated Hospital of Zhejiang University, Zhejiang, P.R. China

Summary

Objective. To study the relationship of serum sodium levels and brain ventricle size after aneurysmal subarachnoid hemorrhage (SAH).

Methods. Serum sodium levels and brain computed tomography (CT) scans were obtained simultaneously and within 21 days from onset of SAH in 69 patients. Serum sodium levels were compared with brain ventricle size on CT. The index of third ventricle was calculated from brain CT, and we studied its relationship to GOS (Glasgow Outcome Scale) scores.

Results. There was obvious correlation between serum sodium levels and index of third ventricle ($r = -0.753$). GOS scores correlated with serum sodium levels in patients with hypernatremia.

Conclusion. There was a negative correlation between serum sodium levels and cerebral ventricle size in SAH patients. Hypernatremia is one factor leading an unfavorable prognosis in SAH patients.

Keywords: Subarachnoid hemorrhage; serum sodium level; third ventricle index; aneurysm.

Introduction

Subarachnoid hemorrhage (SAH) is usually caused by the rupture of an intracranial aneurysm. SAH patients often have changes in serum sodium levels, including hypernatremia or hyponatremia [1, 11], which could have an important effect on prognosis. Some research [2, 7] had indicated that hypernatremia is an independent factor that could produce an unfavorable prognosis. In fact, hyponatremia occurs more frequently than hypernatremia and is considered to contribute to cerebral vasospasm following SAH [10]. Diabetes insipidus could induce hypernatremia and syndrome of inappropriate (secretion of) antidiuretic hormone (SIADH) could induce hyponatremia. These fluid-electrolyte metabolic

disturbances are related to hypothalamus injury following SAH [6, 9]. Hypothalamus injury has no characteristic manifestation on imaging [12]. But because the base of the third ventricle is hypothalamus, it is prudent to determine whether the size of the third ventricle could indirectly reflect hypothalamus injury. Clinically, hydrocephalus patients often experience hyponatremia, and hypernatremia often occurs in patients with intracranial hypertension causing disappearance of the third ventricle. Further research is required to investigate whether changes in the size of the third ventricle correlate to changes in serum sodium levels.

Materials and methods

Patients

We analyzed 69 patients with SAH who were admitted to our hospital between August 2004 and August 2006, which included 32 males and 37 females ranging age from 22 to 65 years. Careful research was undertaken to rule out patients with significant systemic disease such as cardiac disease, renal disease, endocrine disorders, and past neurological disease. Our study was approved by the Committee for Clinical Trials and Research on Humans at Zhejiang University of Medicine. All patients provided written informed consent.

SAH in all patients was confirmed by brain computed tomography (CT) scan and cerebral vessels were examined by digital subtraction angiography (DSA). Patient treatment methods included direct surgery in 46 patients, endovascular embolization in 11 patients, external ventricular drainage in 2 patients, and medical treatment in 10 patients.

Serum sodium levels

Serum sodium levels were obtained twice daily from each SAH patient. We averaged serum sodium levels every 3 days to obtain variances in serum sodium levels.

The presence of hypernatremia (serum sodium concentration >145 mmol/L), hyponatremia (serum sodium concentration <135 mmol/L), or normonatremia (serum sodium concentration $135 \sim 145$ mmol/L)

Correspondence: Dr. Chen Gao, 88 Jie-fang Road, Hangzhou, Zhejiang 310009, P.R. China. e-mail: d.chengao@163.com

was determined by serum sodium measurements obtained twice daily after SAH. We assigned patients into 3 groups by the maximum, minimum, and average of each patient's serum sodium level within 21 days after SAH.

Brain CT

In conjunction with serum sodium levels, brain CT was simultaneously obtained every 3 days to observe intra-calvarium changes. On computer scans of patient brain CTs, we calculated: A) maximum width of the third ventricle; and B) the maximum endo-meridians of the skull on caudate nucleus plane. According to the method used by Mataró *et al.* [3], we calculated the index of third ventricle, and then evaluated the correlation between serum sodium levels and index of third ventricle.

After patients were admitted to our hospital, GCS (Glasgow Coma Scale) scores were evaluated on the third day after admittance, and GOS (Glasgow Outcome Scale) scores were evaluated at the 3-month follow-up visit.

SPSS version 11.0 software (SPSS, Inc., Chicago, IL) was used for statistical analysis. According to the type of data property, Spearman rank correlation analysis or Pearson correlation analysis were used. The level of significance was denoted as $p < 0.05$.

Results

Serum sodium levels following SAH

Serum sodium levels changed in a majority of patients following SAH: 25 patients had hyponatremia (36%), 14 patients had hypernatremia (21%), and 30 patients had normal levels (43%). Both GCS and GOS scores correlated to serum sodium levels ($p < 0.001$, Pearson; Table 1).

Relationship between serum sodium levels and brain ventricle size

Brain ventricles of the SAH patients with hypernatremia had shrunken, excluding 2 patients who had obstructive hydrocephalus resulting from cerebroventricular hemorrhage. In addition, all 16 patients with communicating hydrocephalus had hyponatremia; however, the brain ventricle size in some hyponatremia patients had no change. The patients with obstructive hydrocephalus were excluded and those left were divided into 3 groups by serum sodium level. Third ventricle indices of the 3 groups were compared to each other by Spearman's rank correlation analysis. Third ventricle indices also corre-

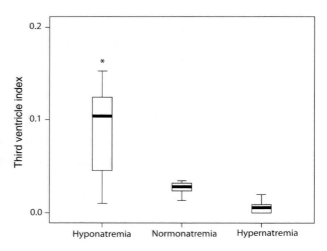

Fig. 1. Third ventricle index of different groups. $^*p < 0.05$ vs. the other groups

Table 2. *Comparison of serum sodium levels before and after ventriculoperitoneal shunt surgery*

	Serum sodium level (mmol/L)	t	p-value
Before surgery	127.11 ± 6.39	5.832	<0.001
After surgery	138.97 ± 4.03		

lated with serum sodium levels ($r = -0.753$; $p < 0.001$) (Fig. 1).

Changes in serum sodium levels after ventriculoperitoneal shunt

The 16 patients with communicating hydrocephalus received a ventriculoperitoneal shunt, and experienced increased serum sodium levels following the surgery (Table 2).

Discussion

Patients with aneurysmal SAH often have changes in serum sodium levels, and in our experience, hyponatremia occurred more frequently than hypernatremia. Our study of 69 patients found 25 hyponatremia patients (36%) and 14 hypernatremia patients (21%). The average serum sodium level of the hypernatremia patients in this study was 163.8 ± 15.3 mmol/L. The serum sodium level of most hypernatremia patients increased in the early stage and their GCS scores descended 3–5 points following the increase. If the serum sodium level persisted at 165 mmol/L or beyond, it progressively increased, even to 185 mmol/L. The third ventricle in patients with severe hypernatremia disappeared and its index was zero. GOS scores of such patients were very

Table 1. *Serum sodium levels, and GCS and GOS scores for 3 patient groups ($p < 0.001$)*

	No. of patients	Serum sodium level	GCS scores	GOS scores
Hypernatremia	14	163.8 ± 15.3	4 ± 1	1.4 ± 0.6
Normonatremia	30	138.7 ± 4.5	13 ± 2	4.3 ± 0.6
Hyponatremia	25	124.5 ± 5.9	8 ± 1	4.4 ± 0.7

GCS Glasgow Coma Scale; *GOS* Glasgow Outcome Scale

low, and 90% died within 6–15 days and the remaining 10% incurred severe brain impairment. Pearson analysis demonstrated an obvious correlation between GOS scores and serum sodium level with hypernatremia ($r = -0.757$), but no correlation with hyponatremia or normal levels. Therefore, hypernatremia could predict poor outcomes in SAH patients, which confirms research by Qureshi et al. [7]. Qureshi et al. also report that the mechanism involved in this phenomenon is yet unknown. In our study, brain CT showed that patients with hypernatremia were complicated by obvious intracerebral hematoma, intraventricular hemorrhage, cerebral infarction of a large area, or obstructive hydrocephalus. In these patients, the third ventricle was pressed and transformed, except in cases of obstructive hydrocephalus where the ventricle was enlarged. The average index of third ventricle was 0.0061 ± 0.0058, which was homochronous with hypernatremia. If the serum sodium level did not exceed 165 mmol/L and furthermore did not last a long time, the prognosis obviously improved.

More commonly, SAH patients were complicated by hyponatremia. In our study, 21 patients (30%) had hyponatremia in the early phase. As the illness progressed, 4 patients with normal serum sodium levels had hyponatremia after 14 days, with an average level of 124.5 ± 5.9 mmol/L. In the hyponatremia group, 16 patients had an enlarged brain ventricle with an average third ventricle index of 0.1188 ± 0.02527. Such patients often had some clinical manifestation, such as cognitive disorder, instability of gait, urinary incontinence, hypermyotonia, etc. The average serum sodium level recovered from 127.11 ± 6.39 mmol/L to 138.97 ± 4.03 mmol/L after all 16 patients received a ventriculoperitoneal shunt. Twelve patients experienced an obvious improvement in gait and cognition, while the size of brain ventricle and the third ventricle's index had no changes. This result corresponded with some of the research by Sorteberg et al. [8] on normal pressure hydrocephalus (NPH). At present, it is still unknown why hyponatremia and hydrocephalus concur.

In our study, 30 patients (43%) had a normal level of serum sodium, with an average level of 138.7 ± 4.5 mmol/L. Of these patients, 84% had normal brain ventricle with a third ventricle index of 0.0295 ± 0.0074; 16% had slightly-enlarged brain ventricle with a third ventricle index of 0.0499. The GCS scores of these patients ranged from 11 to 15, and GOS scores were normal except in 4 patients who had NPH with hyponatremia in the late stage. By analyzing the 3 groups with different serum sodium levels, it was dis-

covered that serum sodium level had little correlation with GCS scores ($r = -0.413$; $p < 0.001$) and an obvious correlation with the third ventricle index ($r = -0.753$; $p < 0.001$). Therefore, it could be concluded that the size of brain ventricle is negatively correlated with serum sodium level.

Following SAH, changes in serum sodium level involved different pathophysiological mechanisms. Most of the patients with hypernatremia had diabetes insipidus and the serum sodium level continued to increase, even though intake of sodium was forbidden and enough non-electrolyte fluid was supplied according to urine volume and central venous pressure (CVP). Intracranial pressure in these patients was very high, resulting in decrease of cerebral blood flow. The third ventricle transformed by compression and nucleus hypothalamus, which is near the third ventricle, was damaged. As a result, secretion of antidiuretic hormone decreased, which could produce a great deal of hypobaric urine. Synchronously, the serum sodium level persistently increased, which could lead to poor outcome. The third ventricle of patients with normal serum sodium levels had no change or minimal enlargement, and the hormone secretion of hypothalamus was normal, so there was no effect on water-electrolyte metabolism. When arachnoid granulations were blocked following SAH, the secretion-absorption balance of cerebrospinal fluid was disturbed and the enlargement of brain ventricle would damage hypothalamus. By SIADH or cerebral salt wasting syndrome, water-electrolyte embolism was affected, resulting in hyponatremia. The patients with communicative hydrocephalus in this group had normal CVP and no hypotension, so hyponatremia might be caused by SIADH. But McGirt et al. [4] discovered that brain natriuretic peptide (BNP) increased in patients with hydrocephalus and considered cerebral salt wasting syndrome a mechanism of hyponatremia. Further research is required to determine the mechanism involved. It is still unknown why the serum sodium level recovered but the size of brain ventricle had no change after ventriculoperitoneal shunt. Novak et al. [5] ascertained that the brain ventricle system has hysteresis similar to that of the blood vascular system, and it is hard for brain ventricle to recover after enlargement. Further research should be carried out to study this phenomenon.

In our pilot study, we investigated the correlation between serum sodium levels and the size of the third ventricle following SAH. The pathophysiological mechanism involved remains unclear, and further study is required.

References

1. Citerio G, Gaini SM, Tomei G, Stocchetti N (2007) Management of 350 aneurysmal subarachnoid hemorrhages in 22 Italian neurosurgical centers. Intensive Care Med 33: 1580–1586

2. Fisher LA, Ko N, Miss J, Tung PP, Kopelnik A, Banki NM, Gardner D, Smith WS, Lawton MT, Zaroff JG (2006) Hypernatremia predicts adverse cardiovascular and neurological outcomes after SAH. Neurocrit Care 5: 180–185

3. Mataró M, Poca MA, Sahuquillo J, Cuxart A, Iborra J, de la Calzada MD, Junqué C (2000) Cognitive changes after cerebrospinal fluid shunting in young adults with spina bifida and assumed arrested hydrocephalus. J Neurol Neurosurg Psychiatry 68: 615–621

4. McGirt MJ, Blessing R, Nimjee SM, Friedman AH, Alexander MJ, Laskowitz DT, Lynch JR (2004) Correlation of serum brain natriuretic peptide with hyponatremia and delayed ischemic neurological deficits after subarachnoid hemorrhage. Neurosurgery 54: 1369–1374

5. Novak P, Glikstein R, Mohr G (1996) Pulsation-pressure relationship in experimental aneurysms: observation of aneurysmal hysteresis. Neurol Res 18: 377–382

6. Powner DJ, Boccalandro C, Alp MS, Vollmer DG (2006) Endocrine failure after traumatic brain injury in adults. Neurocrit Care 5: 61–70

7. Qureshi AI, Suri MF, Sung GY, Straw RN, Yahia AM, Saad M, Guterman LR, Hopkins LN (2002) Prognostic significance of hypernatremia and hyponatremia among patients with aneurysmal subarachnoid hemorrhage. Neurosurgery 50: 749–756

8. Sorteberg A, Eide PK, Fremming AD (2004) A prospective study on the clinical effect of surgical treatment of normal pressure hydrocephalus: the value of hydrodynamic evaluation. Br J Neurosurg 18: 149–157

9. Tsubokawa T, Shiokawa Y, Kurita H, Kaneko N (2004) High plasma concentration of brain natriuretic peptide in patients with ruptured anterior communicating artery aneurysm. Neurol Res 26: 893–896

10. Uygun MA, Ozkal E, Acar O, Erongun U (1996) Cerebral salt wasting syndrome. Neurosurg Rev 19: 193–196

11. Wong GK, Poon WS, Chan MT, Boet R, Gin T, Lam CW (2007) The effect of intravenous magnesium sulfate infusion on serum levels of sodium and potassium in patients with aneurysmal subarachnoid hemorrhage. Magnes Res 20: 37–42

12. Zucchini S, di Natale B, Ambrosetto P, De Angelis R, Cacciari E, Chiumello G (1995) Role of magnetic resonance imaging in hypothalamic-pituitary disorders. Horm Res 44(Suppl 3): 8–14

Acta Neurochir Suppl (2008) 105: 233–236
© Springer-Verlag 2008
Printed in Austria

Lack of association between apolipoprotein E promoters in ε4 carriers and worsening on computed tomography in early stage of traumatic brain injury

Y. Jiang[1,2], X. C. Sun[1], L. Gui[2], W. Y. Tang[1], L. P. Zhen[1], Y. J. Gu[2], H. T. Wu[1]

[1] Department of Neurosurgery, The First Affiliated Hospital of Chongqing Medical University, Chongqing, P.R. China
[2] Department of Neurosurgery, The First Affiliated Hospital of Luzhou Medical College, Luzhou, P.R. China

Summary

We investigated the relationship between apolipoprotein E (APOE) promoters (G-219T, C-427T, A-491T) polymorphisms, and worsening CT results in early stage of traumatic brain injury (TBI) in a previously reported cohort of Chinese patients.

Radiographic evidence of hemorrhage extension or delayed hemorrhage in acute stage (<7 days after TBI) was judged by serial CT scanning compared to that on admission. APOE genotyping was performed by means of PCR-RFLP. χ^2 test and logistic regression analyses were done using SPSS software.

Of 110 Chinese patients, 19 presented with deteriorated clinical condition in acute stage after hospitalization. Among these 19 patients, serial CT scanning revealed 3 cases with hemorrhage extension and 2 cases with delayed hemorrhage. χ^2 test showed no statistical differences in radiographic worsening/stabilization between the APOE ε4(+) and APOE ε4(−) groups ($p = 0.170 > 0.05$). Furthermore, no significant correlation between intracranial bleeding based on CT scanning with genotype or with haplotype frequencies for A-491T, C-427T, or G-219T was found by χ^2 test ($p > 0.05$).

In Chinese population, our data do not support the hypothesis that genetic variations within the APOE gene are associated with CT worsening in early stage of TBI.

Keywords: Apolipoprotein E; traumatic brain injury; early response; intracranial hematoma.

Introduction

Traumatic brain injury (TBI) is an important global public health problem and a leading cause of morbidity and mortality in the neurosurgery field. Posttraumatic intracranial hematoma is one of the major causes of fatal injuries that complicate 25–45% of severe TBI (Glasgow Coma Score (GCS) 3–8), 3–12% of moderate TBI (GCS 9–13), and 1–3% of mild TBI (GCS 14–15) [2]. One of the key factors affecting the clinical course of patients in acute phase of TBI is the change in hematoma volume. The hematoma itself sometimes can lead to secondary brain injury resulting in severe neurological deficits, even delayed fatality. It is important to predict the development of intracranial hematoma following TBI. But the considerable variability is only partly explained by known prognostic features such as patient's sex, age, protective pathways, and therapeutic targets. It has now been demonstrated that genetic polymorphism may play a key role in the susceptibility to TBI, even outcome after TBI.

Recently, most studies on the relationship between genetics and TBI have focused on apolipoprotein E. Apolipoprotein E (apoE = protein), an important mediator of cholesterol and lipid transport in the brain, is coded by a polymorphic gene (APOE = gene). More and more study groups have shown that these APOE alleles, especially ε4 allele, are associated with predisposition to the outcome following TBI [3, 4, 9, 11, 15]. The ε4 allele not only influences poor long-term rehabilitation [9], but also severity in the acute phase after TBI [5, 6]. Furthermore, a few studies focusing on the regulation of apoE expression, have directed their attention to the association between APOE promoter (-491A/T transversion, -427T/C transversion, and -219G/T transversion) and TBI [6, 7]. But the effect of genetics on the formation of posttraumatic intracranial hematoma has not been investigated.

In our previous studies, we have found that not only is APOE ε4 a risk factor, but also the APOE -491AA

Correspondence: Prof. Xiaochuan Sun, Department of Neurosurgery, The First Affiliated Hospital of Chongqing Medical University, Chongqing 400016, P.R. China. e-mail: sunxch1445@gmail.com

promoter in $\varepsilon4$ carriers is a likely factor for clinical deterioration in Chinese population [5, 6]. The aim of this study was to determine the association between APOE promoters in $\varepsilon4$ carriers and worsening on computed tomography (CT), showing the radiographic evidences of either hemorrhage extension or delayed hemorrhage in early stage of TBI.

Materials and methods

Patient population

In this study, we used the cohort of the Chinese patients reported previously [5, 6]. A total of 110 medical records from patients with TBI admitted to 2 neurosurgery departments (First Affiliated Hospitals of Chongqing Medical University and Luzhou Medical College) from December 2003 to May 2004 were collected and studied prospectively. Information extracted from clinical records included age, sex, smoking or not, alcohol-drinking or not, injury cause, initial clinical severity by GCS, and CT findings.

Management was determined by the attending physician, blinded to APOE genotyping. TBI patients' conditions were monitored in ICU continuously for 24 h. CT scanning was performed on admission and repeated every 4–8 h, or at any time necessary during the first 24 h after TBI, and every day or every other day according to clinical status.

CT findings were dichotomized into deterioration or stabilization for this study. Worsening on CT (<7 days after TBI) was judged by either of the following criteria: increase in hematoma volume or delayed hematoma, both detected by serial CT scanning and compared to scans taken at time of admission.

This study was approved by the Ethics Committee of the Department of Medical Research. An informed consent was obtained from patients directly or from a family member.

APOE genotyping

Determinations of APOE genotype and promoter polymorphisms were performed blinded to the diagnosis and clinical condition of patients. Venous blood was collected from patients on admission, then frozen and stored for extraction of DNA by standard techniques. APOE genotype and promoter polymorphisms were determined using a previously described polymerase chain reaction method [5, 6].

Statistical analysis

SPSS software was used. Univariate analysis was performed using the Pearson χ^2 test and the Fisher Exact test when necessary. In the multivariate analysis, we coded the genotypes of each APOE promoter polymorphism as dummy variables according to the hypothesis for a recessive model. Finally, logistic regression analysis was performed to control other factors (including age, sex, GCS, smoking, alcohol-drinking, pattern of TBI, treatments, injury mechanisms), as well as to test interactions between promoter genotypes and worsening on CT after TBI.

Results

In this study, we used the cohort of Chinese patients reported previously, where we found an association between deterioration of clinical condition and APOE -491AA promoter [5, 6]. In this cohort, the distribu-

Table 1. *Comparison between number of patients with/without hematoma and apolipoprotein E allel*

Hematoma	$\varepsilon2$ allel		$\varepsilon3$ allel		$\varepsilon4$ allel	
	$\varepsilon2(+)$	$\varepsilon2(-)$	$\varepsilon3(+)$	$\varepsilon3(-)$	$\varepsilon4(+)$	$\varepsilon4(-)$
Yes	5	24	28	1	4	25
No	13	68	80	1	13	68
p-value	0.882		0.460		0.773	

tions of APOE genotypes and alleles matched Hardy-Weinberg law. Of 110 patients, 29 presented with intracranial hematomas detected by the first CT scan after hospitalization (<7 days). χ^2 test showed no statistical differences in APOE allele frequencies between the 29 patients with intracranial hematomas and the other 81 cases (Table 1).

Of 110 patients, 19 presented with deteriorated clinical condition after hospitalization (<7 days). Decrease in GCS was detected in all worsening patients, including those who were found to have radiographic evidence of either hemorrhage extension or delayed hemorrhage. Among the 19 patients, repeated CT scanning revealed 3 cases with hemorrhage extension and 2 cases with delayed hemorrhage. Data were analyzed by statistics using SPSS software and Fisher's exact probability test to compare the genotype frequencies. χ^2 test showed no statistical differences in radiographic worsening/stabilization between the APOE $\varepsilon4(+)$ and APOE $\varepsilon4(-)$ groups ($p = 0.170 > 0.05$). Furthermore, no significant correlation between worsening on CT scans with genotype or with haplotype frequencies for A-491T or C-427T or G-219T were found by χ^2 test ($p > 0.05$) (Table 2). After the adjustment by further multiple logistic regression for general information (age, sex, smoking or not, alcohol-drinking or not), the injury causes, GCS, CT findings, treatments, and injury mecha-

Table 2. *Comparison between number of patients with/without worsening on CT scans and apolipoprotein E genotype*

APOE genotype	CT worsening	CT stabilization	p-value
$\varepsilon2(+)$	1	17	1.000
$\varepsilon2(-)$	4	88	
$\varepsilon3(+)$	4	104	0.089
$\varepsilon3(-)$	1	1	
$\varepsilon4(+)$	2	15	0.170
$\varepsilon4(-)$	3	90	
-219TT	2	50	1.000
-219GT + GG	3	58	
-427TT	3	93	0.121
-427TC + CC	2	12	
-491AA	3	77	0.612
-491AA + AT	2	28	

nisms, APOE $\varepsilon4$ and APOE promoter were not found to be risk factors for worsening on CT scans ($p > 0.05$).

Discussion

In the general population, genetic polymorphism occurs as the result of mutation and can be defined as a genetic locus. The single nucleotide polymorphisms (SNPs) resulting from a single base variation are the most common polymorphisms. ApoE is one of the most important cholesterol transport proteins and an important mediator of cholesterol and lipid transport in the brain. ApoE is a polymorphic protein with 3 common isoforms (apoE2, E3, E4), encoded by three alleles ($\varepsilon2$, $\varepsilon3$, $\varepsilon4$) of a single gene on chromosome 19q13.2. Furthermore, several polymorphisms within the promoter region of the APOE gene have been identified at -491 (A/T transversion), -427 (T/C transversion), and -219 (G/T transversion), which may affect the transcriptional activity of the APOE gene [1].

Recently, APOE has been implicated as influencing outcome following TBI. In our previous studies, we reported that APOE $\varepsilon4$ is a risk factor that predisposes to clinical deterioration in acute phase after TBI [5]. And our further research focusing on APOE promoter also has shown that APOE -491AA promoter in $\varepsilon4$ carriers is apt to influence clinical deterioration in Chinese population [6]. These findings may suggest that APOE genotype plays a role in early responses to TBI and contributes to poor outcome after TBI.

Intracranial hematomas are known to occur more commonly in patients who have sustained brain injuries. Although posttraumatic intracranial hematoma may be one of the factors associated with deterioration, the effect of APOE genotype on posttraumatic intracranial hematoma has not been studied as much as that on the outcome of TBI. So far, there is only one investigation [8] reporting that larger hematomas were found in head-injured patients with one or more APOE $\varepsilon4$ alleles than in patients without the allele.

In this study, χ^2 test showed no statistical differences in the APOE allele frequencies between the 29 patients with intracranial hematomas and the other 81 cases without it. Furthermore, no significant correlation of intracranial bleeding based on CT scanning with genotype or with haplotype frequencies for A-491T, C-427T, or G-219T was found by χ^2 test ($p > 0.05$). These results suggest that not only the APOE genotype but also APOE promoter may not be risk factors for an intracranial hematoma after TBI, although APOE

might affect vitamin K-dependent coagulation, as suggested by Shearer [12].

In our study, worsening on CT (<7 days after TBI) was defined as either hemorrhage extension or delayed hematoma. Hemorrhage extension means increase in hematoma volume, and delayed hematoma can be defined as an intracranial hematoma that is insignificant or not present on initial head CT scan at admission, but revealed by subsequent CT scanning and showing sizeable epidural, subdural, or intracerebral bleeding. Among 19 patients who showed deterioration during the first 7 days, only 5 cases showed radiographic evidence of either hemorrhage extension or delayed hematoma. There was no statistical difference in CT worsening/stabilization between the APOE $\varepsilon4(+)$ and APOE $\varepsilon4(-)$ groups, which indicated that APOE $\varepsilon4$ has no distinct effect on hemorrhage extension or delayed hematoma following TBI. And according to further statistic analysis, APOE promoter does not influence the CT worsening in this study. These results suggest that not only the APOE genotype but also APOE promoter may not predict radiographic evidence of hemorrhage extension or delayed hematoma after TBI. Stein et al. [14] tried to determine whether the ApoE $\varepsilon4$ genotype predisposes patients to coagulopathy and intravascular microthrombosis after TBI, and reported that ApoE genotype was not associated with intravascular coagulation in TBI. Their finding may partly support our results.

As mentioned above, there is only 1 investigation [8] reporting that APOE $\varepsilon4$ does predict a larger hematoma, which is contrary to our findings. The difference may be that we have focused on the association between allele frequencies and CT worsening in the early stage after TBI, while Liaquat et al. analyze the relationship between APOE $\varepsilon4$ and the size of the intracranial hematoma. Ethnic and sample size differences may also influence the association between gene and intracranial hematoma.

In brief, although more and more studies are interested in APOE gene, there are few reports focusing on the relationship between APOE genotype and intracranial hematoma. There is some evidence showing that ApoE isoforms have differential influences on blood coagulation or cerebrovascular pathology [10, 13, 16]. Our study failed to support the hypothesis that APOE genotype and promoter polymorphism may be a risk factor for posttraumatic intracranial hematoma after TBI or to predict worsening on CT scans. Larger cohort studies are needed to elucidate the relationship between genotype and coagulopathy to vascular complications of TBI.

References

1. Artiga MJ, Bullido MJ, Sastre I, Recuero M, García MA, Aldudo J, Vázquez J, Valdivieso F (1998) Allelic polymorphisms in the transcriptional regulatory region of apolipoprotein E gene. FEBS Lett 421: 105–108

2. Bullock MR, Chesnut R, Ghajar J, Gordon D, Hartl R, Newell DW, Servadei F, Walters BC, Wilberger JE (2006) Guidelines for the surgical management of traumatic brain injury: Chapter 1. Neurosurgery 58: S1–S3

3. Chiang MF, Chang JG, Hu CJ (2003) Association between apolipoprotein E genotype and outcome of traumatic brain injury. Acta Neurochir (Wien) 145: 649–654

4. Friedman G, Froom P, Sazbon L, Grinblatt I, Shochina M, Tsenter J, Babaey S, Yehuda B, Groswasser Z (1999) Apolipoprotein E-epsilon4 genotype predicts a poor outcome in survivors of traumatic brain injury. Neurology 52: 244–248

5. Jiang Y, Sun X, Xia Y, Tang W, Cao Y, Gu Y (2006) Effect of APOE polymorphisms on early responses to traumatic brain injury. Neurosci Lett 408: 155–158

6. Jiang Y, Sun X, Gui L, Xia Y, Tang W, Cao Y, Gu Y (2007) Correlation between APOE -491AA promoter in ε4 carriers and clinical deterioration in early stage of traumatic brain injury. J Neurotrauma 24: 1802–1810

7. Lendon CL, Harris JM, Pritchard AL, Nicoll JA, Teasdale GM, Murray G (2003) Genetic variation of the APOE promoter and outcome after head injury. Neurology 61: 683–685

8. Liaquat I, Dunn LT, Nicoll JA, Teasdale GM, Norrie JD (2002) Effect of apolipoprotein E genotype on hematoma volume after trauma. J Neurosurg 96: 90–96

9. Lichtman SW, Seliger G, Tycko B, Marder K (2000) Apolipoprotein E and functional recovery from brain injury following post-acute rehabilitation. Neurology 55: 1536–1539

10. Loktionov A, Bingham SA, Vorster H, Jerling JC, Runswick SA, Cummings JH (1998) Apolipoprotein E genotype modulates the effect of black tea drinking on blood lipids and blood coagulation factors: a pilot study. Br J Nutr 79: 133–139

11. Millar K, Nicoll JA, Thornhill S, Murray GD, Teasdale GM (2003) Long term neuropsychological outcome after head injury: relation to APOE genotype. J Neurol Neurosurg Psychiatry 74: 1047–1052

12. Shearer MJ (1995) Vitamin K. Lancet 345: 229–234

13. Smith C, Graham DI, Murray LS, Stewart J, Nicoll JA (2006) Association of APOE e4 and cerebrovascular pathology in traumatic brain injury. J Neurol Neurosurg Psychiatry 77: 363–366

14. Stein SC, Graham DI, Chen XH, Dunn L, Smith DH (2005) Apo E genotype not associated with intravascular coagulation in traumatic brain injury. Neurosci Lett 387: 28–31

15. Teasdale GM, Murray GD, Nicoll JA (2005) The association between APOE epsilon4, age and outcome after head injury: a prospective cohort study. Brain 128: 2556–2561

16. Weir CJ, McCarron MO, Muir KW, Dyker AG, Bone I, Lees KR, Nicoll JA (2001) Apolipoprotein E genotype, coagulation, and survival following acute stroke. Neurology 57: 1097–1100

Author index

Index of keywords

SpringerNeurosurgery

Talat Kiris, John H. Zhang (eds.)

Cerebral Vasospasm

New Strategies in Research and Treatment

2008. XIII, 450 pages. 128 figures.
Hardcover **EUR 199,95***
Reduced price for subscribers to "Acta Neurochirurgica": EUR 179,95
ISBN 978-3-211-75717-8
Acta Neurochirurgica, Supplement 104

More than 90 papers give a summary of clinical and basic studies on cerebral vasospasm, including reviews by leading researchers in this field. Several new frontiers are proposed for future research directions that will not only promote research from neurosurgery and neurology but also from other interconnecting fields of emergency medicine, electrophysiology, molecular biology, and vascular biology.

Contents:

Vasospasm Pathogenesis • Vasospasm Biochemistry • Vasospasm Electrophysiology • Vasospasm Pharmacology • Vasospasm Molecular • Vasospasm Molecular Biology • Vasospasm Modeling and Remodeling

* All prices are recommended retail prices. Net-prices subject to local VAT.

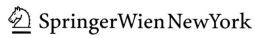 SpringerWien NewYork

P.O. Box 89, Sachsenplatz 4–6, 1201 Vienna, Austria, Fax +43.1.330 24 26, books@springer.at, **springer.at**
Haberstraße 7, 69126 Heidelberg, Germany, Fax +49.6221.345-4229, SDC-bookorder@springer.com, springer.com
P.O. Box 2485, Secaucus, NJ 07096-2485, USA, Fax +1.201.348-4505, service@springer-ny.com, springer.com
Prices are subject to change without notice. All errors and omissions excepted.

SpringerNeurosurgery

Yasuhiro Yonekawa, Tetsuya Tsukahara,
Anton Valavanis, Nadia Khan (eds.)

Changing Aspects in Stroke Surgery: Aneurysms, Dissection, Moyamoya angiopathy and EC-IC Bypass

2008. VIII, 141 pages, 65 partly coloured figures.
Hardcover **EUR 149,95**
Reduced price for subscribers to "Acta Neurochirurgica": EUR 134,95
ISBN 978-3-211-76588-3
Acta Neurochirurgica, Supplement 103

What is arterial dissection? What is Moyamoya angiopathy? What is the state of art of AVM treatment? Readers will find answers to these questions in this book. But they will also be informed about the state of the art treatment in the daily stroke therapy.

Contents:
Part 1: Aneurysms, Arteriovenous malformations and fistulas
Part 2: Dissection of cerebral arteries
Part 3: Revascularisation procedures, EC-IC Bypass revisited
Part 4: Moyamoya Angiopathy, History

* All prices are recommended retail prices. Net-prices subject to local VAT.

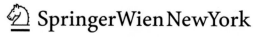 Springer Wien New York

P.O. Box 89, Sachsenplatz 4–6, 1201 Vienna, Austria, Fax +43.1.330 24 26, books@springer.at, **springer.at**
Haberstraße 7, 69126 Heidelberg, Germany, Fax +49.6221.345-4229, SDC-bookorder@springer.com, springer.com
P.O. Box 2485, Secaucus, NJ 07096-2485, USA, Fax +1.201.348-4505, service@springer-ny.com, springer.com
Prices are subject to change without notice. All errors and omissions excepted.